P9-BYC-974

Atlas of
INTERVENTIONAL
CARDIOLOGY

Atlas of
INTERVENTIONAL
CARDIOLOGY

Jeffrey J. Popma, M.D.
Washington Hospital Center
Washington, D.C.

Martin B. Leon, M.D.
Washington Hospital Center
Washington, D.C.

Eric J. Topol, M.D.
The Cleveland Clinic Foundation
Cleveland, OH

W.B. SAUNDERS COMPANY
A Division of Harcourt Brace & Company
Philadelphia   London   Toronto   Montreal   Sydney   Tokyo

W.B. SAUNDERS COMPANY
A Division of
Harcourt Brace & Company

The Curtis Center
Independence Square West
Philadelphia, Pennsylvania 19106

Library of Congress Cataloging-in-Publication Data

Popma, Jeffrey J.

Atlas of interventional cardiology / Jeffrey J. Popma, Martin B. Leon,
Eric J. Topol.

p. cm.

ISBN 0–7216–3569–5

1. Coronary heart disease—Surgery—Atlases.   2. Coronary heart
disease—Atlases.   I. Leon, Martin B.   II. Topol, Eric J.
III. Title.

[DNLM: 1. Cardiovascular Diseases—therapy—atlases.
2. Angioplasty, Balloon—atlases. WG 166 P828a 1994]

RD598.P56 1994

617.4′12—dc20

DNLM/DLC   94–1694

Atlas of Interventional Cardiology   ISBN 0–7216–3569–5

Copyright © 1994 by W.B. Saunders Company

All rights reserved. No part of this publication may be reproduced or transmitted in any form or by any
means, electronic or mechanical, including photocopy, recording, or any information storage and retrieval
system, without permission in writing from the publisher.

Printed in the United States of America.

Last digit is the print number: 9   8   7   6   5   4   3   2

To my wife, Theresa
and my children, Jessica, Nicole *and* Christopher

—JJP

INTRODUCTION

For the first 10 years that percutaneous coronary intervention was performed, there was just "plain ole balloon angioplasty." Although the lesions intially treated were often quite complex, the concept of achieving a larger arterial lumen by means of catheter-based balloon dilatation was relatively uniform. Since the mid-1980s, however, growth of novel methods of nonsurgical coronary revascularization has been explosive. Most of these methods, including directional, rotational, and extraction atherectomy as well as stenting and excimer laser angioplasty, are now approved by the United States Food and Drug Administration for general use. As a result of expanded use of these techniques, this field of coronary management has been transformed from what was once was called "balloon angioplasty" to what now is termed "coronary intervention," a much broader, catch-all concept of nonsurgical coronary revascularization. The new terminology does not imply that balloon angioplasty has been replaced but rather that it has been supplemented with a variety of new techniques that address the underlying atherosclerotic plaque in a different fashion. Rather than "compressing and stretching" the diseased coronary segment and vessel wall, which often occurs at the expense of balloon-induced barotrauma, the plaque can now be resected, debulked, emulsified, or vaporized or the vessel itself can be scaffolded. This diverse array of technologies, which has been built upon a strong foundation of many refinements in balloon technology, comprises the contemporary tools available to the contemporary interventional cardiologist. The most important future challenges relate to how the various technologies can best be applied, either in a stand-alone or integrated fashion.

To date, a major outgrowth of the use of new devices has been an expansion of the proportion of patients and of the diversity of lesions that can be effectively treated by percutaneous transcoronary techniques. In the past, patients with lesions that were highly complex owing to ulceration or angulation may have been preferentially referred for coronary artery bypass surgery. With the expanded armamentarium of coronary devices, it is now possible to apply nonsurgical approaches more broadly.

A second and important "windfall" of the era of new devices and techniques has been the improvement in the overall safety of percutaneous transcoronary procedures. This increase in safety margin can result from an improved primary approach to the vessel and lesion (or as an ad hoc strategy) to address a disrupted segment. Examples include active resection of an intimal tear via atherectomy or stenting of a vessel to promote stable recanalization and to maximize lumen caliber. The net effect of having all of the devices available has been to reduce the need for emergency bypass surgery from historical levels of 4% to 5% to levels now less than 2% to 3%. Since emergency surgery is such a significant complication, with its high attendant mortality, myocardial infarction rate of at least 50%, and urgent use of a suboptimal conduit (saphenous vein rather than internal mammary vein access), these new techniques represent an important step forward in improving the overall safety of standard balloon angioplasty and new device angioplasty.

The "frontier" for coronary intervention will be to address the critical and vexing problem of restenosis, which currently results in a need for repeat revascularization procedures in more than 25% of patients. Two recent large-scale randomized trials have demonstrated reductions in both angiographic and clinical restenosis parameters using one device (tubular-slotted stent), whereas other trials have demonstrated only partial effects in angiographic but not in clinical indices after plaque debulking (by directional atherectomy).

Most of this book focuses on acute procedural success or complications, with the understanding that there is a pivotal interplay between the end result in the cardiac catheterization laboratory and the follow-up angiographic results months later. Thus, a cardinal goal of coronary intervention is for clinicians to achieve as ideal a result as possible, yet duly recognizing that at times striving for perfection can result in a complication.

Our approach is not to think of the balloon or any particular new technology in an isolated fashion, but rather in a highly integrated fashion. This lesion-specific approach to intervention does not rely on any device or balloon technique exclusively but rather on the composite set of alternatives. It is clear that for any given lesion, vessel, or patient, a variety of techniques or strategies can be used with adequate success and avoidance of complications. Unfortunately, little hard data exists for the appropriate selection of balloons and devices; thus, for the most part, we must use rational, cost-effective strategies that not only provide the optimal acute-phase result but also the greatest long-term benefit. In situations in which few randomized trial data are available, it may be important to rely on observational results and the experience of today, with the hope that more rigorous, meaningful data are forthcoming. Although it is clear that data are just beginning to emerge from large-scale balloon and new device trials (e.g., CAVEAT, CCAT, BENESTENT, and STRESS), we are a long way from having technique-to-technique comparisons (e.g., rotational atherectomy versus excimer laser angioplasty) that can be useful when considering management for a calcified ostial lesion.

The *Atlas* is divided into two sections. The first presents the lesion-specific, integrated approach to coronary intervention. For each category of lesion, some balloon cases are presented, and many of the alternative technologies are demonstrated. Whenever possible, a lesion-specific treatment algorithm is presented that summarizes the options and the major points in the decision tree for selecting a particular technique. In some cases, new technologies are used in tandem. These cases illustrate key practical points about complex lesions and attempt to provide a comprehensive "menu" approach to the various catheter and device choices available for the treatment of individual types of lesions. The straightforward type A lesion of the American Heart Association/American College of Cardiology classification scheme (Table 1) is not covered in this book in detail, since this type of lesion is particularly well suited for balloon angioplasty. The first section addresses each of the characteristics of type B and type C lesions, pointing out the potential to address each and every lesion class with balloon angioplasty, per se, or alternatively, with various other devices and with the possibility of using balloon dilatation as an adjunctive or "finishing" step. Possible mechanisms for the lack of full efficacy with a technique are offered. Indeed, if there is a better understanding of the complexity of the type B and C lesions, the appreciation for the relative simplicity of Type A lesions will be enhanced. Nevertheless, it bears noting that even if balloons and new devices show equivalent acute results in type A

lesions, current and future studies may demonstrate differences in restenosis frequency, which may impact operator device choice strategies.

In the second section of the *Atlas,* a discussion of technique-specific management is given with a review by technique, including the background, a brief description, and case examples of each procedure to highlight its potential applications and, in some cases, the boundaries. In a sense, the whole "pie" is cut into separate pieces. The technique-specific presentation is intended to provide a more detailed understanding of each catheter and device but also to attempt to preserve the concept that balloons and each of the new devices should be considered in a highly integrated approach. In order for this to develop, however, understanding of the capabilities and limitations of each tool is necessary. It must be pointed out that for virtually all of the new devices there continues to be evolution in technique and equipment. For example, it is unclear how quickly to burr through a lesion with a rotational atherectomy device or whether a specific stent should be overexpanded according to the stent-artery ratio. Similarly, the directional atherectomy cutters, like most of the new device equipment, continue to be iteratively refined.

It is hoped that the angiographic case examples and high-quality images provided herein—each of which has been carefully selected for a particular educational purpose—will be helpful from the practical standpoint of promoting successful coronary intervention and in the graphic conveyance of a balanced view of how to integrate several different revascularization technologies. We firmly believe that a "picture is worth thousands of words," and recognize that interventional cardiologists, by nature, are especially graphically oriented. Therefore, the text has been kept to a minimum. We have also attempted to avoid references to specific balloon products or to guide wire and guiding catheter brands in order to give an impartial assessment of the options available for balloon and new device technology.

The field of percutaneous coronary intervention will

Table 1   Lesion-Specific Characteristics

Type A Lesions (High Success, >85%; Low Risk)

• Discrete (<10 mm)	• Little or no calcium
• Concentric	• Less than totally occlusive
• Readily accessible	• Not ostial in locations
• Nonangulated segment, <45°	• No major side branch involvement
• Smooth contour	• Absence of thrombus

Type B Lesions (Moderate Success, 60–85%; Moderate Risk)

• Tubular (10–20 mm in length)	• Moderate to heavy calcification
• Eccentric	• Total occlusions <3 months old
• Moderate tortuosity of proximal segment	• Ostial in location
• Moderately angulated segment, ≥45°, <90°	• Bifurcation lesions requiring double guide wire
• Irregular contour	• Some thrombus present

Type C Lesions (Low Success, <60%; High Risk)

• Diffuse (≥20 mm in length)	• Total occlusion >3 months old
• Excessive tortuosity of proximal segment	• Inability to protect major side branches
• Extremely angulated segments, ≥90°	• Degenerated vein grafts with friable lesions

(Data adapted with permission from Ryan T, Faxon D, Gunnar R, et al. Guidelines for percutaneous transluminal coronary angioplasty. J Am Coll Cardiol 1988; 12:529–545.)

clearly continue to evolve in a dynamic way over the years ahead. Beyond appearance of new alternative devices that will further complement the current armamentarium and potentially make catheter and device selection even more difficult, the techniques of intravascular imaging will become increasingly important. By incorporating angioscopy, echocardiography (2- and 3-dimensional), and Doppler techniques, a greatly enhanced awareness of the diseased segment will become routinely possible. At the beginning of an intervention, ''full disclosure'' of the vessel's extent and localization of calcium, thickness of the media, and eccentricity as well as of echolucent or echodense constituency of the plaque and of the diffuseness of the disease in the vessel (including distal or side branch involvement) will all become routinely available and will clearly influence device selection. For example, an angiogram may reveal extensive calcification, but an intravascular ultrasound can demonstrate that the calcification is all deep and periadventitial; this may change selection of technique from rotational atherectomy to balloon angioplasty.

Following the intervention, it is important that lumen caliber be restored to the maximum. It is frequently sobering to view ultrasonographically the extent of persistent, significant atherosclerotic plaque left behind at the time when the angiogram suggests a satisfactory (or even excellent) result. Surely, the various imaging devices will be of great assistance to us in the future in determining when to stop and when to press on as well as in selecting the tool or tools to use for specific arterial lesions.

Finally, it will always be important to incorporate new data on balloon angioplasty and new devices as they become available. Rather than relying on the experience of a particular operator or hospital site, results from large-scale registries, in which data are carefully collected with core laboratory angiographic review, and results from randomized trials using rigorous methodology will always be extremely helpful in the overall approach to device selection and the optimal application of the tools of interventional cardiology.

JEFFREY J. POPMA, M.D.
MARTIN B. LEON, M.D.
ERIC J. TOPOL, M.D.

ACKNOWLEDGMENTS

With deepest admiration we thank our colleagues and friends at the Washington Hospital Center who have provided us with such a vast amount of clinical material: Augusto D. Pichard, M.D., Kenneth M. Kent, M.D., Lowell F. Satler, M.D., and Gary S. Mintz, M.D. We have identified many of the unique clinical scenarios presented within this *Atlas* only as a result of their innovation and commitment to the identification of optimal transcather treatment strategies.

We also thank our former colleagues at the University of Michigan for allowing us to review their excellent interventional work during our tenure there (JJP, EJT): Stephen G. Ellis, M.D., Eric R. Bates, M.D., Joseph A. Walton, M.D., David W. Muller, M.D., Elizabeth G. Nabel, M.D., and Stephen W. Werns, M.D. We also acknowledge the expert graphics support of Christopher Burke.

We greatly appreciate the contributions of the other interventional cardiologists who have allowed us to review their challenging cases and have provided their advisory expertise: Cass A. Pinkerton, M.D. (St. Vincent's Hospital, Indianapolis, IN), Bernhard Meier, M.D. (University Hospital, Bern, Switzerland), Ulrich Sigwart, M.D. (Royal Brompton National Heart and Lung Hospital, London, England), Christopher J. White, M.D. (Oschner Clinic, New Orleans, LA), and Dean J. Kereiakes, M.D. (Christ Hospital, Cincinnati, OH).

We also appreciate the expert editorial assistance of Margaret Felker, the technical assistance of Moshe Mehlman and Darrell Debowey, and the supportive efforts of the staff at the Angiographic Core Laboratory of the Washington Hospital Center: Theresa A. Bucher, Michael B. Keller, Alan J. Merritt, Christine A. Ditrano, Teraza Y. Conway, Robert A. DeFalco, Luella T. Lewis, Lisa A. Sokolowicz, Benjamin Kleiber, Ya Chien Chuang, and Kristina Clark.

This work was supported, in part, by a grant from the Cardiology Research Foundation.

CONTENTS

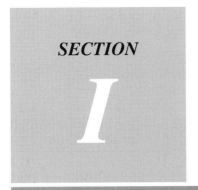

SECTION

I

A LESION-SPECIFIC APPROACH TO CORONARY INTERVENTION

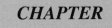

CHAPTER

1

Lesion Eccentricity and Irregularity

LESION ECCENTRICITY

Intravascular ultrasound studies suggest that asymmetric plaque accumulation occurs in most coronary atherosclerotic lesions. Lesion asymmetry or "eccentricity" (Table 1–1) is a commonly noted adverse morphologic feature and is reported in nearly 60% of lesions in some series. The independent risk for an unfavorable outcome resulting from lesion eccentricity is somewhat controversial. Although researchers in some series have suggested that balloon angioplasty in the treatment of patients with eccentric lesions is not associated with an increased procedural risk, the authors of other studies who used semiquantitative criteria for grading lesion eccentricity have suggested that eccentric lesions are associated with a less favorable angiographic and procedural outcome. Asymmetric balloon expansion of a normal vessel wall that occurs in eccentric as opposed to concentric lesions may increase the degree of elastic recoil or the frequency of coronary dissections. Some authors have also noted that eccentric lesions may lead to an increased tendency for a patient to develop restenosis after balloon angioplasty. In addition, eccentricity is commonly found in association with other morphologic features, such as calcium deposition, thrombus, bend points, and diffuse lesions, which may have an important influence on specific treatment strategies. It is likely that the use of intravascular ultrasound is helpful in selecting and tailoring device interventions in patients with this complex and diverse group of lesions.

Table 1–1 Definitions

Feature	Definitions
Eccentricity	Stenosis noted to have one of its lumen edges in the outer one-quarter of the apparent normal lumen
Irregular Lesions	Lesions with an abnormal lumen contour
Ulceration	Lesions with a small crater consisting of a discrete lumen widening in the area of the stenosis that does not extend beyond the normal arterial lumen
Saw tooth	Multiple, sequential jagged lumen irregularities
Aneurysmal	Segment of arterial dilatation larger than the dimensions of the normal arterial segment
Intimal flap	An extension of the vessel wall into the arterial lumen

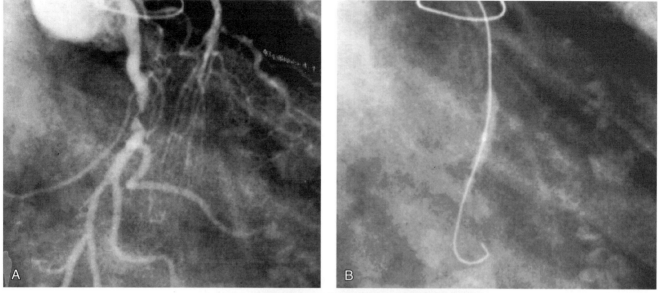

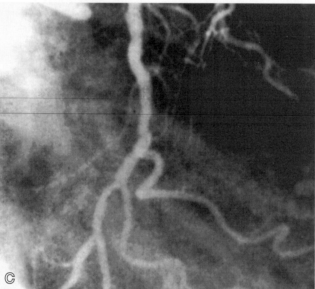

Figure 1–1
An eccentric lesion in the midportion of the left circumflex was noted to contain a moderate amount of lesion calcium fluoroscopically *(Panel A)*. Standard balloon angioplasty was performed with a 3.0-mm noncompliant balloon *(Panel B)*. Despite high balloon inflation pressures (12 atm), a residual "waist," attributable to lesion rigidity, was observed. After balloon deflation, a 30% residual stenosis was obtained *(Panel C)*.

To improve the angiographic and procedural outcome observed after balloon angioplasty in patients with eccentric lesions, a number of alternative balloon procedures and new device strategies have been applied. For example, longer (5- to 15-minute) balloon inflations have been performed to optimize the immediate angiographic result. Angioplasty with perfusion balloons may be used to minimize the degree of ischemia in lesions that supply large amounts of blood to myocardium.

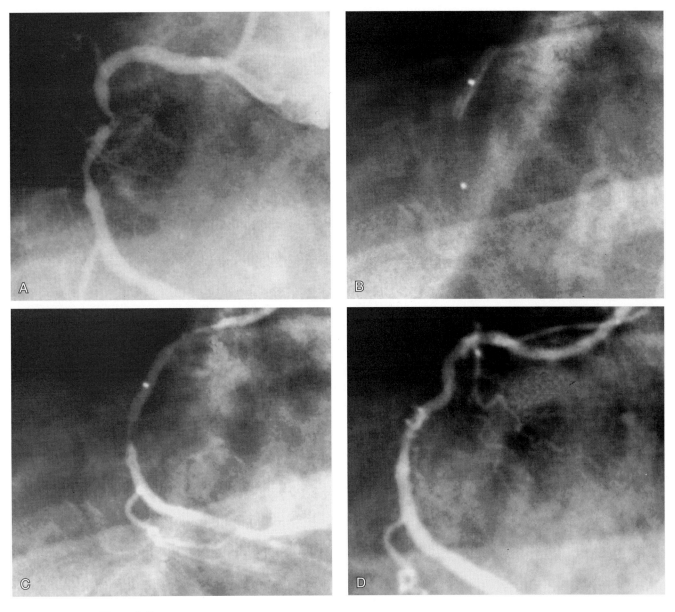

Figure 1–2
This angulated, eccentric stenosis of the midportion of a tortuous right coronary artery *(Panel A)* was dilated with a 3.0-mm Rx perfusion balloon catheter *(Panel B)*. Excellent anterograde flow was demonstrated during balloon inflation *(Panel C)*. After a 10-minute balloon inflation period, a <10% residual stenosis was achieved without evidence of dissection or intimal disruption, despite significant straightening of the vessel *(Panel D)*.

In patients with eccentric lesions located in large (≥3.0 mm), noncalcified coronary arteries, directional atherectomy has been used to selectively excise biopsy-sized fragments of atherosclerotic plaque. Notably, some degree of mechanical dilatation via balloon stretching and device "dottering" may also occur with directional atherectomy. Quantitative angiographic studies have suggested that partial plaque excision with directional atherectomy may alter lesion compliance and reduce the degree of elastic recoil when adjunct dilatation balloon is required.

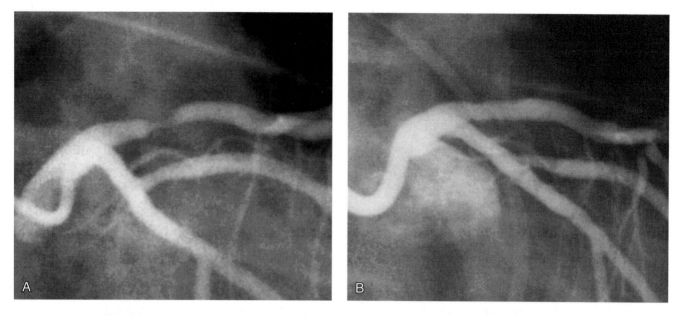

Figure 1–3
An eccentric stenosis of the proximal segment of the left anterior descending artery *(Panel A)* was treated using directional atherectomy. Plaque excision was performed with the cutting window preferentially rotated superiorly toward the arterial surface characterized by eccentricity. After retrieval of an abundant amount of tissue, a <10% residual stenosis was obtained. Note the smooth lumen contour without dissection, the presence of intimal flaps, or intraluminal haziness *(Panel B).*

Rotational coronary atherectomy has also been used in patients with eccentric lesions, particularly those that contain significant intralesion superficial (abluminal) calcium.

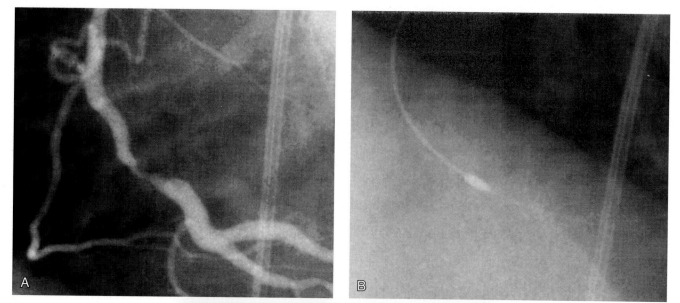

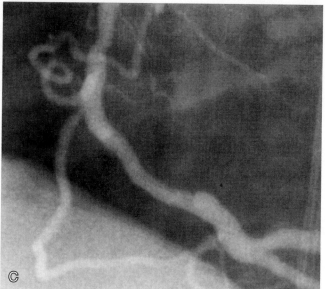

Figure 1–4

Rotational coronary atherectomy of a calcified, eccentric lesion in the distal segment of the right coronary artery *(Panel A)* was performed using 1.50-mm and 1.75-mm burrs *(Panel B)*. After two passes, a 50% residual stenosis was noted; a 2.5-mm perfusion balloon was used to dilate the residual stenosis. After balloon deflation, a 20% residual stenosis was obtained. Notably, in this calcified, eccentric lesion, a smooth lumen resulted without evidence of dissection or distal embolization *(Panel C)*.

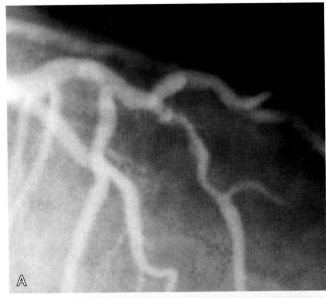

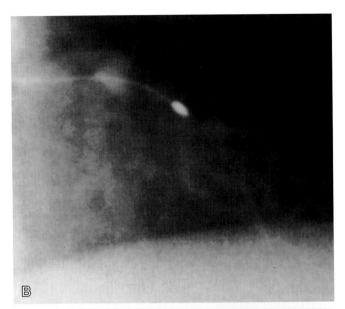

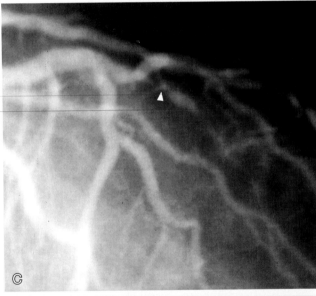

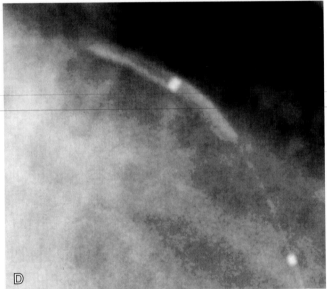

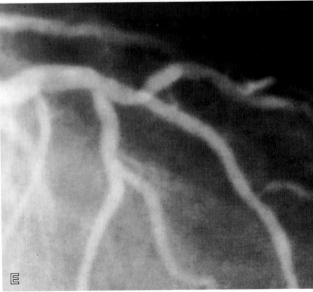

Figure 1–5

A calcified, eccentric lesion was demonstrated in the midportion of the left anterior descending artery *(Panel A)*. Owing to the artery's excess length (15 mm) and to intralesion calcification, rotational atherectomy was selected for revascularization. Two 30-second passes were performed across the stenosis using a 1.75-mm burr *(Panel B)*. Repeat angiography after the second pass demonstrated abrupt closure at the treatment site *(arrow)*, probably secondary to coronary vasospasm *(Panel C)*. Intracoronary nitroglycerin, 200 μg, was administered, and a 3.0-mm Rx perfusion balloon catheter was inflated across the occlusion for 3 minutes *(Panel D)*. After two inflations, anterograde flow was restored, and an excellent angiographic result was obtained *(Panel E)*.

Intracoronary stenting has been used in patients with focal and some tubular lesions (<12 mm) with severe eccentricity located in larger vessels (≥3.0 mm in diameter), particularly in those with recalcitrant restenosis. The internal scaffolding effect of the intracoronary stent lessens the degree of elastic recoil that occurs in eccentric lesions after balloon deflation and usually achieves excellent acute angiographic results.

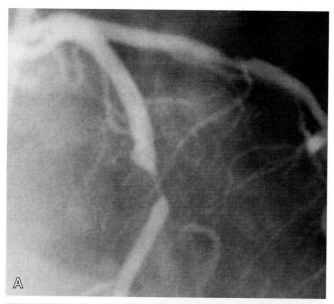

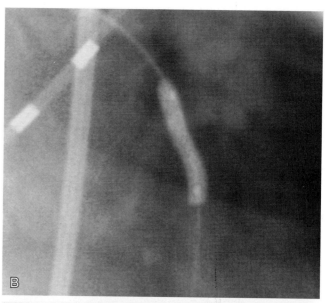

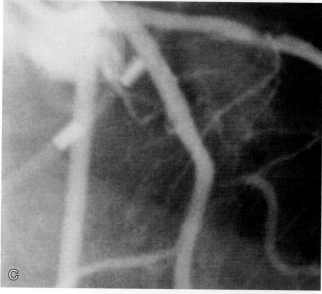

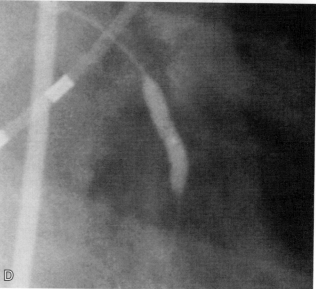

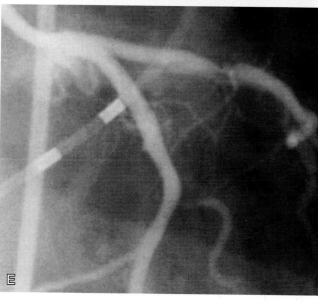

Figure 1–6

The eccentric stenosis in the midsegment of the left circumflex was treated on two prior occasions with standard balloon angioplasty *(Panel A)*. After predilatation with a 2.0-mm balloon catheter, a 3.0-mm, tubular, slotted Palmaz-Schatz stent was fully expanded to 6 atm *(Panel B)*. After balloon deflation, a 10% residual stenosis was noted at the distal aspect of the stent *(Panel C)*. A 3.5-mm dilatation balloon catheter was then used to further dilate the distal portion of the stent *(Panel D)*. Although little change in the residual stenosis was demonstrated angiographically (10% residual stenosis) *(Panel E)*, adjunct balloon dilatation presumably served to fully implant the stent into the vessel wall, potentially reducing the risk of subacute thrombosis and late restenosis.

LESION IRREGULARITY

Irregular lesions include those lesions with ulceration, a saw-tooth pattern (suggesting lesion friability), aneurysmal dilatation, and intimal flaps (Table 1–1). These somewhat heterogeneous angiographic features suggest that the underlying atherosclerotic plaque may be complex, potentially containing an abnormal surface morphology and superimposed thrombus. Lesions with ulceration, particularly those with haziness and filling defects, indicate that recent plaque rupture has occurred. Standard balloon dilatation in this setting may be associated with more severe elastic recoil and thrombotic complications than balloon angioplasty in nonulcerated lesions.

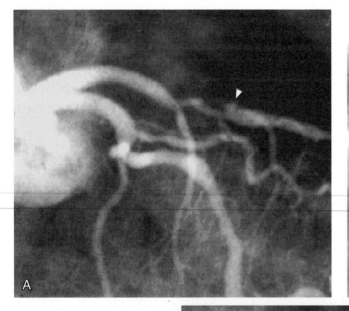
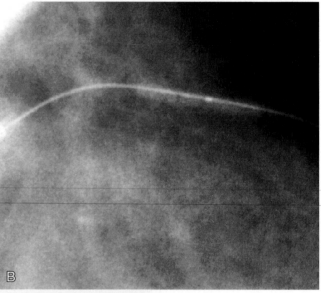
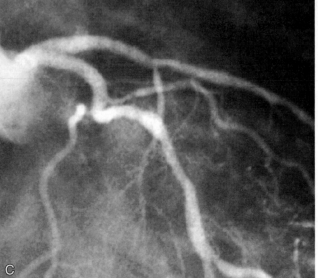

Figure 1–7
A tubular stenosis was noted in the midportion of the left anterior descending artery *(Panel A)*. At the distal aspect of the lesion, an ulceration was seen *(arrow)*. A 3.0-mm balloon catheter was inflated to 6 atm; this resulted in full balloon expansion *(Panel B)*. After balloon deflation, the ulcerated lesion was no longer visualized; however, a marked degree of elastic recoil occurred, and a 30% residual stenosis was obtained *(Panel C)*. To avoid balloon oversizing relative to the reference artery size, a larger balloon was not used.

Because experienced investigators have subjectively associated irregular lesions with more frequent procedural complications and suboptimal angiographic results after balloon angioplasty, a variety of new angioplasty devices have been used in the subset of patients with such lesions.

Directional coronary atherectomy has been applied to ulcerated lesions, particularly those located in larger vessels. Intracoronary stents have been used to internally compress ulceration and expand the atherosclerotic and normal vessel segment.

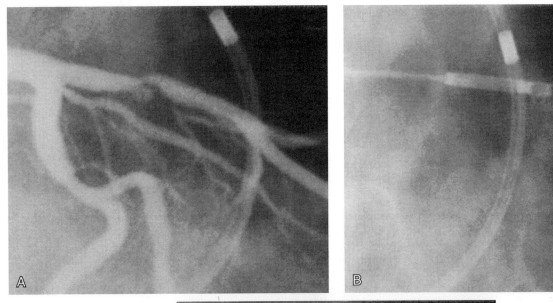

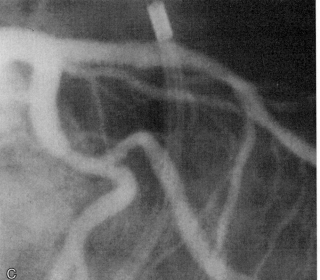

Figure 1–8
An ulcerated lesion was demonstrated in the proximal segment of the left anterior descending artery *(Panel A)*. A 7-French DVI EX atherectomy device was positioned across the lesion *(Panel B)*, and cuts favoring an inferior orientation with greatest plaque accumulation were obtained. After directional atherectomy, the ulceration was no longer visible, and mild ectasia at the atherectomy site was observed *(Panel C)*. The appearance of a smaller vessel distally was attributable to overexpansion of the proximal segment and mild vasoconstriction distal to the treatment site.

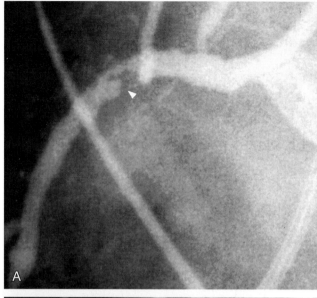

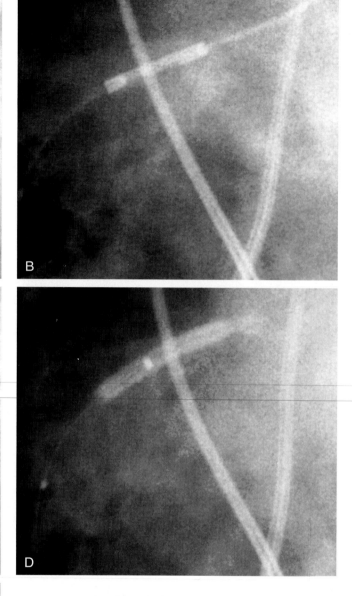

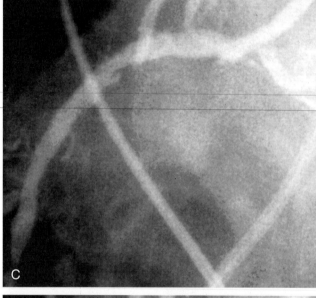

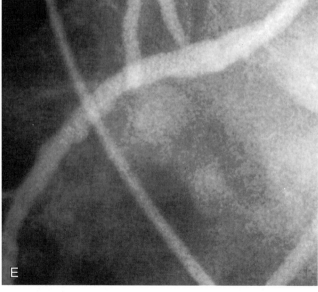

Figure 1–9

A focal eccentric stenosis was noted *(arrow)* in the proximal segment of the right coronary artery with ulceration in the distal portion of the lesion *(Panel A)*. Directional coronary atherectomy was performed with a 6-French DVI SCA atherectomy device *(Panel B)*; after several cuts, a persistent intimal flap was noted *(Panel C)*. A 3.0-mm Rx perfusion catheter was advanced across the stenosis *(Panel D)*. After a prolonged (5-minute) balloon inflation period, smoothing of the lumen contour occurred; however, some persistent minor irregularity in the distal aspect of the lesion remained *(Panel E)*.

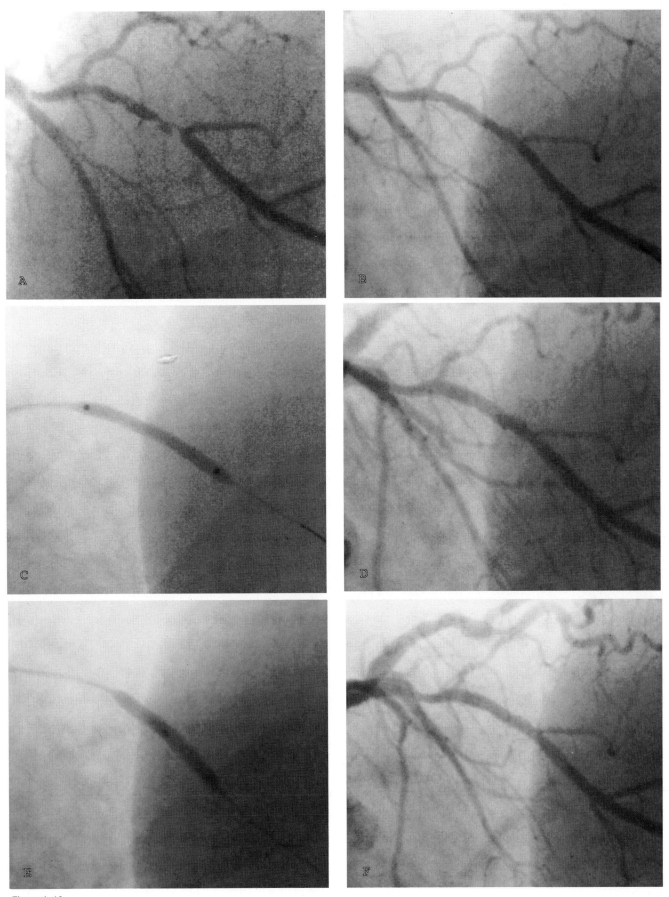

Figure 1–10
An ulcerated lesion was demonstrated in the midsegment of the left anterior descending artery *(Panel A)*. Predilatation of the lesion was performed with a 2.0-mm balloon catheter; compression of the ulcerated lesion resulted *(Panel B)*. Progressive elastic recoil developed, and a 2.5-mm Gianturco-Roubin stent was positioned across the lesion *(Panel C)*. Marked improvement of the vessel diameter was demonstrated *(Panel D)*, and adjunct balloon angioplasty was performed with a 3.0-mm balloon catheter *(Panel E)*. After final balloon inflation, a <10% residual stenosis was obtained, with mild ectasia occurring within the stented segment *(Panel F)*. (Courtesy of C. Pinkerton, MD.)

Post-stenotic aneurysmal dilatation is an infrequent morphologic finding before coronary angioplasty but does suggest thinning of the media and adventitial walls as well as expansion of the post-stenotic arterial segment. Coronary angioplasty is generally performed with caution in the presence of aneurysmal lesions so that coronary perforation or rupture can be avoided.

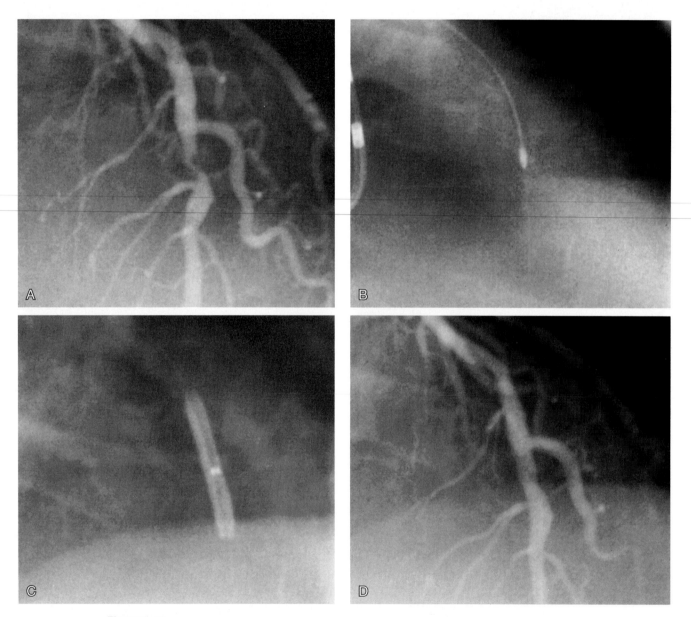

Figure 1–11
Mild post-stenotic dilatation was demonstrated distal to the calcified, concentric lesion of the midportion of the left anterior descending artery *(Panel A)*. Rotational atherectomy with 1.25-mm and 1.75-mm burrs was performed *(Panel B)*. Because of a 40% residual stenosis, a 2.5-mm perfusion balloon was inflated *(Panel C)*, and a 20% residual stenosis was obtained *(Panel D)*. Mild intraluminal haziness at the treatment site was noted.

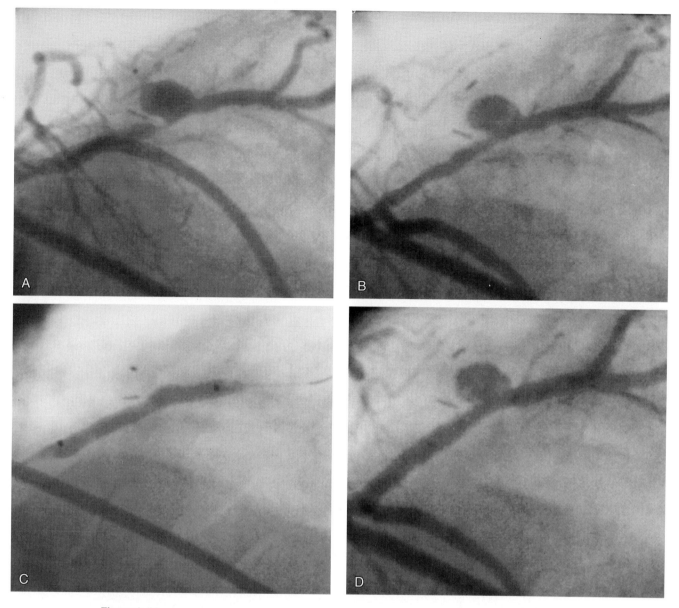

Figure 1–12
An eccentric lesion of the midportion of the left anterior descending artery was located just proximal to the anastomotic insertion of a saphenous vein into the left anterior descending artery *(Panel A)*. The saphenous vein graft had become totally occluded, and intracoronary stent placement in the native left anterior descending artery was recommended. After predilatation with a 2.5-mm dilatation balloon catheter *(Panel B)*, a 3.0-mm Gianturco-Roubin stent was deployed across the residual lesion *(Panel C)*, resulting in a 20% residual stenosis *(Panel D)*. (Courtesy of C. Pinkerton, MD.)

Disruption of the normal vessel architecture and atherosclerotic plaque occur in some patients after balloon angioplasty, resulting in protrusion of intimal flaps into the arterial lumen. The intimal flaps are often difficult to treat with standard balloon methods owing to an increased degree of elastic recoil of the vessel, to mobile or avulsed plaque components that continue to protrude into the lumen, and to a propensity for extensive dissection with overly aggressive mechanical barotrauma. Prolonged balloon inflation, directional coronary atherectomy, and intracoronary stenting are important new device options for treating the subset of patients with such lesions.

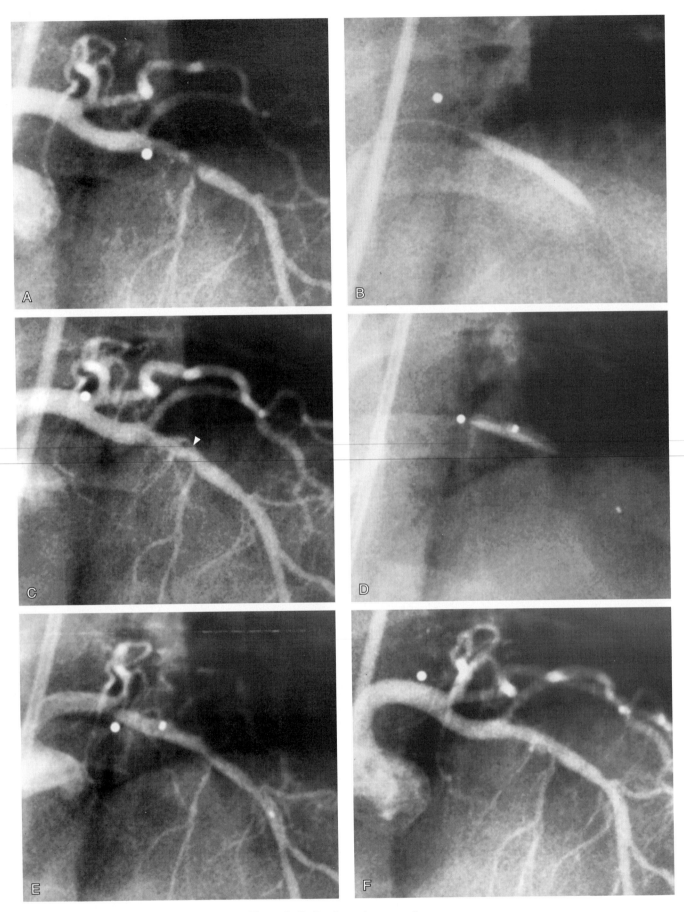

Figure 1–13. *See legend on opposite page*

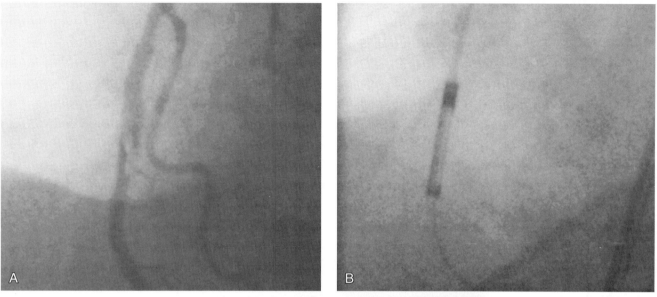

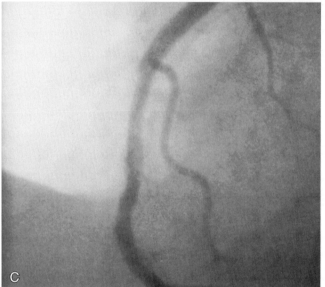

Figure 1–14
After standard balloon angioplasty, a residual dissection flap persisted in the midportion of the right coronary artery despite prolonged balloon inflations with a perfusion balloon *(Panel A)*. A 6-French DVI EX catheter was positioned across the intimal flap, and directed cuts were performed *(Panel B)*. After atherectomy, the lumen contour was markedly improved *(Panel C)*.

Figure 1–13
A calcified, eccentric plaque was demonstrated in the midportion of the left anterior descending artery *(Panel A)*. Initial balloon inflation was performed with a 2.5-mm dilatation balloon catheter *(Panel B)*. After balloon deflation, a residual intimal flap developed along the anterior surface of the artery *(arrow, Panel C)*. Despite additional balloon inflations, the intimal flap persisted, and a 3.0-mm perfusion balloon catheter was inflated across the residual stenosis for 10 minutes *(Panel D)*. Anterograde flow was demonstrated *(Panel E)*, and the intimal flap was adequately compressed *(Panel F)*.

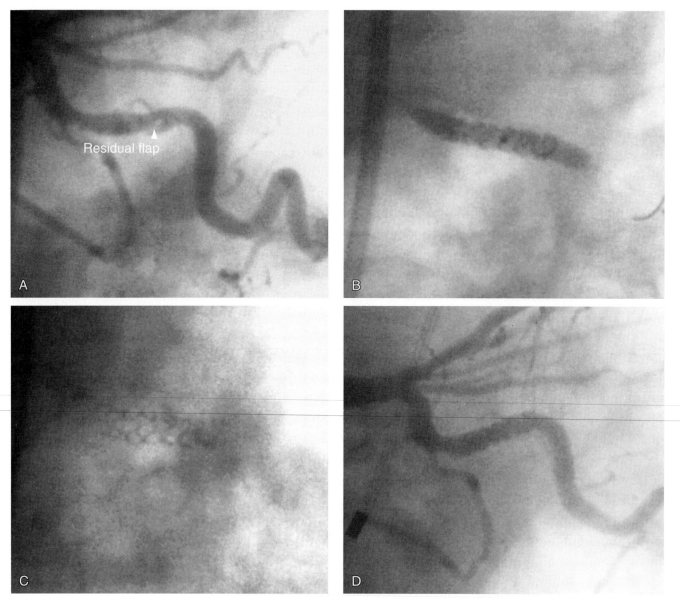

Figure 1–15
After balloon angioplasty of the midsegment of the left circumflex, an intimal flap persisted *(Panel A)*.
Additional balloon inflations were performed, but substantial improvement in the lesion morphology
did not occur. A 3.5-mm Wiktor stent was deployed *(Panel B)*, with the tantalum filaments of the stent
clearly visible *(Panel C)*. After stent placement, the intimal flap was no longer visualized *(Panel D)*.

SELECTED REFERENCES

Ambrose J, Winters S, Stern A, et al. Angiographic morphology and the pathogenesis of unstable angina pectoris. J Am Coll Cardiol 1985; 5:609–616.

Bell M, Garratt K, Bresnahan J, et al. Relation of deep arterial resection and coronary artery aneurysms after directional coronary atherectomy. J Am Coll Cardiol 1992; 20:1474–1481.

Cowley M, DiSciascio G, Rehr R, Vetrovec G. Angiographic observations and clinical relevance of coronary thrombus in unstable angina. Am J Cardiol 1989; 63:108E–113E.

Freeman M, Williams A, Chisholm R, et al. Intracoronary thrombus and complex morphology in unstable angina: Relation to timing of angiography and in-hospital cardiac events. Circulation 1989; 82:439–447.

Ghazzal Z, Hearn J, Litvack F, et al. Morphologic predictors of acute complications after percutaneous excimer laser coronary angioplasty. Results of a comprehensive angiographic analysis: Importance of the eccentricity index. Circulation 1992; 86:820–827.

Hinohara T, Rowe M, Robertson G, et al. Directional coronary atherectomy for the treatment of coronary lesions with abnormal contour. J Invasive Cardiol 1990; 2:57–63.

Kalbfleisch S, McGillem M, Simon S, et al. Automated quantitation of indexes of coronary lesion complexity: Comparison between patients with stable and unstable angina. Circulation 1990; 82:439–447.

Krolick M, Bugni W, Walsh J. Coronary artery aneurysm formation following directional coronary atherectomy. Cathet Cardiovasc Diagn 1992; 27:117–121.

Meier B, Gruentzig A, Hollman J, et al. Does the length or eccentricity of coronary stenoses influence the outcome of transluminal dilatation? Circulation 1983; 1983:497–499.

Preisack M, Voelker W, Haase K, Karsch M. Case report: Formation of vessel aneurysm after stand alone excimer laser angioplasty. Cathet Cardiovasc Diagn 1992; 27:122–124.

Rab S, King S III, Roubin G, et al. Coronary aneurysms after stent placement: A suggestion of altered vessel wall healing in the presence of anti-inflammatory agents. J Am Coll Cardiol 1991; 18:1524–1528.

Schryver T, Popma J, Kent K, et al. Use of intracoronary ultrasound to identify the "true" coronary lumen in chronic coronary dissection treated with intracoronary stenting. Am J Cardiol 1992; 19:1107–1108.

Walford G, Midei M, Aversano T, et al. Coronary artery aneurysm formation following percutaneous transluminal coronary angioplasty: Treatment of associated restenosis with repeat percutaneous transluminal coronary angioplasty. Cathet Cardiovasc Diagn 1990; 20:77–83.

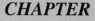
Ostial Lesions

Balloon angioplasty in patients with aorto-ostial lesions or of lesions that originate within the first 3 mm of the left anterior descending or circumflex coronary arteries (or their major branches) may be associated with reduced procedural success rates and more frequent complications (e.g., coronary dissection and the need for emergency bypass surgery) than balloon angioplasty of nonostial lesions. Factors that account for the reduced procedural success rates include difficulties with guide catheter support, lesion rigidity (which precludes complete balloon expansion), extensive plaque accumulation, and elastic recoil (which necessitates the use of oversized balloon catheters). Moreover, angiographic and clinical recurrences of ischemia are common, occurring in 50% of treated patients.

Selection of the appropriate method for coronary revascularization of ostial lesions using various forms of transcatheter therapy depends on a number of factors, including vessel size and location, extent of lesion calcification, and takeoff angulation of the vessel. In patients with uncompli-

cated ostial lesions, preliminary reports have suggested that acceptable procedural success rates can be achieved with the use of new device or balloon angioplasty approaches. A treatment algorithm for ostial disease is proposed in Figure 2–1.

Device selection for the treatment of ostial lesions is based on a vessel's size, its distal angulation, and the degree of calcification. In the presence of moderate to severe lesion calcium, rotational atherectomy is the preferred approach. Once multiple passes have been performed using a suitably sized burr, balloon angioplasty, directional atherectomy, or intracoronary stenting can be performed to treat a residual (>30%) stenosis. In the presence of mild lesion calcium and a reference vessel size of <3 mm, rotational atherectomy or excimer laser angioplasty (concentric or directional) can be used. If a residual stenosis of >30% persists, adjunct balloon angioplasty may be performed to optimize the angiographic result. If the diameter of the reference artery is >3.0 mm and without moderate or severe calcifi-

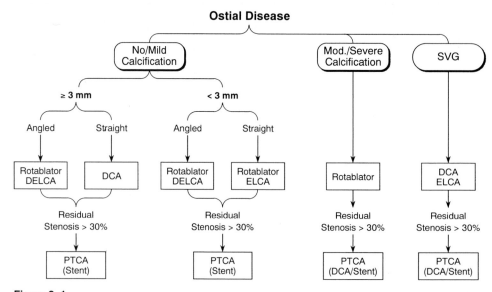

Figure 2–1
A treatment algorithm for ostial disease.

cation at the lesion site, directional atherectomy is recommended, provided that the takeoff angle of the ostium is not severe (≥45°). If marked angulation is present, rotational atherectomy or directional laser angioplasty is the preferred approach. In the event of a significant residual stenosis (>30%), adjunct balloon angioplasty or possibly intracoronary stenting can be performed to optimize procedural results.

On occasion, the sequential use of multiple devices (rotational and directional atherectomy excimer laser angioplasty or directional atherectomy) may be needed to optimize the final angiographic result.

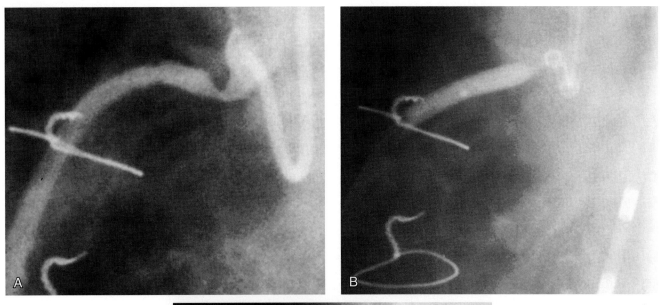

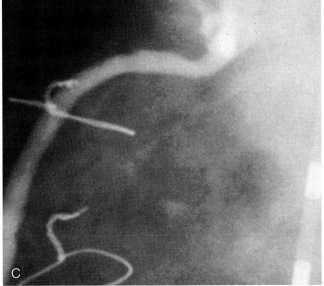

Figure 2–2
An eccentric, ostial stenosis of the right coronary artery was without fluoroscopic calcium *(Panel A)*. Directional atherectomy was not considered owing to the presence of severe peripheral vascular disease, and therefore standard balloon angioplasty was performed. With an Amplatz guiding catheter slightly withdrawn to allow balloon inflation across the ostium, a 3.5-mm balloon catheter was fully inflated to 8 atm *(Panel B)*. Afterwards, a 20% residual stenosis was obtained *(Panel C)*.

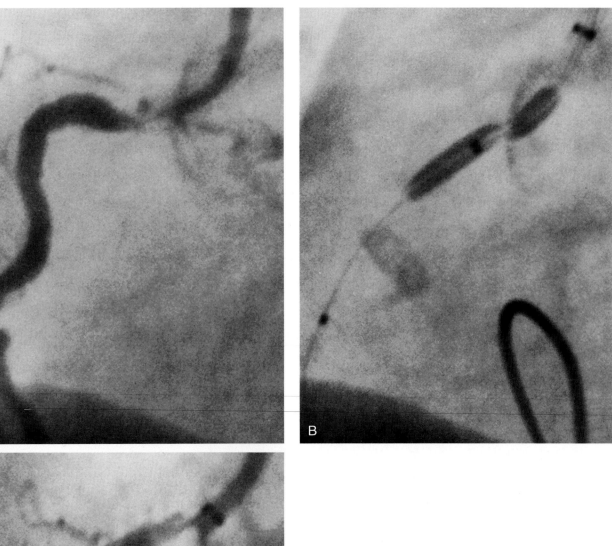

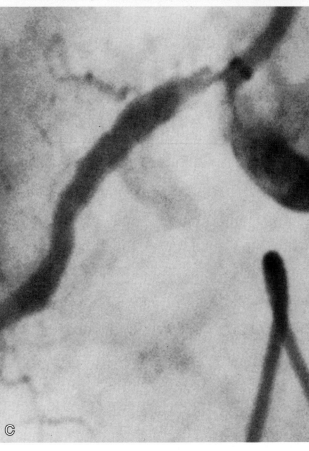

Figure 2–3
A heavily calcified stenosis involving the origin of the right coronary artery *(Panel A)* was treated with a 3.0-mm balloon catheter *(Panel B)*. Despite inflations to 6 atm, a residual "waist" was present. A prolonged balloon inflation was performed, but a suboptimal angiographic result was obtained *(Panel C)*. The patient was referred for elective coronary bypass surgery.

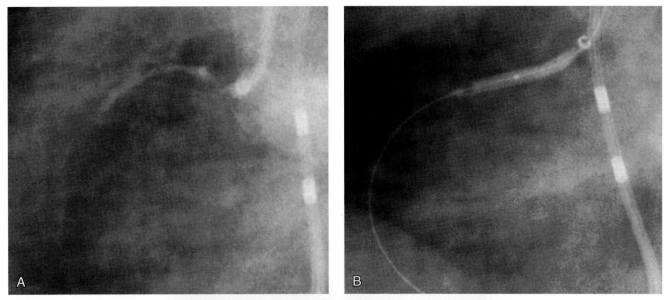

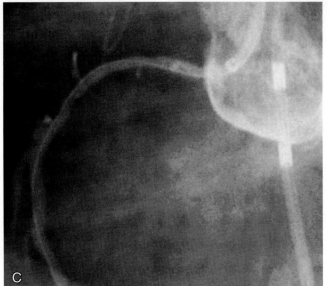

Figure 2–4
The ostial lesion of the right coronary artery resulted in subtotal occlusion of the vessel *(Panel A)*, rendering estimation of the reference vessel size difficult. No fluoroscopic calcium was visualized. A 2.5-mm balloon catheter was advanced across the ostial lesion, and the guiding catheter was gently withdrawn. Complete balloon expansion was obtained at 6 atm *(Panel B)*, and an acceptable angiographic result (a 10% residual stenosis) was achieved using balloon angioplasty *(Panel C)*.

Encouraging initial results have also been reported using directional coronary atherectomy in patients with ostial lesions involving larger coronary arteries (>3.0 mm) that are without significant calcium. Intravascular ultrasound studies suggest that a substantial degree of residual plaque remains after directional atherectomy is performed in patients with ostial lesions, despite the appearance of marked angiographic improvements.

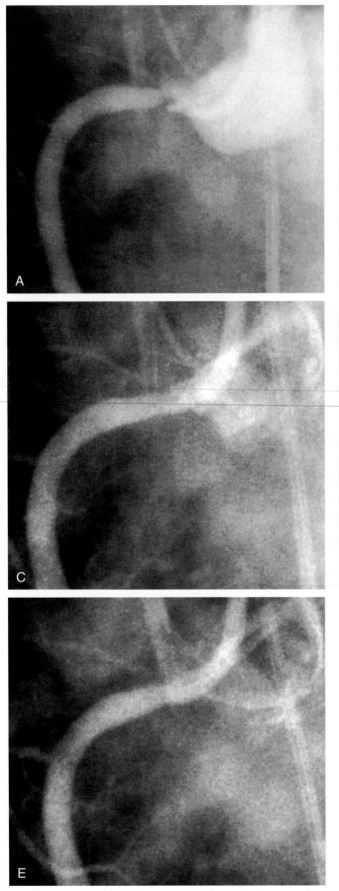

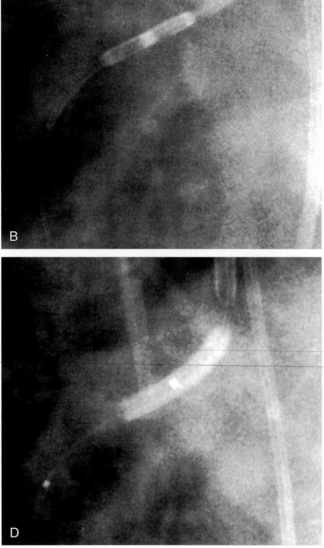

Figure 2–5

An ulcerated, ostial lesion involving the right coronary artery *(Panel A)* was treated with a 7-French DVI EX directional atherectomy device. After the guiding catheter was withdrawn into the aorta, directed, inferior cuts of the lesion were performed *(Panel B)*. Following atherectomy, the ulceration was no longer visualized; however, the superior surface of ostium appeared somewhat irregular *(Panel C)*. For this reason, a 3.5-mm balloon catheter was inflated *(Panel D)*, yielding a 20% residual stenosis and a smooth lumen contour *(Panel E)*.

The relatively high profile and rigidity of the directional atherectomy device may make the procedure more difficult in some ostial lesions.

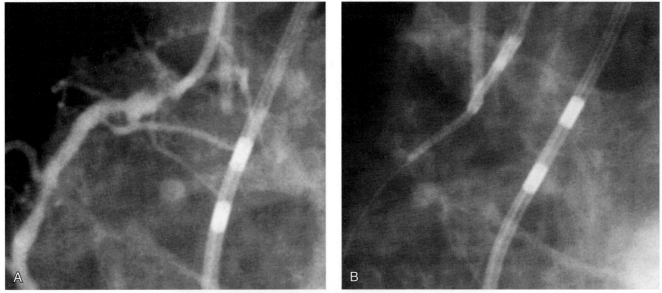

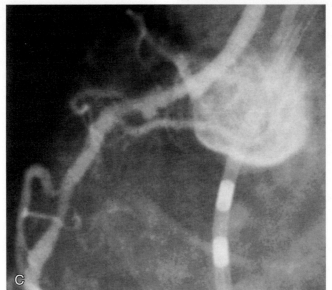

Figure 2–6
An irregular ostial lesion of the right coronary artery was found to have moderate calcification in the proximal segment of the artery, even though no intralesion calcium was identified ultrasonographically *(Panel A)*. Despite excellent guide catheter support, a 6-French DVI EX directional atherectomy device could not be advanced across the ostium *(Panel B)*. The directional atherectomy catheter was removed, and standard balloon angioplasty was performed, resulting in an adequate but suboptimal 30% residual stenosis *(Panel C)*.

In patients with calcified right coronary artery lesions, rotational atherectomy selectively ablates fibrocalcific plaque. Once plaque debulking has occurred, either adjunct balloon angioplasty or directional atherectomy may be performed in selected patients.

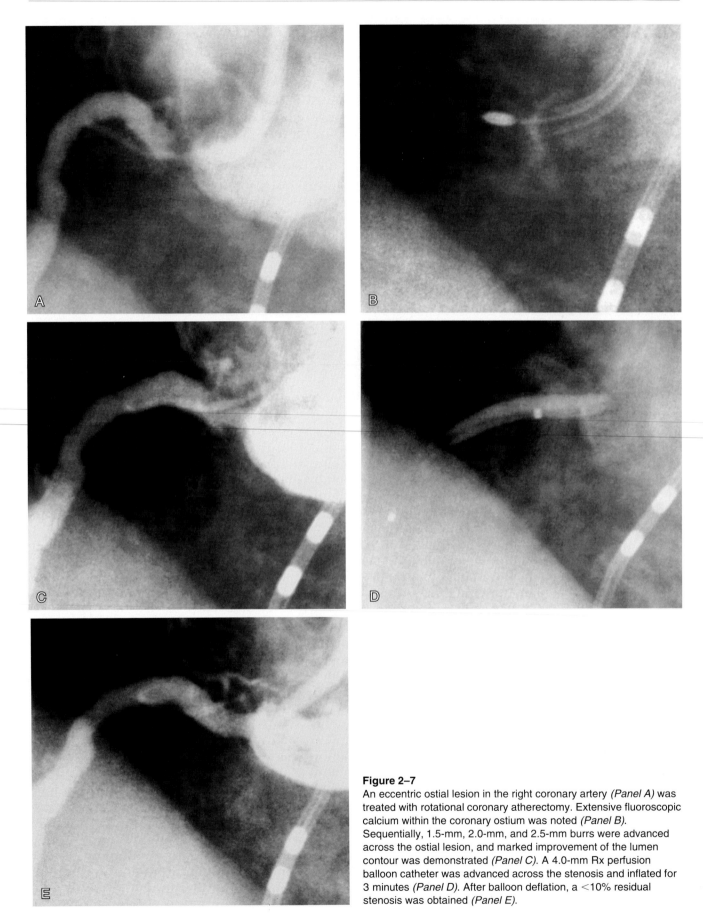

Figure 2–7
An eccentric ostial lesion in the right coronary artery *(Panel A)* was treated with rotational coronary atherectomy. Extensive fluoroscopic calcium within the coronary ostium was noted *(Panel B)*. Sequentially, 1.5-mm, 2.0-mm, and 2.5-mm burrs were advanced across the ostial lesion, and marked improvement of the lumen contour was demonstrated *(Panel C)*. A 4.0-mm Rx perfusion balloon catheter was advanced across the stenosis and inflated for 3 minutes *(Panel D)*. After balloon deflation, a <10% residual stenosis was obtained *(Panel E)*.

In patients with nonangulated ostial lesions of the right coronary artery, excimer laser angioplasty may represent an alternative to rotational atherectomy for the ablation of lesions with moderate lesion calcium. Although the 308-nm excimer laser effectively ablates calcific plaque, its ablative effect on severe lesion calcification is less certain.

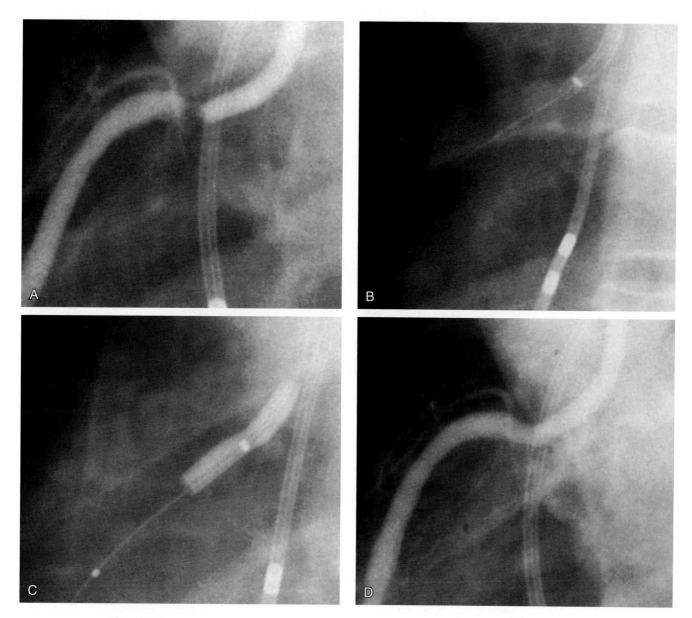

Figure 2–8
An eccentric ostial stenosis of the right coronary artery *(Panel A)* contained a moderate degree of intralesion calcium by intravascular ultrasound *(Panel B)*. A 1.3-mm excimer (308-nm) laser catheter was advanced across the stenosis using a single-pass technique. A 50% residual stenosis was obtained. With the guiding catheter withdrawn into the aorta, balloon angioplasty using a 3.0-mm perfusion catheter was performed *(Panel C)*. A residual waist was noted at the ostium, suggesting the presence of residual lesion rigidity. After balloon deflation, a 20% residual stenosis was obtained *(Panel D)*.

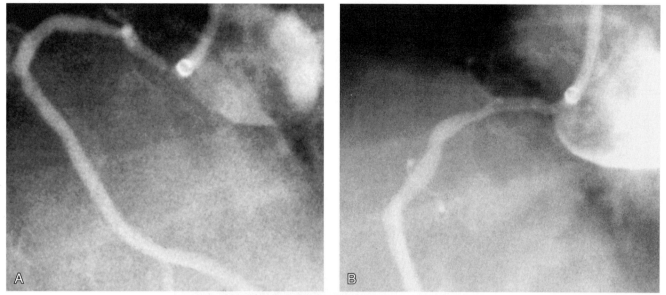

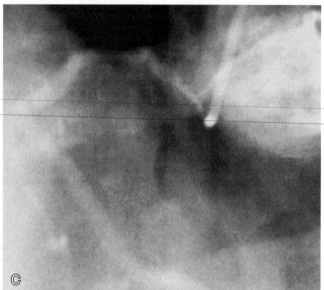

Figure 2–9
A noncalcified ostial stenosis of the right coronary artery *(Panel A)* was treated with a 1.3-mm excimer laser (308 mm) catheter and a 2.5-mm adjunct balloon catheter. After final balloon deflation, a 20% residual stenosis was obtained *(Panel B)*. Despite an acceptable initial result, the patient's symptoms recurred 2 months later. Repeat angiography demonstrated a recurrent ostial stenosis *(Panel C)*. This highlights the dual challenge of treating ostial lesions; not only is primary success in their ablation more difficult, but also their recurrence rate is higher.

Ostial lesions involving the origin of a saphenous vein graft may have a greater degree of lesion rigidity than do lesions located within the body of a saphenous vein graft. At times, they exhibit the characteristics of aortic wall lesions rather than those of saphenous vein lesions. In patients with lesions of this complex subset, new angioplasty devices that reduce residual atherosclerotic plaque (atherectomy/ ablation devices) and diminish elastic recoil (intracoronary stents) may be useful in obtaining an improved initial angiographic result. Undoubtedly, this lesion subset presents one of the highest risks for restenosis, again underscoring the need for achieving optimal final lumen dimensions.

Directional atherectomy has been used in patients with ostial lesions of larger saphenous vein grafts (≥3.0 mm) with encouraging initial results; however, late recurrence has been reported. The principal advantage of directional atherectomy in this lesion subset is that partial plaque resection changes lesion compliance and renders the ostium more amenable to mechanical dilatation by the device or by adjunct balloon. All interventions should be performed with utmost caution in ostial lesions that are located within aged or degenerated saphenous vein grafts owing to the potential risk of distal embolization.

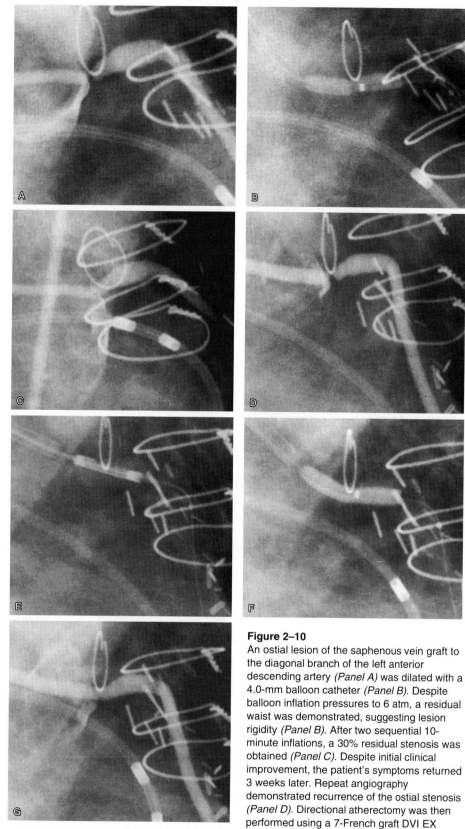

Figure 2–10

An ostial lesion of the saphenous vein graft to the diagonal branch of the left anterior descending artery *(Panel A)* was dilated with a 4.0-mm balloon catheter *(Panel B)*. Despite balloon inflation pressures to 6 atm, a residual waist was demonstrated, suggesting lesion rigidity *(Panel B)*. After two sequential 10-minute inflations, a 30% residual stenosis was obtained *(Panel C)*. Despite initial clinical improvement, the patient's symptoms returned 3 weeks later. Repeat angiography demonstrated recurrence of the ostial stenosis *(Panel D)*. Directional atherectomy was then performed using a 7-French graft DVI EX catheter *(Panel E)*, and abundant tissue removal was achieved. Adjunct balloon angioplasty using a 4.0-mm balloon catheter resulted in almost complete balloon expansion *(Panel F)*. Although the angiographic result after directional atherectomy was improved compared with that obtained using balloon angioplasty alone, a 30% residual stenosis persisted *(Panel G)*. The patient's symptoms recurred 3 months later, and repeat angiography demonstrated restenosis at the directional atherectomy site.

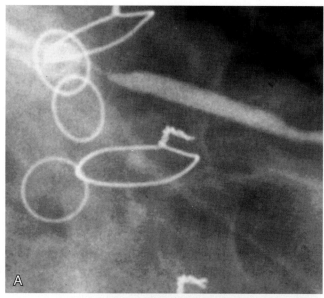

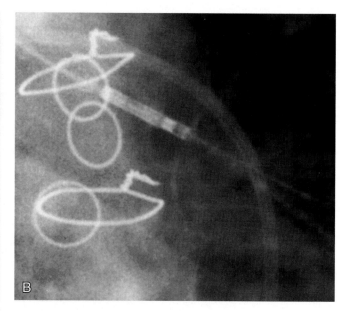

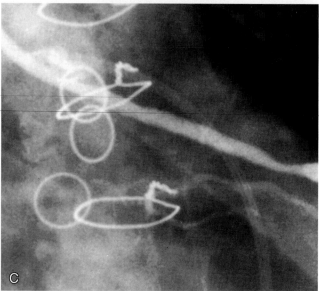

Figure 2–11

An eccentric stenosis of the ostium of a saphenous vein graft to the left anterior descending artery *(Panel A)* was treated using a 7-French DVI EX directional atherectomy device *(Panel B).* Circumferential cuts were performed; however, cuts were preferentially made toward the superior surface. Notably, an intermediate lesion in the distal segment of the graft could not be crossed with the nose cone. After 6 excisions were performed, a 10% residual stenosis was obtained without evidence of distal embolization *(Panel C).*

Two additional new devices have been used in the treatment of patients with ostial lesions of saphenous vein grafts. Transluminal extraction atherectomy has demonstrated excellent initial results in ostial saphenous vein graft lesions, particularly those with degeneration. For recalcitrant restenotic lesions that involve the ostium of larger saphenous vein grafts (>3.0 mm), intragraft stenting has also been used.

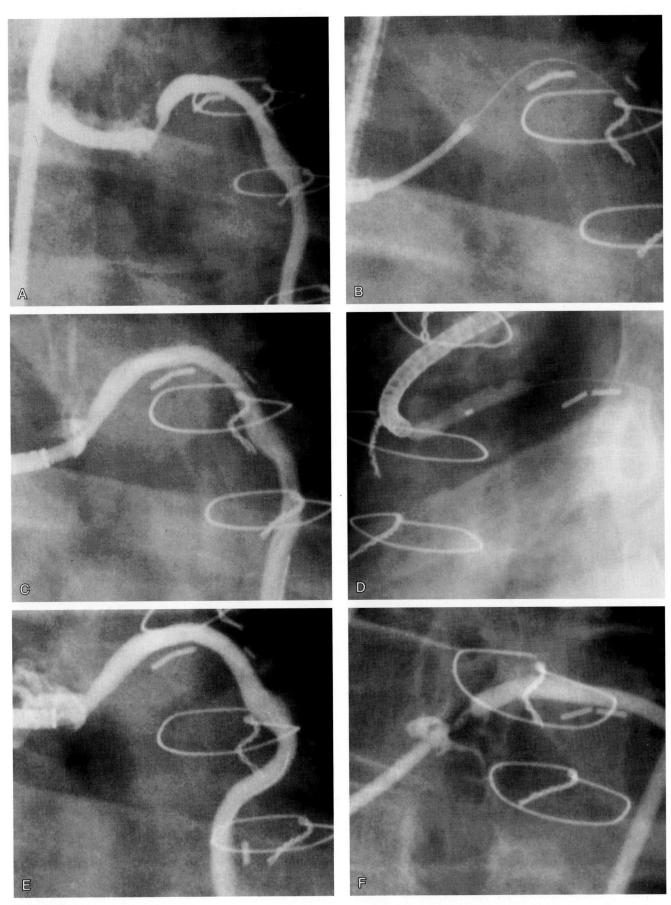

Figure 2–12
An eccentric ostial lesion of a nondegenerated saphenous vein graft to the obtuse marginal branch *(Panel A)* was treated with a 7-French transluminal extraction atherectomy catheter *(Panel B)*. Four passes were performed across the lesion, and the atheromatous debris was collected using vacuum suction *(Panel B)*. After atherectomy, a 30% residual stenosis and mild lumen irregularities were noted *(Panel C)*. For this reason, a 3.5-mm balloon catheter was inflated across the lesion *(Panel D)*; this improved the lumen diameter and smoothed the roughened surface *(Panel E)*. Despite an excellent initial angiographic result, restenosis occurred 4 months later *(Panel F)*.

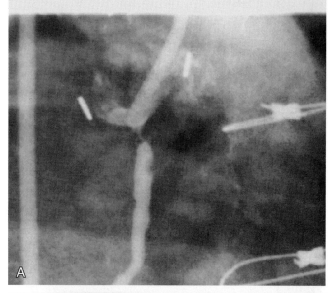

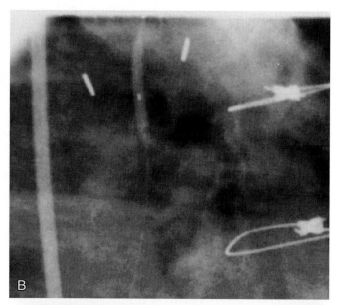

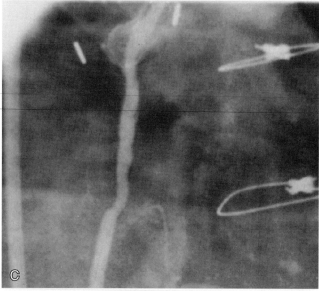

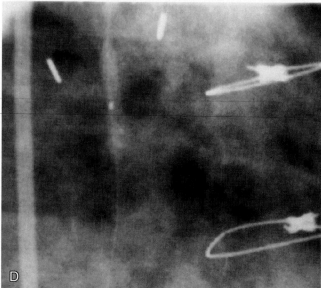

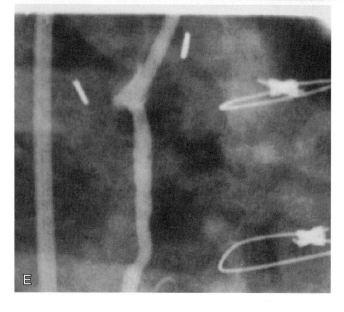

Figure 2–13

The ostial lesion of the saphenous vein graft to the posterior descending branch had been treated with standard balloon angioplasty on two prior occasions *(Panel A)*. On both occasions, the initial angiographic result was limited owing to elastic recoil. Therefore, intragraft stenting was recommended. Predilatation using a 2.5-mm balloon catheter *(Panel B)* resulted in a lumen of sufficient diameter *(Panel C)* to allow passage of a 3.5-mm Palmaz-Schatz tubular slotted stent across the ostial lesion. With the multipurpose guiding catheter slightly withdrawn into the aorta, almost complete balloon inflation was achieved at 6 atm *(Panel D)*. After stent deployment, a 10% residual stenosis was obtained *(Panel E)*.

Few series have reported the results of balloon angioplasty of ostial lesions that involved the left anterior descending or circumflex arteries, presumably because of the infrequent use of conventional balloon angioplasty in this setting. Clinical impressions of experienced investigators suggest that (1) incomplete dilation is a frequent obstacle and that (2) coronary dissections may occur more commonly with ostial lesions than with nonostial lesions in these locations when standard balloon angioplasty is used.

The procedural risk of left main artery occlusion with retrograde propagation of a dissection from the ostium of the left anterior descending or left circumflex coronary arteries must be considered carefully. Directional and rotational atherectomy have been used as alternatives in patients with ostial lesions involving the left anterior descending and circumflex coronary arteries. Device selection depends on the degree of calcification within the vessel, lesion length, vessel tortuosity, and the reference vessel size.

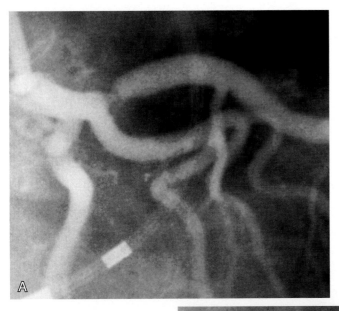
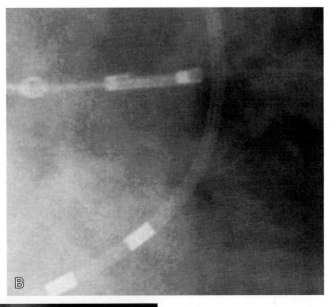
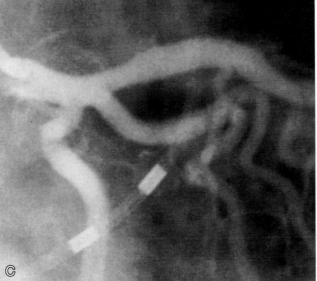

Figure 2–14
The noncalcified ostial lesion of the proximal segment of the left anterior descending artery *(Panel A)* was treated with a 7-French DVI EX atherectomy catheter *(Panel B)*. Because of the large caliber of the left anterior descending artery (3.8 mm), higher balloon inflation pressures were used (40 psi). An abundant amount of tissue was retrieved, and a 20% residual stenosis was achieved using stand-alone atherectomy *(Panel C)*.

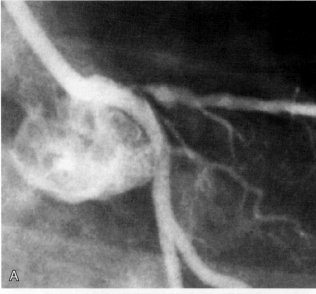

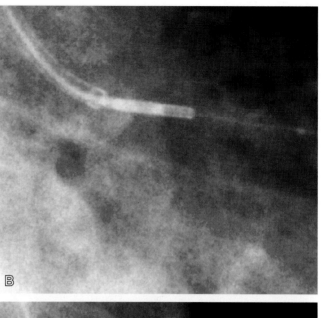

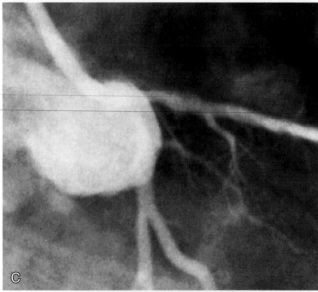

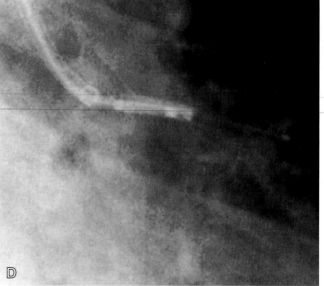

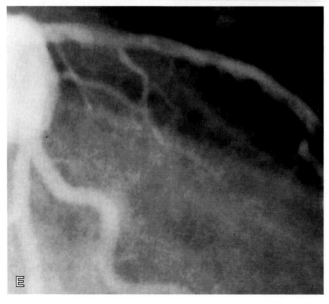

Figure 2–15

An eccentric, mildly calcified and irregular lesion of the ostial left anterior descending artery *(Panel A)* was treated using a 6-French DVI EX directional atherectomy device *(Panel B)*. After directed, inferior cuts were performed, a 30% residual stenosis was obtained *(Panel C)*. A 7-French DVI EX atherectomy device was then positioned across the residual stenosis, and additional preferential cuts were obtained along the inferior aspect of the left anterior descending artery *(Panel D)*. After further atherectomy, a <10% residual stenosis was obtained *(Panel E)*.

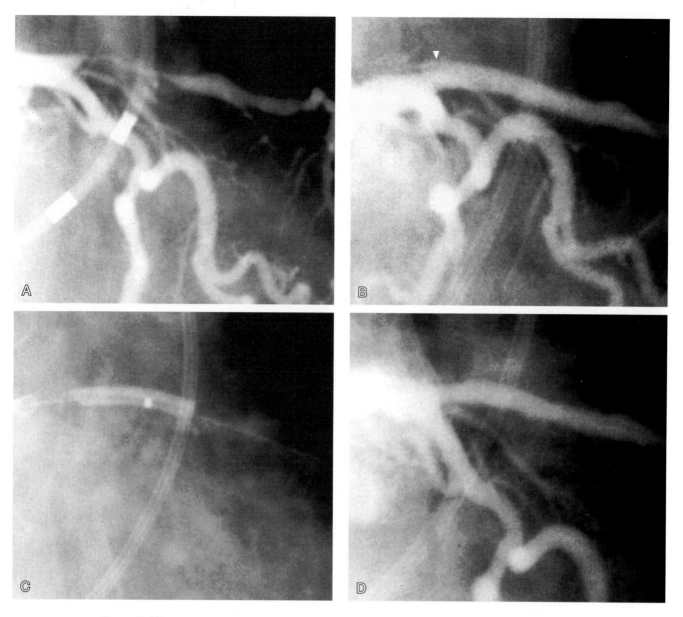

Figure 2–16

A long (15-mm) ostial lesion of the left anterior descending artery *(Panel A)* was treated with a 7-French DVI EX atherectomy device. After circumferential cuts were performed, an excellent angiographic result was obtained, and an abundant amount of tissue was removed *(Panel B)*. A local dissection (<5 mm) was noted *(arrow)* and treated with inflation of a 3.0-mm balloon catheter *(Panel C)*. This resulted in a 20% residual stenosis *(Panel D)*.

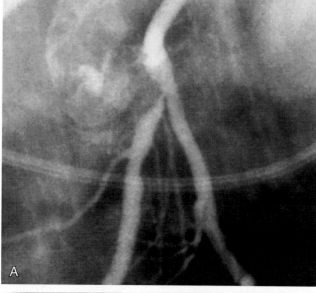

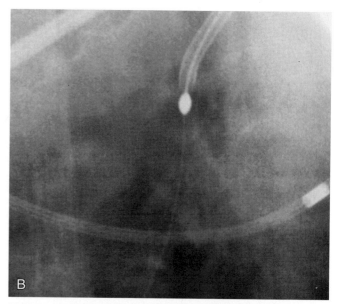

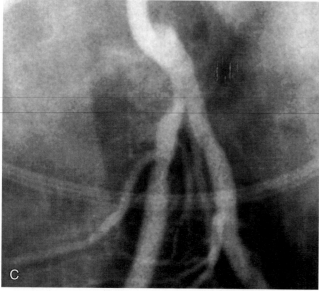

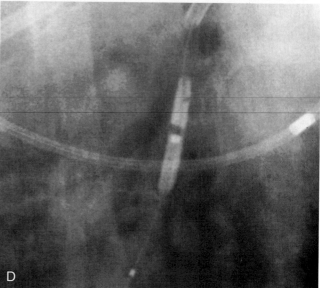

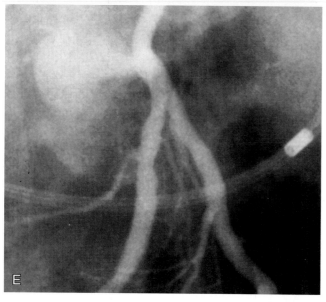

Figure 2–17
The heavily calcified ostial lesion of the left circumflex coronary artery *(Panel A)* was treated using 1.5-mm and 1.75-mm burrs *(Panel B)*. After two passes, a 40% residual stenosis was obtained *(Panel C)*. A 3.0-mm balloon catheter was inflated across the residual stenosis *(Panel D)*, resulting in a 10% residual stenosis *(Panel E)*. (Reprinted from Popma J, Brogan W, Pichard A, et al. Rotational atherectomy of ostial stenoses. Am J Cardiol 1993; 71:436, with permission.)

Coronary angioplasty of the ostia of branch vessels of the epicardial coronary arteries has been associated with reduced procedural success compared with that attained with nonostial stenoses. Reduced success rates are probably a result of the same factors that characterize true ostial lesions—that is, lesion rigidity due to fibrosis and extensive plaque accumulation and further complicated by smaller vessel size. In many patients, standard balloon angioplasty is sufficient to treat these ostial branch vessel lesions. On occasion, however, this intervention fails to achieve a successful result, particularly when lesion calcification is present. In such cases, new device angioplasty using directional or rotational atherectomy or excimer laser angioplasty may be useful.

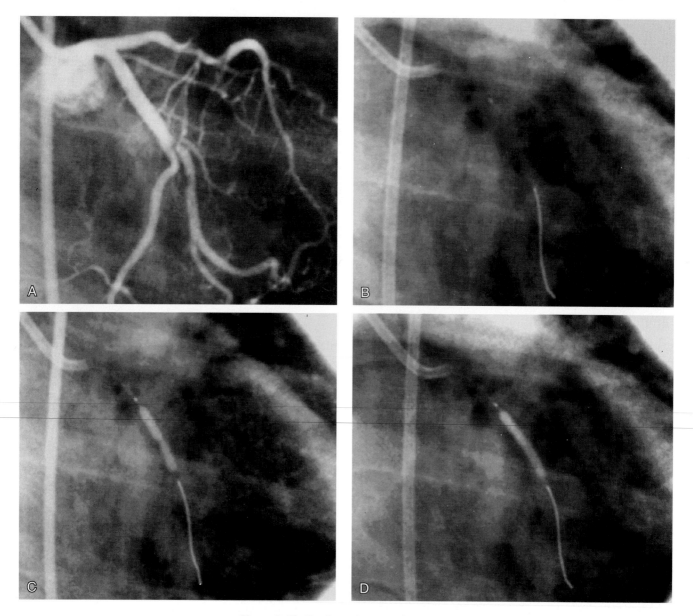

Figure 2–18. *See legend on opposite page*

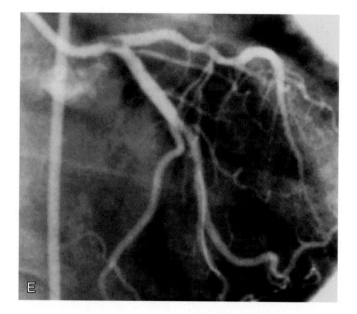

Figure 2–18
An ostial stenosis of the obtuse marginal branch *(Panel A)* had mild fluoroscopic calcium. A 2.5-mm balloon catheter was advanced across the lesion and inflated to 6 atm *(Panel C)*. On account of lesion rigidity, a residual waist was noted; oscillating inflations to 12 atm were performed, resulting in full balloon expansion *(Panel D)*. An acceptable angiographic result was obtained without evidence of coronary dissection of the parent branch (left circumflex) *(Panel E)*.

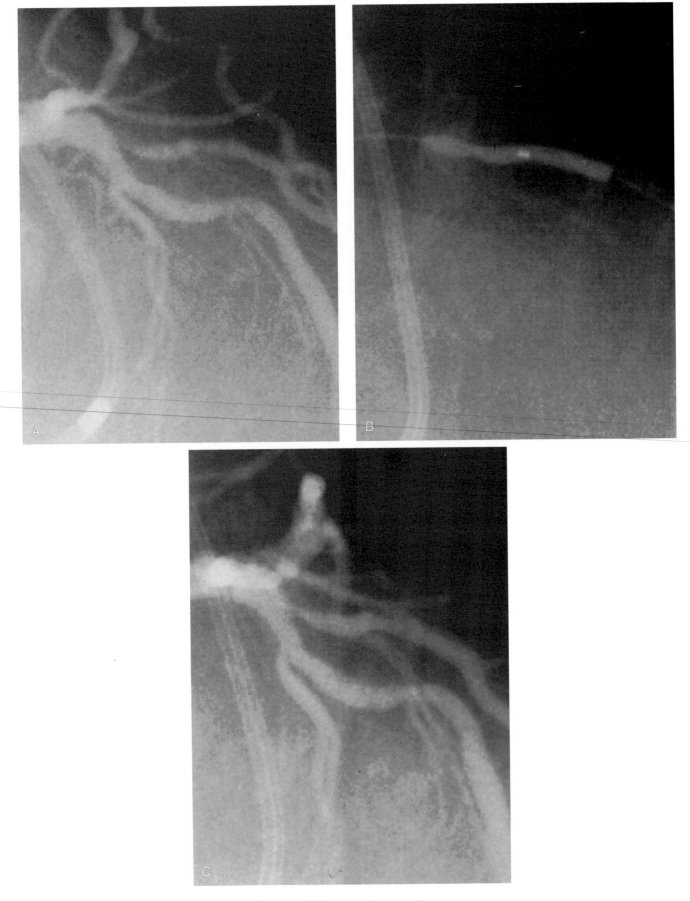

Figure 2–19. *See legend on opposite page*

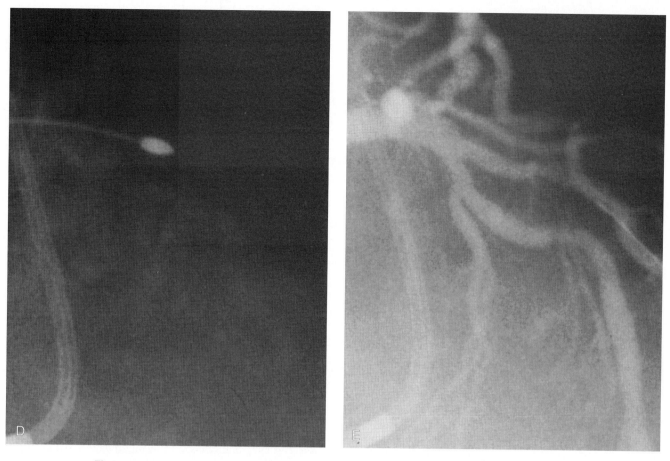

Figure 2–19

A 90% stenosis of the ostium of the first diagonal branch of the left anterior descending artery *(Panel A)* was treated with a 2.5-mm balloon dilatation catheter. Despite inflation to 10 atm, a residual waist was noted *(Panel B)*. After two inflations, a 70% residual stenosis persisted *(Panel C)*. A 2.0-mm rotational atherectomy device burr was used to treat the residual stenosis *(Panel D)*. After two passes, an excellent result was obtained *(Panel E)*; distal spasm of the midportion of the vessel was treated with nitroglycerin administration.

SELECTED REFERENCES

Kuntz R, Piana R, Schnitt S, et al. Early ostial vein graft stenosis: Management by atherectomy. Cathet Cardiovasc Diagn 1991; 24:41–44.

Mathias D, Mooney F, Lange H, et al. Frequency of success and complications of coronary angioplasty of stenoses at the ostium of side-branches. Am J Cardiol 1991; 67:491–495.

Popma J, Brogan W, Pichard A, et al. Rotational coronary atherectomy of ostial stenoses. Am J Cardiol 1993; 71:436–438.

Popma J, Dick R, Haudenschild C, et al. Atherectomy of right coronary ostial stenoses: Initial and long-term results, technical features and histologic findings. Am J Cardiol 1991; 67:431–433.

Popma J, Leon M, Mintz G, et al. Results of coronary angioplasty using the transluminal extraction catheter. Am J Cardiol 1992; 70:1526–1532.

Stewart J, Ward D, Davies M, Pepper J. Isolated coronary ostial stenosis: Observations on the pathology. Eur Heart J 1987; 8:917–920.

Topol E, Ellis S, Fishman J, et al. Multicenter study of percutaneous transluminal angioplasty for right coronary artery ostial stenoses. J Am Coll Cardiol 1987; 9:1214–1218.

Total Coronary Occlusions

Total coronary occlusions are a frequent cause of failure of standard balloon angioplasty; failure which is most often due to the inability to pass a coronary guide wire across the occluded segment or, if a guide wire has been advanced, to the inability to successfully dilate the segment using standard balloon methods. Often, the presence of one or more total occlusions in a patient with multivessel coronary artery disease dictates referral for coronary artery bypass surgery.

A number of new devices have been used as adjuncts or alternatives to balloon dilatation of recanalized total occlusions. The potential advantages of new devices in patients with this lesion subset include the ability to (1) debulk the plaque without causing severe disruption to the intima and media; (2) alter plaque compliance, rendering the underlying plaque segment amenable to balloon dilatation; and (3) provide internal scaffolding to reduce elastic recoil.

A strategic algorithm for the use of the various technologies for total occlusions has been proposed (Figure 3–1).

In general, after the totally occluded segment has been crossed by a coronary guide wire, predilatation using an undersized balloon (≤2.0 mm) may be performed. Once the segment has been recanalized, the length of the occlusion can be more accurately determined. In shorter (<10 mm) segments of occlusion in vessels >3.0 mm in diameter, directional atherectomy has been successful. Calcific lesions may be treated with rotational atherectomy, although the extent of distal run-off for the ablative microparticulate must be assessed. In patients with refractory restenosis, intracoronary stenting has been attempted. Long diffusely diseased segments (≥20 mm) may be treated by balloon angioplasty (using long balloons) or by excimer laser coronary angioplasty in an attempt to "debulk" the underlying atherosclerotic plaque. In virtually all patients who have undergone excimer laser angioplasty, a residual stenosis persists, and adjunct balloon dilatation can be performed using long (30–40 mm) balloons.

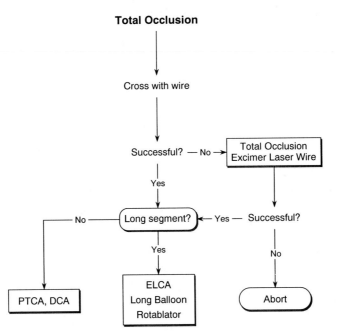

Figure 3–1
A proposed strategic algorithm for the management of total occlusions.

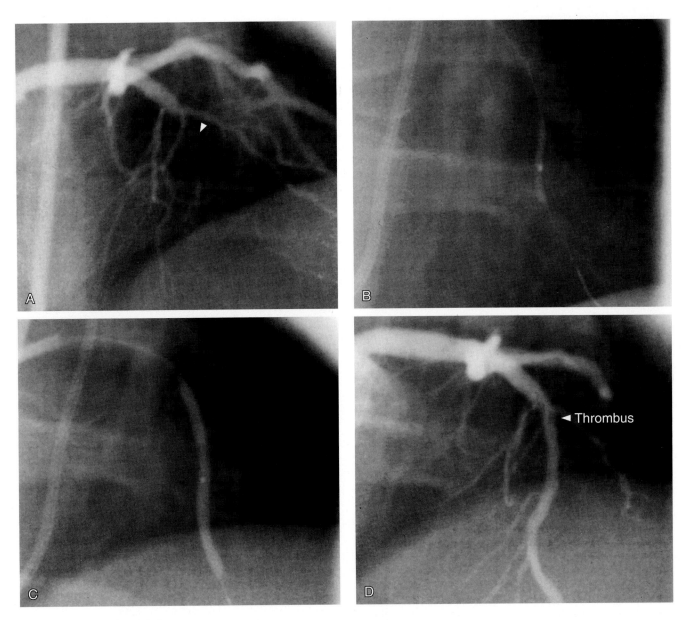

Figure 3–2
Coronary angiography was performed in this patient 3 weeks after an anterior wall myocardial infarction. It demonstrated a total occlusion in the midsegment of the left anterior descending artery *(arrow, Panel A)*. A 0.014-inch intermediate guide wire was advanced through a probing sheath across the occluded segment, and initial dilatation was performed using a 2.0-mm balloon catheter *(Panel B)*. Recanalization of the left anterior descending artery demonstrated a diffusely (25-mm) diseased segment in its midportion. Subsequent balloon dilatation was performed using a 2.5-mm long (40-mm) balloon *(Panel C)*. After balloon deflation, a 30% residual stenosis was obtained; however, a moderate degree of residual intraluminal haziness consistent with thrombus persisted *(Panel D)*.

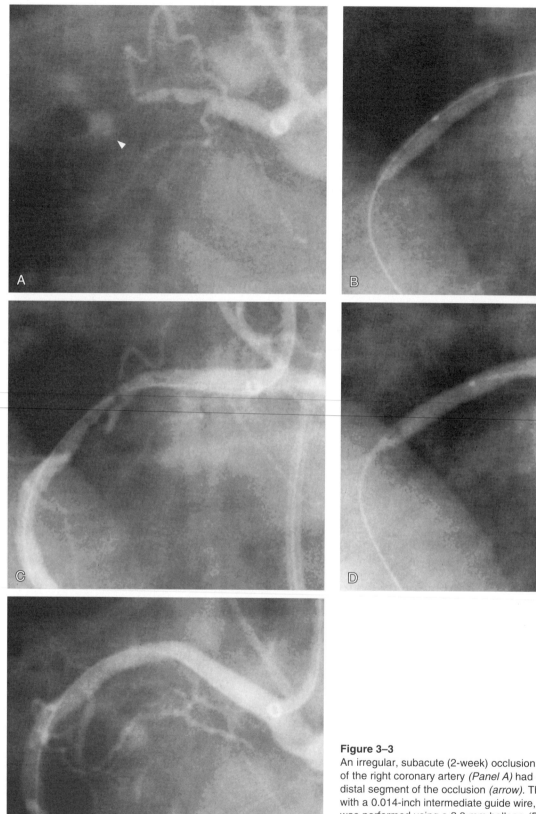

Figure 3–3

An irregular, subacute (2-week) occlusion of the proximal segment of the right coronary artery *(Panel A)* had contrast staining in the distal segment of the occlusion *(arrow)*. The occlusion was crossed with a 0.014-inch intermediate guide wire, and balloon dilatation was performed using a 3.0-mm balloon *(Panel B)*. After vessel recanalization, a linear dissection and intimal flap were demonstrated *(Panel C)*. Balloon dilatation using a 3.5-mm long (30-mm) balloon was subsequently performed *(Panel D)*. After a prolonged (3-minute) balloon inflation, a <10% residual stenosis was obtained *(Panel E)*.

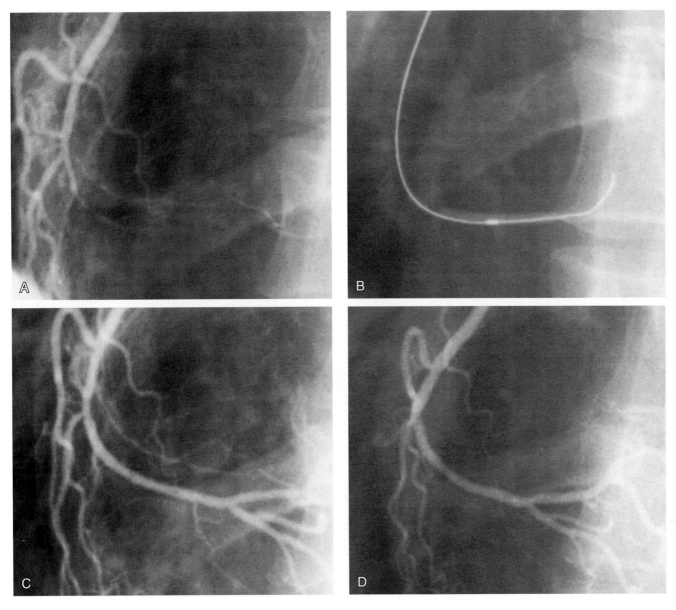

Figure 3–4
A chronic total occlusion of the midsegment of the right coronary artery *(Panel A)* was crossed with a
0.014-inch standard coronary guide wire. Balloon dilatation in the proximal and distal segments
(Panel B) of the lesion using a 2.5-mm balloon catheter resulted in a <10% residual stenosis *(Panel
C)*. Symptoms recurred 4 months later, and repeat angiography demonstrated a widely patent
dilatation site *(Panel D)* with disease progression in the left coronary artery.

A number of predictors of failure for coronary angioplasty in patients with chronic occlusions have been identified, including the presence of bridging collateral vessels,
long (≥2 cm) occlusions, the absence of a discrete pouch
or entry funnel, severe proximal vessel tortuosity, and a
long duration of occlusion (>3 months). Refinements in
angioplasty techniques have led to improved results in re-
canalizing and, subsequently, treating total occlusions.
These include the use of stiff hydrophilic guide wires as
well as enhanced imaging of the occlusion entry site (bi-
plane angiography) and distal parent neolumen via collateral vessels (simultaneous ipsilateral and contralateral coronary injections).

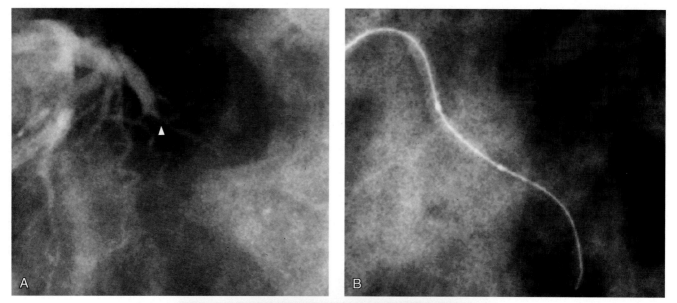

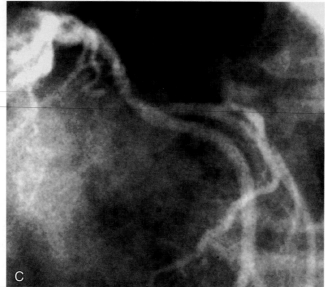

Figure 3–5
Three days after this patient experienced a posterior wall myocardial infarction, a total occlusion of
the midsegment of the left circumflex coronary artery was demonstrated *(Panel A)*. A discrete pouch
was noted in the left anterior oblique projection *(arrow)*. A 0.014-inch high-torque intermediate
coronary guide wire was advanced across the stenosis, and a 3.0-mm balloon dilatation catheter was
inflated to 6 atm *(Panel B)*. After balloon deflation, a 30% residual stenosis was demonstrated *(Panel
C)*. To avoid oversizing additional balloon catheters relative to the reference vessel segment,
additional, larger balloon inflations were not performed.

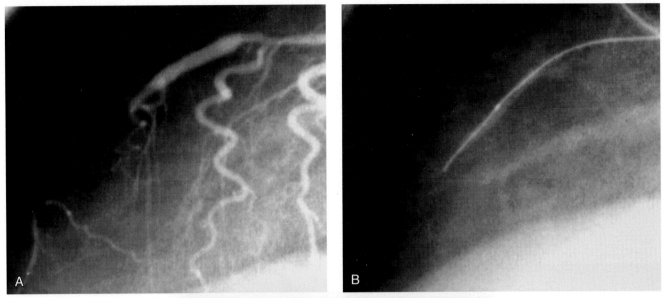

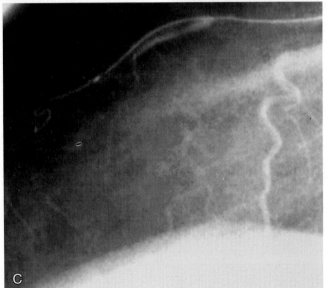

Figure 3–6
A long (35-mm) chronically occluded segment of the midportion of the left anterior descending artery
was approached with standard balloon angioplasty *(Panel A)*. A variety of 0.014- and 0.018-inch
guide wires were advanced within a 2.5-mm balloon dilatation catheter for support, but the guide
wires did not reach the distal segment of the left anterior descending artery. In an attempt to provide a
larger channel for balloon passage, the 2.5-mm balloon catheter was inflated to 4 atm *(Panel B)*,
resulting in a long spiral dissection in the midsegment *(Panel C)*. Further attempts to recanalize the
left anterior descending artery were abandoned.

Complications are relatively infrequent after coronary an-gioplasty of total occlusions, particularly when collateral vessels to the occluded segment are present. On occasion, however, reocclusion may result in recurrent ischemia, po-tentially due to derecruitment of collateral vessels or embo-lization of collateral vessels to the occluded segment.

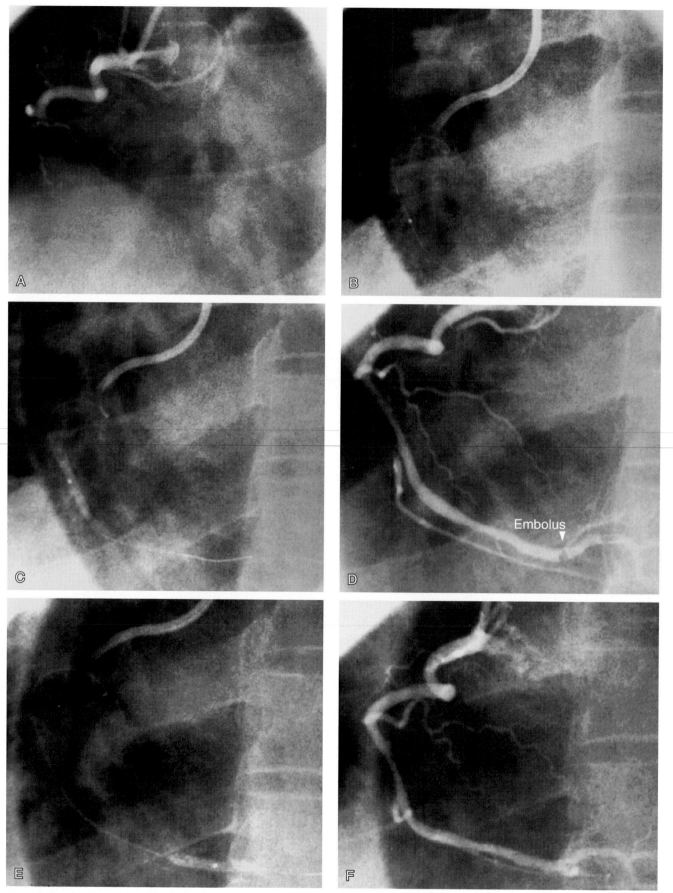

Figure 3–7
A total occlusion was noted in the midsegment of the right coronary artery distal to severe proximal vessel tortuousity *(Panel A)*. Using a left Amplatz soft-tipped guiding catheter, the right coronary artery was deeply engaged to allow sufficient backup support to permit passage of a 0.014-inch intermediate guide wire across the total occlusion *(Panel B)*. A 2.5-mm balloon dilatation catheter was advanced across the occluded segment and inflated to 6 atm *(Panel C)*. A moderate degree of elastic recoil occurred, and a 40% tubular residual stenosis persisted. After balloon deflation, the patient developed chest pain, inferior electrocardiographic changes, and diminished flow into the posterior descending branch. Repeat angiography demonstrated a coronary embolus *(Panel D)* in the distal portion of the right coronary artery and posterior descending branch. Balloon dilatation was performed using a low-pressure 2.5-mm balloon *(Panel E)* with resolution of the distal embolus and restoration of distal coronary perfusion *(Panel F)*.

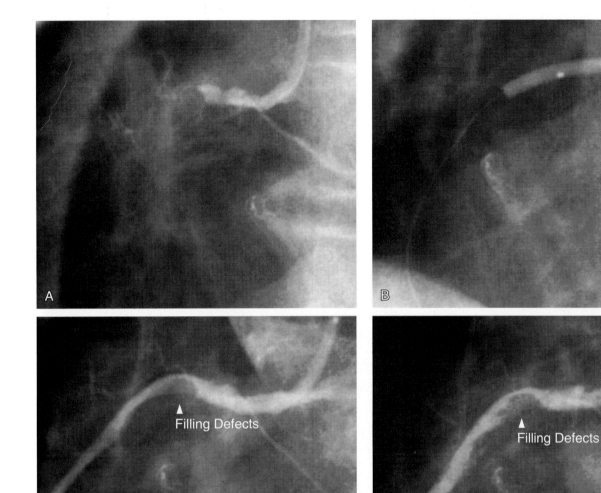

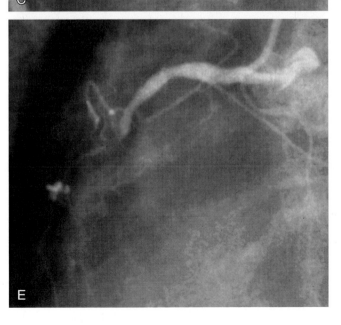

Figure 3–8

Seven days after this patient experienced an inferior wall myocardial infarction, a total occlusion of the proximal segment of the right coronary artery was demonstrated *(Panel A)*. Balloon angioplasty was performed using a 0.014-inch high-torque floppy wire and a 3.0-mm balloon catheter *(Panel B)*. After initial recanalization, a filling defect in the proximal segment was noted *(Panel C)*; this defect persisted despite prolonged balloon inflations and intracoronary administration of urokinase, 500,000 U *(Panel D)*. Twelve hours later, the patient developed recurrent chest pain associated with electrocardiograhic changes suggestive of ischemia, and repeat angiography demonstrated thrombotic reocclusion just distal to the angioplasty site *(Panel E)*.

Direct coronary angioplasty has been used in patients with acute myocardial infarction in an effort to prevent bleeding complications associated with thrombolytic therapy. Procedural success rates in excess of 95% have been reported with the use of direct angioplasty, and direct angioplasty may be the treatment of choice in selected patients presenting within 6 hours of symptom onset of acute myocardial infarction.

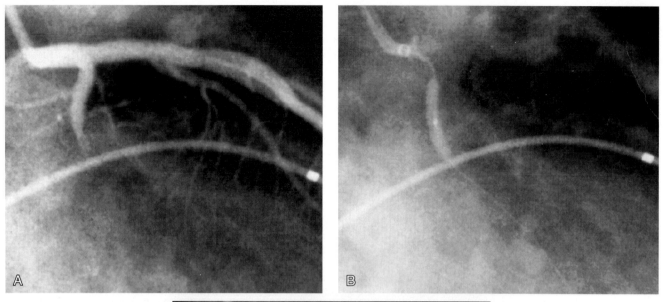

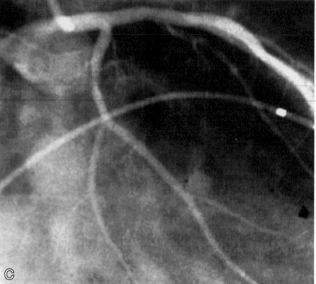

Figure 3–9
Emergency coronary angiography was performed in this patient with electrocardiographic evidence of an acute posterolateral myocardial infarction, which demonstrated an acute occlusion of the proximal segment of the left circumflex artery. A 0.018-inch high-torque exchange coronary guide wire was advanced across the thrombotic occlusion *(Panel A),* and a 3.0-mm balloon was inflated to 6 atm *(Panel B).* After two balloon inflations, the left circumflex and large (obtuse) marginal branches were recanalized with a <10% residual stenosis *(Panel C).*

Owing to more extensive thrombus burden and other factors, such as distal run-off, thrombolytic therapy is less effective in patients with acutely occluded saphenous vein grafts than in those with thrombotic occlusions in native vessels. As a result, emergent catheterization and angio- plasty may be an acceptable alternative form of therapy in selected coronary bypass patients who present to the hospital within 12 hours of symptom onset of acute myocardial infarction.

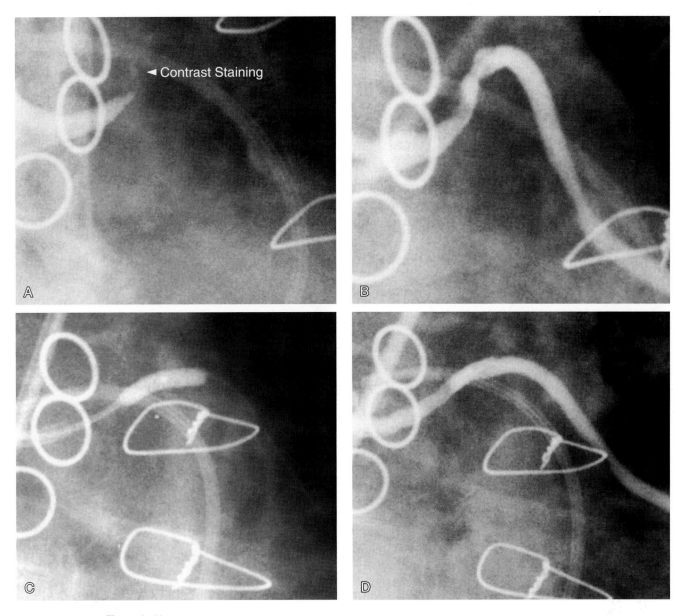

Figure 3–10
An acute thrombotic occlusion of the proximal segment of a saphenous vein graft to the left anterior descending artery was associated with mild contrast staining *(Panel A)*. A 0.018-inch high-torque floppy wire was advanced across the stenosis, and initial balloon dilatations were performed using a 2.5-mm balloon catheter. Although recanalization of the left anterior descending artery was achieved, a 30% residual stenosis associated with a dissection and with filling defects was noted *(Panel B)*. Prolonged balloon inflations using 3.5-mm and 4.0-mm balloons *(Panel C)* resulted in a minimal residual stenosis; however, a mild degree of intraluminal haziness persisted *(Panel D)*. No evidence of distal embolization or reduction in anterograde flow was present once recanalization of the graft had been achieved.

Restenosis after an initially successful procedure occurs in 50% to 60% of patients with lesions causing total occlusion; the stenosis recurs as a total occlusion in 20% of cases. When restenosis occurs as a discrete lesion, it can be easily treated with repeat balloon angioplasty.

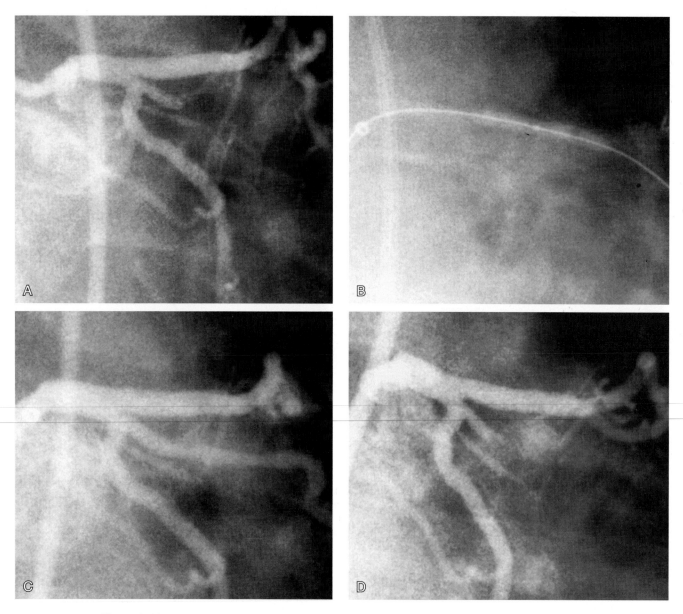

Figure 3–11
A total occlusion of the ramus branch *(Panel A)* was crossed with a 0.014-inch intermediate coronary guide wire, and dilatation with a 2.5-mm balloon catheter was performed *(Panel B)*. After a 3-minute balloon inflation, a minimal residual stenosis (<10%) was demonstrated *(Panel C)*. Despite the excellent initial result, symptoms recurred 6 weeks later, and repeat angiography demonstrated a recurrent total occlusion *(Panel D)*.

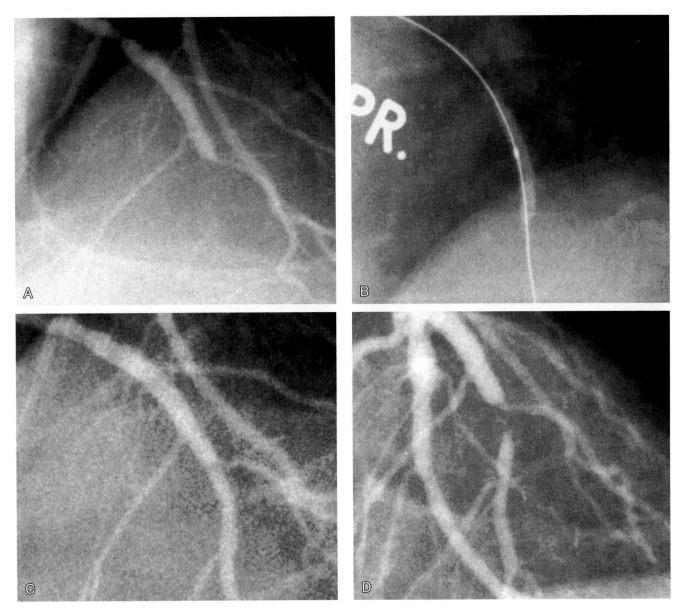

Figure 3–12
A total occlusion of the distal left anterior descending artery *(Panel A)* was crossed with a 0.014-inch intermediate guide wire, and a 2.5-mm balloon catheter was inflated *(Panel B)*. After sequential inflations, a minimal residual stenosis was achieved *(Panel C)*. Symptoms recurred 3 months later, and repeat coronary angiography demonstrated focal restenosis of the midsegment of the left anterior descending artery *(Panel D)*, which was easily treated with standard balloon angioplasty.

To overcome the limitations of standard coronary guide wires (which often can be advanced only with difficulty and which have a tendency to form subintimal tracks), an "olive"-shaped, 1-mm ball tip mounted on a 0.021-inch stainless steel wire—the Magnum wire—has been developed. The methodology for use of the Magnum wire is delineated in Table 3–1.

Table 3–1   Guidelines for the Use of the Magnum Wire

Step	Description
Preparation	After a gentle curve has been placed on the distal 1 cm of the Magnum wire, the wire is introduced retrograde into a dilatation balloon appropriately sized to the reference segment.
Advancement	The distal burr tip should protrude 10 cm from the balloon catheter during advancement through the coronary segment using the J-tip configuration to traverse bends and bifurcations.
Crossing the lesion	The olive tip is positioned at the site of total occlusion, and the catheter is advanced just proximal to the olive tip, splinting the wire. Contrast medium is injected to ascertain the correct position of the olive tip with regard to the stump of the occlusion. The Magnum wire is then thrust forward with half turns if the burr does not advance. With continued pressure, the Magnum wire often passes easily across the site of occlusion.
Advancing the balloon	Once the position of the Magnum wire has been confirmed angiographically, the balloon catheter is advanced across the lesion, and balloon dilatation is performed in the standard fashion.
Exchanges	Because of the short length of the wire (185 cm), usual exchange methods cannot be performed. Due to the rigidity of the wire, the balloon catheter can be retracted without fear of losing distal wire position.

(Adapted from Meier B, Carlier M, Finci L, et al. Magnum wire for balloon recanalization of chronic total coronary occlusions. Am J Cardiol 1989; 64:148–154.)

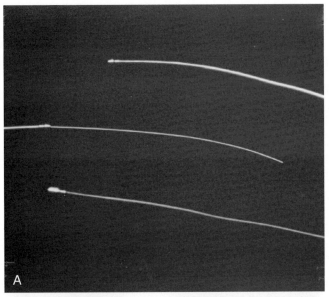

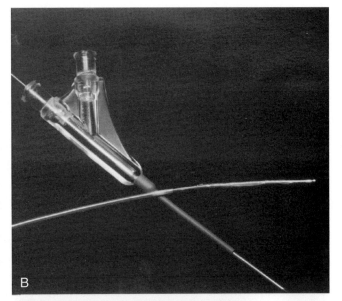

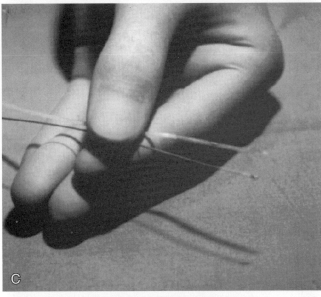

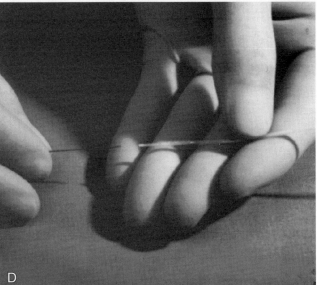

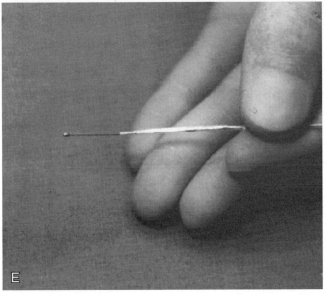

Figure 3–13
The 0.021-inch Magnum wire has a 1-mm olive-shaped tip at its
distal segment *(Panel A)*. Because of the large wire dimensions, the
wire is generally used with a Magnum balloon *(Panels B and C)*.
The wire is introduced in a retrograde fashion into the balloon
catheter *(Panel D)*, and the wire and balloon are advanced as a unit
(Panel E) into the guiding catheter.

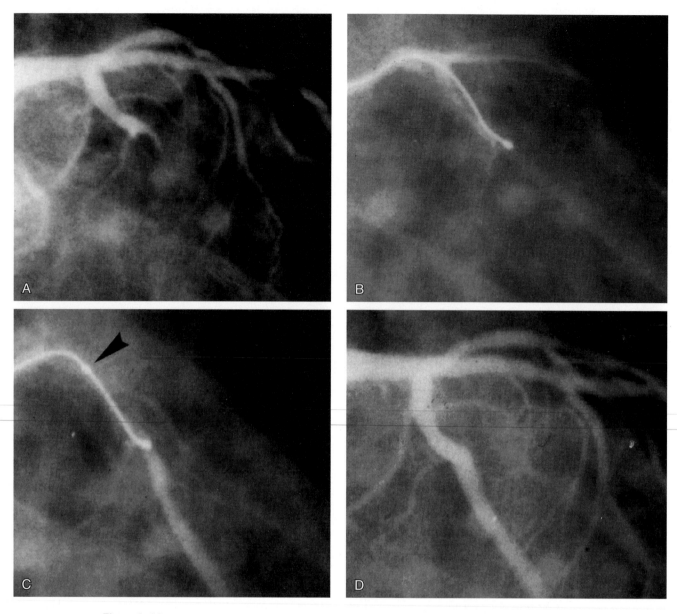

Figure 3–14
A total occlusion of the proximal segment of the left circumflex *(Panel A)* was treated with the
Magnum wire. The 1-mm olive-shaped burr was advanced to the site of occlusion *(Panel B)*, and the
balloon dilatation catheter was advanced to just proximal to the wire *(Panel C)*. With sufficient guiding
catheter support, the Magnum wire crossed the occlusion; balloon angioplasty was performed,
resulting in a <10% residual stenosis and no evidence of dissection *(Panel D)*. (Courtesy of B. Meier,
MD.)

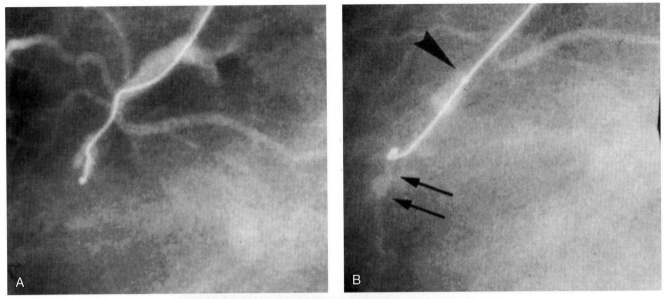

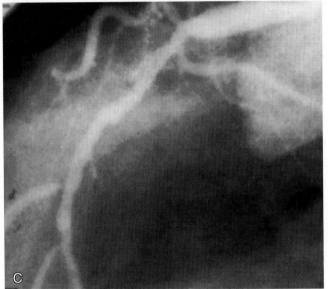

Figure 3–15
A chronic total occlusion of the midportion of the right coronary artery was crossed with the Magnum wire *(Panel A)*. The olive-shaped burr was positioned to avoid a subintimal dissection flap *(Panel B, smaller arrows)*. Contrast injection demonstrated that the balloon catheter was within the lumen *(Panel B, large arrow)*. After balloon dilatation using standard techniques, a 20% residual stenosis was obtained *(Panel C)*. (Courtesy of B. Meier, MD.)

When significant plaque burden is present (usually in larger vessels) or when moderate to severe calcification at the occlusion site is noted, directional or rotational atherectomy may be preferable after initial guide wire recanalization. Stents are also being evaluated to treat focal total occlusions in larger vessels (≥3 mm).

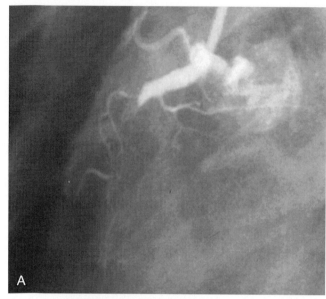

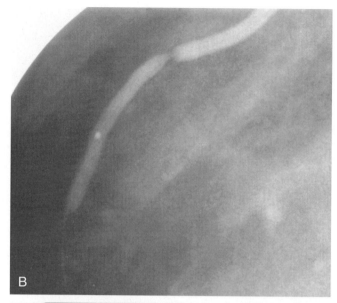

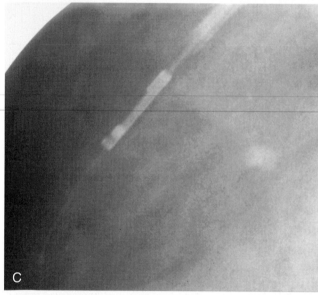

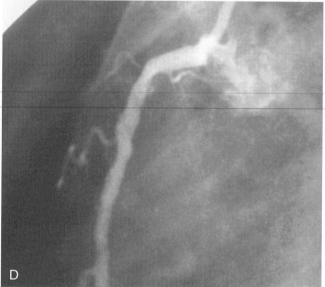

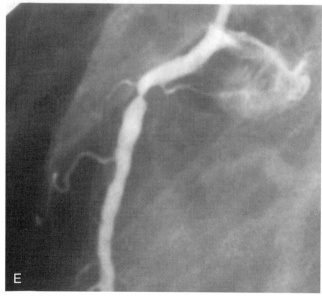

Figure 3–16
The totally occluded proximal segment of the right coronary artery *(Panel A)* was crossed with a 0.014-inch intermediate guide wire, and balloon dilatation with a 2.5-mm long (30-mm) balloon catheter was performed *(Panel B)*. A 6-French directional atherectomy device was advanced across the lesion, and circumferential cuts were performed *(Panel C)*. An excellent anatomic result was obtained with a 10% residual stenosis *(Panel D)*. The patient's symptoms recurred 2 months later; repeat angiography was performed, demonstrating a focal stenosis at the site of prior total occlusion *(Panel E)*. This recurrent stenosis was easily dilated using standard balloon techniques.

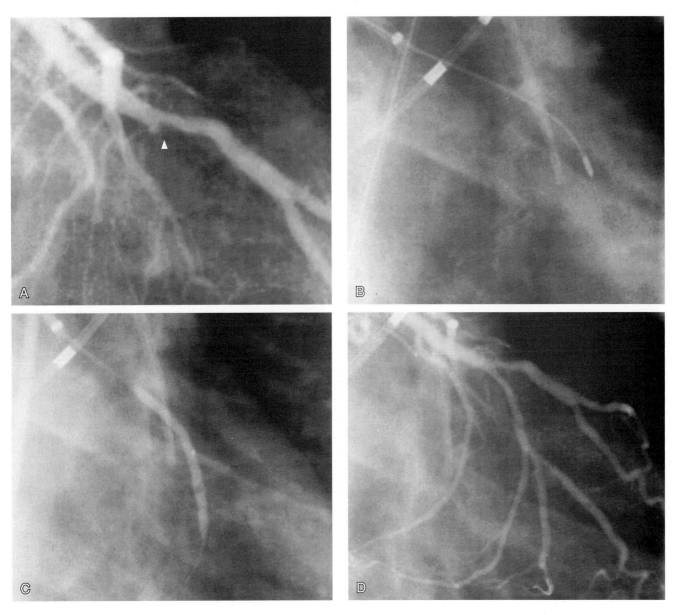

Figure 3–17
A calcified, total occlusion of a large diagonal branch supplying the posterolateral myocardium *(arrow, Panel A)* was crossed with a 0.009-inch HT exchange length guide wire. A 1.5- and a 1.75-mm burr were used to ablate the fibrocalcific plaque and to re-establish coronary perfusion *(Panel B)*. A 2.5-mm long (30-mm) balloon *(Panel C)* was used to treat the residual stenoses. After adjunct balloon dilatation, an excellent angiographic result was obtained *(Panel D)*.

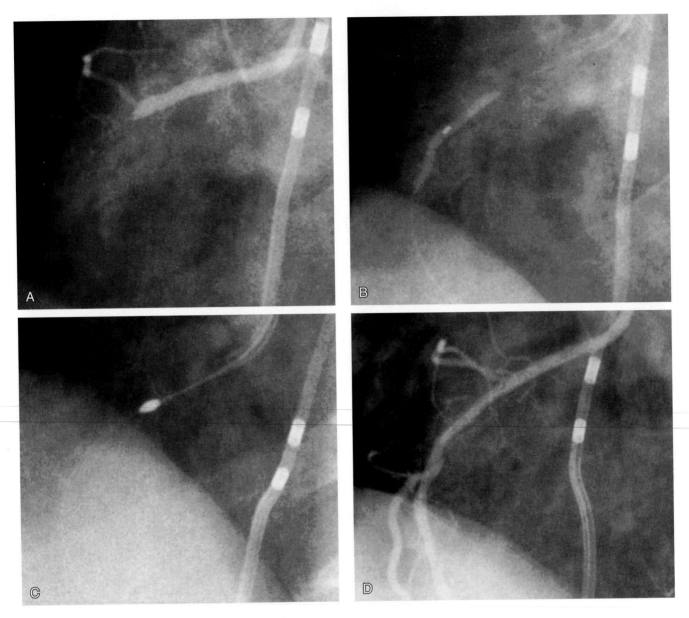

Figure 3–18
The total occlusion of the midportion of the right coronary artery *(Panel A)* was noted to contain moderate fluoroscopic calcium. A 0.014-inch intermediate coronary guide wire was used to cross the lesion, and dilatation was performed using a 2.0-mm balloon catheter *(Panel B)*. A residual 30% stenosis persisted, and rotational coronary atherectomy was performed using 1.75- and 2.0-mm burrs *(Panel C)*. After two passes, an excellent angiographic result was evident *(Panel D)*.

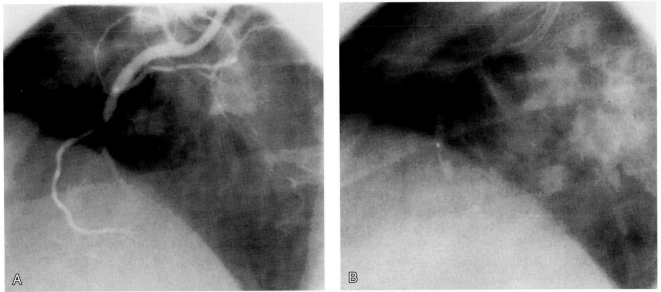

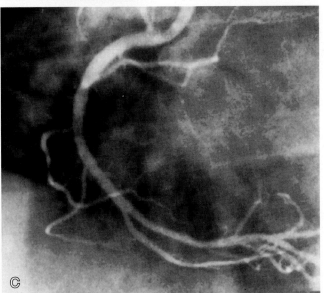

Figure 3–19
A recurrent total occlusion of the midsegment of the right coronary artery *(Panel A)* was treated with a
3.0-mm Palmaz-Schatz tubular slotted stent after pretreatment with a 2.0-mm balloon dilatation
catheter *(Panel B)*. An excellent angiographic result was obtained *(Panel C)*, and no evidence of
restenosis was present at late angiographic follow-up.

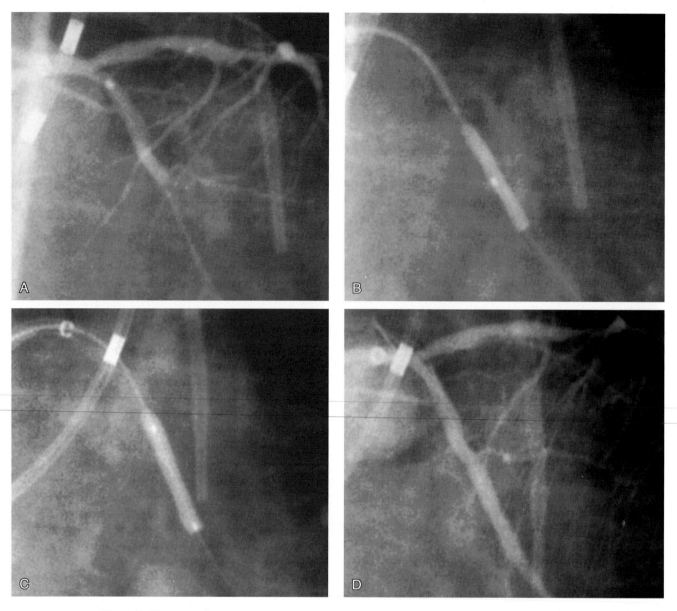

Figure 3–20
A recurrent total occlusion of the proximal segment of the left circumflex *(Panel A)* was predilated with a 2.5-mm balloon catheter *(Panel B)*. A 3.0-mm Palmaz-Schatz stent was deployed across the occluded segment *(Panel C)*, resulting in a <10% residual stenosis *(Panel D)*.

Figure 3–21
A total occlusion of the proximal segment of the right coronary artery *(Panel A)* was crossed with a 0.014-inch intermediate guide wire *(Panel B)*. A 2.0-mm excimer laser (308-nm) catheter was advanced across the lesion *(Panel C)*, resulting in recanalization of the occlusion *(Panel D)*. Adjunct balloon angioplasty was performed, achieving a 30% residual stenosis *(Panel E)*. At control angiography 6 months later, the right coronary artery remained widely patent *(Panel F)*.

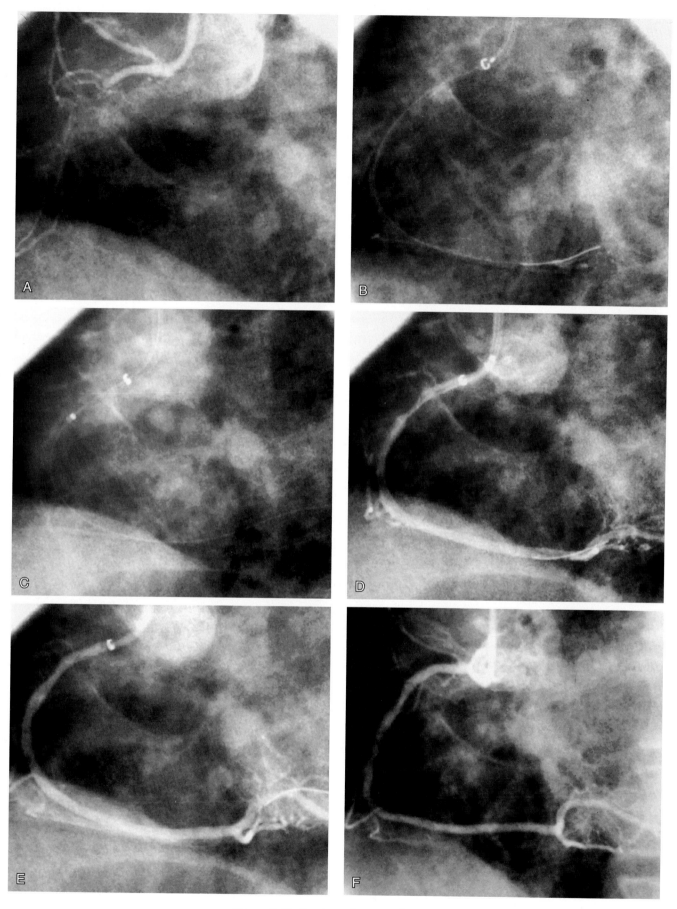

Figure 3–21. *See legend on opposite page*

REFERENCES

Dick R, Haudenschild C, Popma J, et al. Directional atherectomy for total coronary occlusions. Coron Artery Dis 1991; 2:189–199.

Ivanhoe R, Weintraub W, Douglas J, et al. Percutaneous transluminal coronary angioplasty of chronic total occlusions: Primary success, restenosis, and long-term clinical follow-up. Circulation 1992; 85: 106–115.

Kereiakes D, Selmon M, McAuley B, et al. Angioplasty in total coronary artery occlusion: Experience in 76 consecutive patients. J Am Coll Cardiol 1985; 6:526–533.

Maiello L, Colombo A, Almagor Y, et al. Coronary stenting with a balloon-expandable stent after recanalization of chronic total occlusions. Cathet Cardiovasc Diagn 1992; 25:293–296.

Meier B. Chronic total coronary occlusion angioplasty. Cathet Cardiovasc Diagn 1989; 17:212–217.

Meier B, Carlier M, Finci L, et al. Magnum wire for balloon recanalization of chronic total coronary occlusions. Am J Cardiol 1989; 64:148–154.

Serruys P, Umans V, Heyndrickx G, et al. Elective PTCA of totally occluded coronary arteries not associated with myocardial infarction: Short-term and long-term results. Eur Heart J 1985; 6:2–12.

Stone G, Rutherford B, McConahay D, et al. Procedural outcome of angioplasty for total coronary artery occlusion: An analysis of 971 lesions in 905 patients. J Am Coll Cardiol 1990; 15:849–856.

Sugrue D, Holmes D, Smith H, et al. Coronary artery thrombus as a risk factor for acute vessel occlusion during coronary angioplasty: Improving results. Br Heart J 1986; 56:62–66.

Werner G, Buchwald C, Unterberg C, et al. Recanalization of chronic total coronary arterial occlusions by percutaneous excimer-laser and laser-assisted angioplasty. Am J Cardiol 1990; 66:1445–1450.

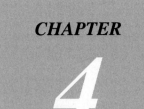

CHAPTER

4

Angulated Lesions

Balloon angioplasty is frequently performed in lesions with moderate to severe vessel angulation. Data from contemporary balloon angioplasty trials indicate that approximately 25% of lesions are moderately angulated (bend ≥45°) and that 2% are severely angulated (bend ≥90°). Prior series have suggested that procedural success is reduced and complications are more common after balloon angioplasty of angulated lesions than after angioplasty of nonangulated ones. Accordingly, lesion angulation may account for 44% of all procedural complications associated with balloon angioplasty. Intravascular ultrasound studies have suggested that coronary dissections often occur at the junction of the atherosclerotic plaque and the normal arterial segment. Angulated lesions are at increased risk for dissection after balloon angioplasty because the balloon dilatation catheter straightens the vessel, tearing the junction of the normal wall and atherosclerotic plaque. This junction is generally more rigid and resistant to axial straightening, particularly in calcified lesions.

Overall procedural failure in the treatment of patients with angulated lesions generally relates to one of three factors: (1) the inability to cross the lesion with a guide wire; (2) the inability to fully dilate the lesion to <50% final diameter stenosis; or (3) the development of an angioplasty-induced dissection that requires stenting or emergent or urgent coronary bypass surgery. The risk for the development of a coronary dissection appears related to clinical and angiographic factors, including the presence of thrombus, excess lesion length (≥10 mm), and advanced patient age (>65 years).

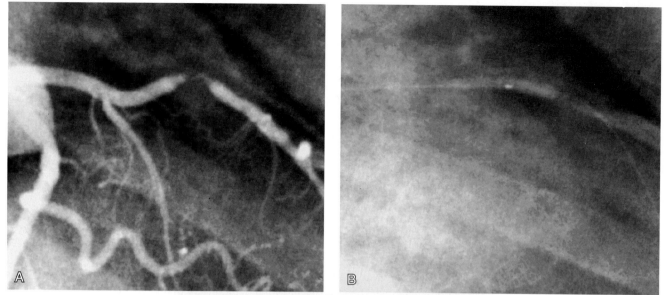

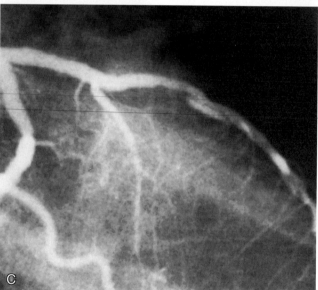

Figure 4–1

A mildly calcified, angulated stenosis of the midsegment of the left anterior descending artery *(Panel A)* was treated with standard balloon angioplasty using a 2.5-mm balloon catheter *(Panel B)*. After two inflations, a localized (10-mm) dissection developed along the inferior surface of the left anterior descending artery *(Panel C)*. Given normal myocardial flow and the absence of clinical symptoms, the patient was managed medically without further intervention.

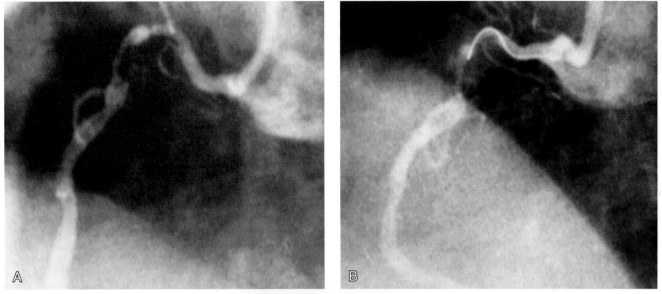

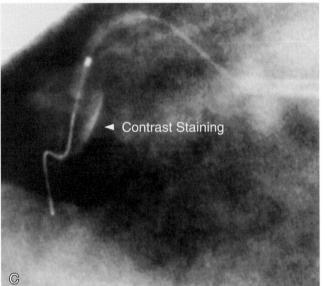

Figure 4–2

A severely angulated stenosis was demonstrated in the proximal segment of the right coronary artery *(Panel A)*. A variety of coronary guide wires were used to cross the diseased segment without success. Further attempts resulted in a subintimal guide wire position and localized contrast staining *(Panel B)*. Subsequently, a wire was passed through the lesion, which was thought to be intraluminal, and balloon inflation was performed within the apparently normal lumen. As a result, further contrast staining and ultimate abrupt closure occurred *(Panel C)*. Note the depth of the perivascular dissection and hematoma as assessed by the distance between the contrast staining and inflated balloon diameter *(arrow)*.

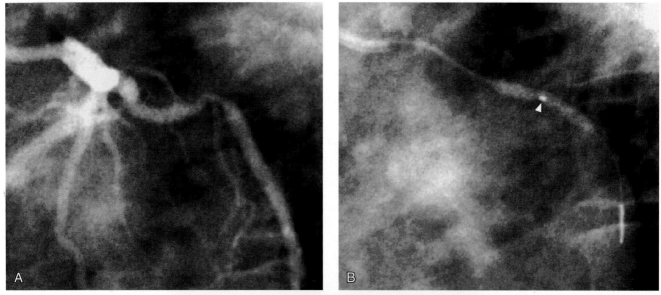

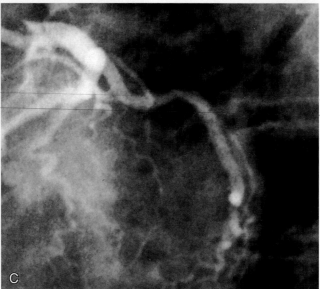

Figure 4–3
An eccentric, angulated stenosis of the midportion of the left circumflex coronary artery *(Panel A)* was treated with standard balloon angioplasty using a 2.5-mm balloon catheter. After balloon inflation to 8 atm, a residual waist of the balloon catheter was demonstrated *(arrow, Panel B)*. After balloon deflation, a 40% residual stenosis was obtained *(Panel C)*. A 3.0-mm balloon dilatation catheter was not used because of the risks of inducing a coronary dissection.

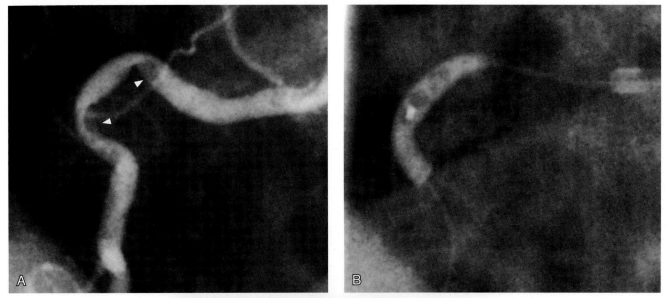

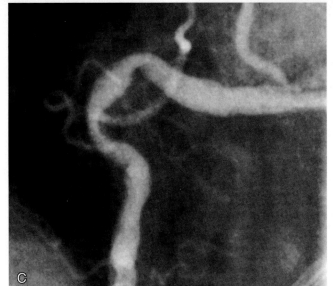

Figure 4–4
Sequential stenoses located in a severely angulated segment of the proximal right coronary artery had intraluminal filling defects consistent with the presence of thrombus *(arrows, Panel A)*. These angulated lesions were dilated with a 2.5-mm and, subsequently, a 3.0-mm balloon catheter *(Panel B)*. Despite complete balloon expansion, a significant degree of elastic recoil developed after balloon deflation, and a minimal improvement in lumen dimensions was obtained *(Panel C)*.

A variety of modifications of standard balloon angioplasty techniques have been used to decrease the complications associated with the treatment of angulated stenoses. Both short (10-mm) and long (30- to 40-mm) balloons have been recommended. A 25-mm balloon with deliberate 135° to 145° angulation has been used in selected patients with excellent initial results; however, the relatively high profile (4.3 French) of this catheter may limit its clinical use. One study has suggested that the use of polyethylene terephthalate balloon material may reduce the incidence of coronary dissection after balloon angioplasty of angulated stenoses. Other studies have suggested that asymmetrically positioned balloon inflations may reduce the degree of vessel straightening that occurs with standard balloon angioplasty. In addition to alterations in the balloon approach, changes in the wire may also be helpful. Stiffer wires, such as the Nitinol, the 0.018-inch wires (rather than 0.14-inch [or 0.10-inch] wires), or extra-support wires may be useful for straightening the diseased segment at the time of inflation. Wire straightening can spuriously affect the appearance of the lesion and of perilesion segments by causing intimal ''wrinkling,'' which some authors have described as an ''accordion'' contour of the lumen.

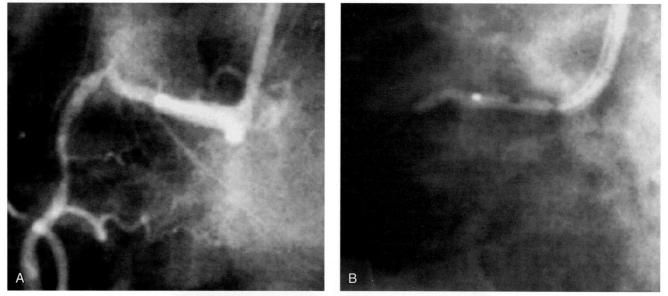

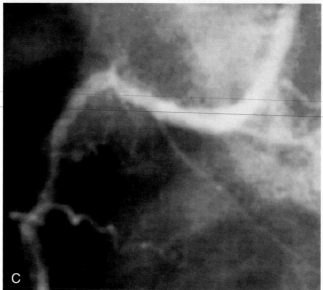

Figure 4–5
An angulated lesion in the proximal segment of the right coronary artery was treated with standard balloon angioplasty *(Panel A)*. Balloon inflation was performed with the balloon catheter positioned proximally within the artery to avoid straightening of the arterial segment *(Panel B)*. After balloon deflation, a 30% residual stenosis persisted *(Panel C)*.

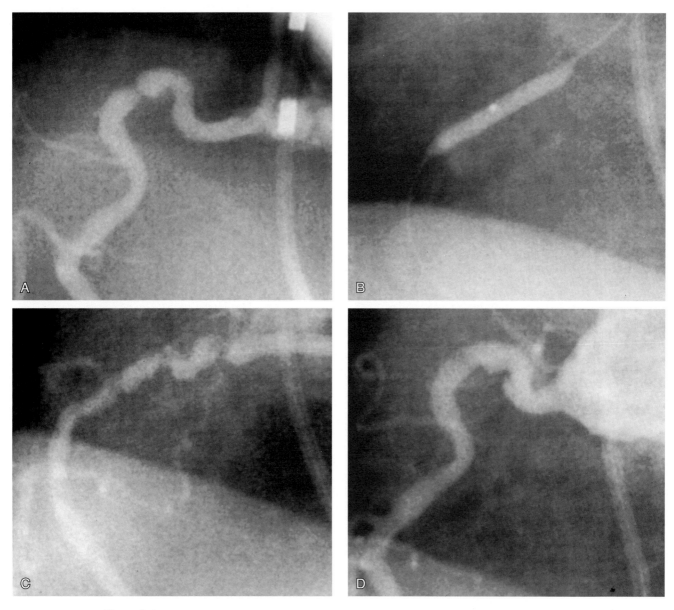

Figure 4–6
A severely angulated stenosis of the proximal segment of the right coronary artery *(Panel A)* was treated with balloon angioplasty. After a 0.014-inch guide wire was positioned in the distal artery, a 2.5-mm balloon dilatation catheter was advanced across the lesion and inflated to nominal pressures *(Panel B)*. After balloon deflation, repeat contrast injection suggested a severely disrupted proximal segment *(Panel C)*. After removal of the coronary guide wire, which had markedly straightened the proximal segment, an acceptable angiographic result was obtained *(Panel D)*.

A select number of new angioplasty devices have been used in angulated lesions. An increase in periprocedural complications has been demonstrated after directional atherectomy of moderately angulated lesions (≥45°); however, a few angulated lesions appear to straighten atraumatically because of the rigidity of the atherectomy device and catheter. It is important to note that calcification proximal to or at the angulated lesion site precludes directional atherectomy catheter advancement and predisposes the vessel to dissections.

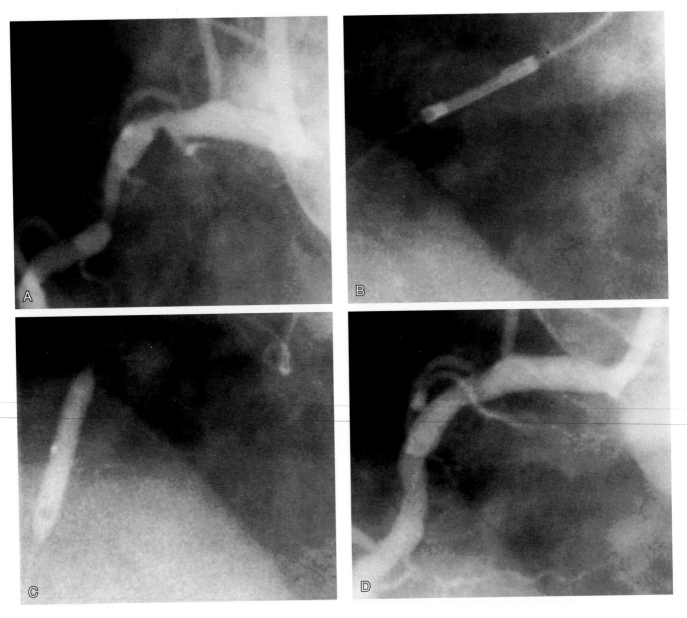

Figure 4–7
Sequential stenoses were noted within the proximal and midsegments of the right coronary artery *(Panel A)*. The eccentric, angulated stenosis of the proximal right coronary artery was treated with a 6-French DVI EX atherectomy device, with circumferential cuts made at a maximum inflation pressure of 30 psi *(Panel B)*. A 3.5-mm balloon catheter was then inflated across the concentric lesion in the midportion of the right coronary artery *(Panel C)*. After balloon deflation, an acceptable angiographic result was obtained in both lesions *(Panel D)*.

Angulated lesions that have significant lesion calcium may be treated with rotational coronary atherectomy because of the flexibility of the rotational atherectomy device's burr over the relatively rigid 0.009-inch coronary guide wire.

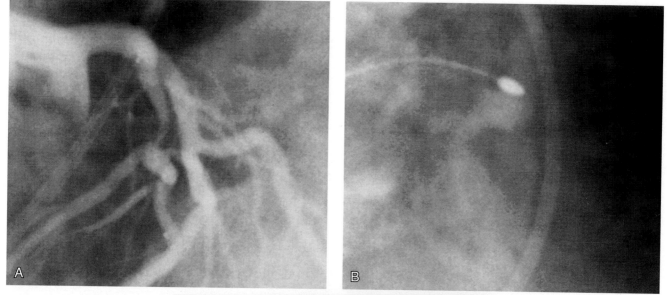

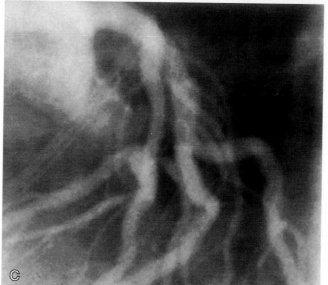

Figure 4–8

The moderately calcified, angulated stenosis of the midsegment of the left anterior descending artery *(Panel A)* was treated with 1.75- and 2.0-mm atherectomy burrs *(Panel B)*. After stand-alone rotational atherectomy, a 20% residual stenosis was obtained without angiographic evidence of dissection or side branch occlusion *(Panel C)*.

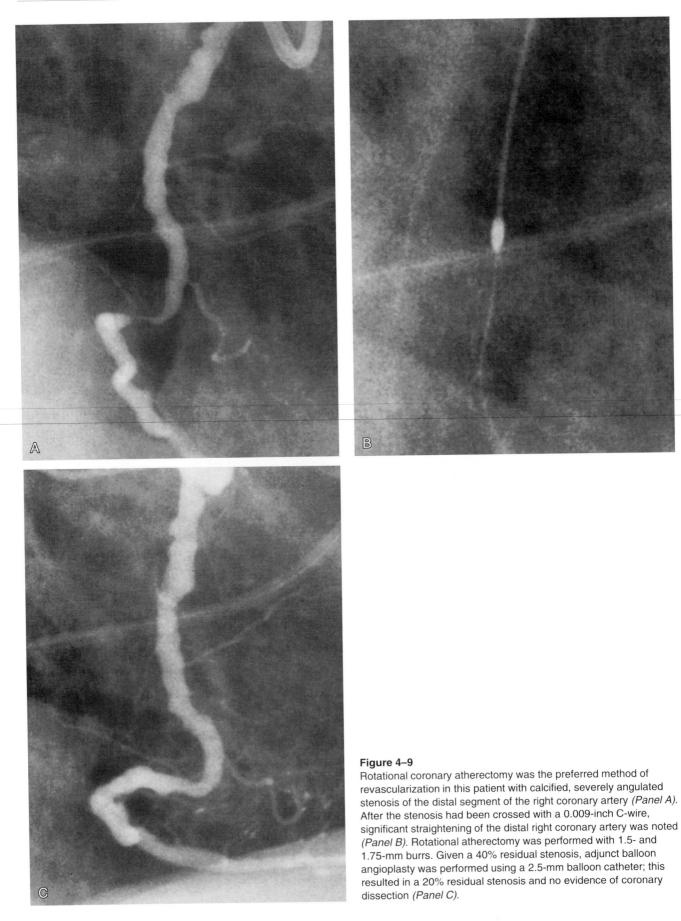

Figure 4–9

Rotational coronary atherectomy was the preferred method of revascularization in this patient with calcified, severely angulated stenosis of the distal segment of the right coronary artery *(Panel A)*. After the stenosis had been crossed with a 0.009-inch C-wire, significant straightening of the distal right coronary artery was noted *(Panel B)*. Rotational atherectomy was performed with 1.5- and 1.75-mm burrs. Given a 40% residual stenosis, adjunct balloon angioplasty was performed using a 2.5-mm balloon catheter; this resulted in a 20% residual stenosis and no evidence of coronary dissection *(Panel C)*.

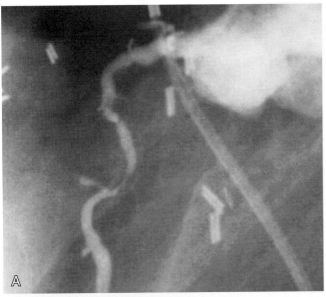

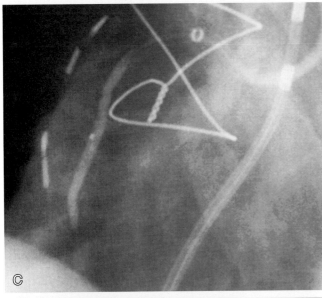

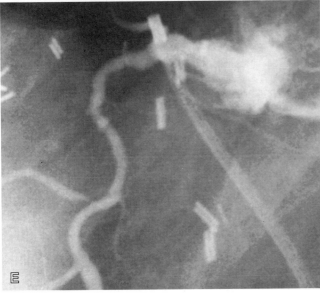

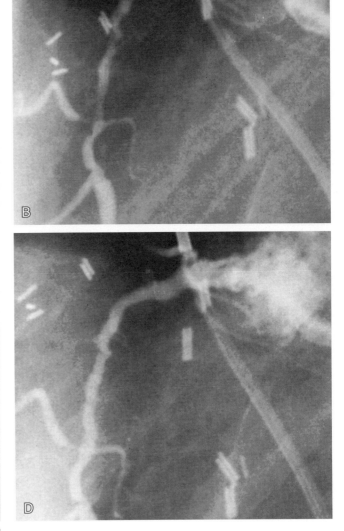

Figure 4–10

A concentric, moderately angulated stenosis of the midsegment of
the right coronary artery was selected for rotational atherectomy
(Panel A). After positioning a 0.009-inch wire into the distal vessel,
the midsegment of the right coronary artery was straightened
substantially, and rotational atherectomy using a 1.75-mm burr was
performed. After two passes, a 40% residual stenosis remained
(Panel B). A 2.5-mm long (40-mm) balloon was used to dilate the
residual stenosis *(Panel C)*. After balloon angioplasty, a moderate
degree of lesion irregularity persisted *(Panel D)*. After guide wire
removal, the curvature of the right coronary artery returned, and a
20% residual stenosis was demonstrated *(Panel E)*.

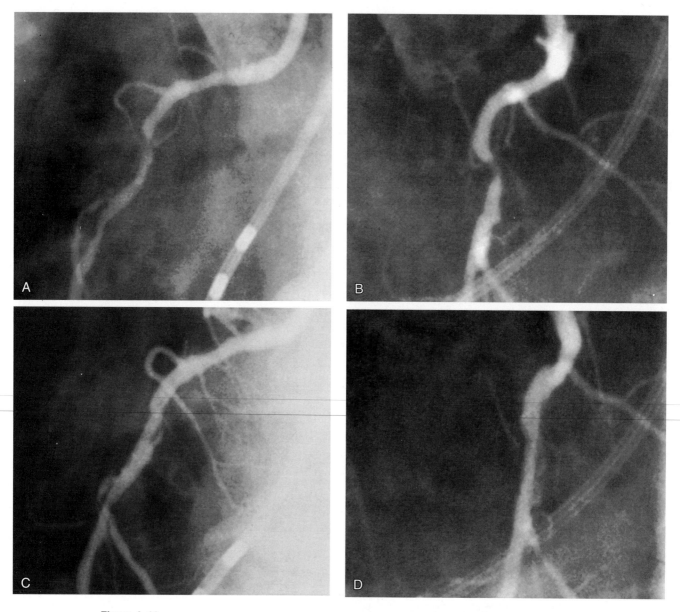

Figure 4–11
A calcified, angulated stenosis of the midportion of the right coronary artery was demonstrated in the left *(Panel A)* and right *(Panel B)* anterior oblique projections. After rotational atherectomy and adjunct balloon angioplasty, a linear dissection was noted in both projections *(Panels C and D).*

SELECTED REFERENCES

Ellis S, De Cesare N, Pinkerton C, et al. Relation of stenosis morphology and clinical presentation to the procedural results of directional coronary atherectomy. Circulation 1991; 84:644–653.

Ellis S, Roubin G, King S III, et al. Angiographic and clinical predictors of acute closure after native vessel coronary angioplasty. Circulation 1988; 77:372–379.

Ellis S, Topol E. Results of percutaneous transluminal coronary angioplasty of high-risk angulated stenoses. Am J Cardiol 1990; 66:932–937.

Ellis S, Vandormael M, Cowley M, et al. Coronary morphologic and clinical determinants of procedural outcome with angioplasty for multi-

vessel coronary artery disease: Implications for patient selection. Circulation 1990; 82:1193–1202.

Ryan T, Faxon D, Gunnar R, et al. Guidelines for percutaneous transluminal coronary angioplasty. J Am Coll Cardiol 1988; 12:529–545.

Slack J, Pinkerton C. Complex coronary angioplasty: Use of extended and angled balloon catheters. Cathet Cardiovasc Diagn 1987; 13:284–287.

Vivekaphirat V, Zapala C, Foschi A. Clinical experience with the use of the angled-balloon dilatation catheter. Cathet Cardiovasc Diagn 1989; 17:121–125.

CHAPTER 5

Bifurcation Lesions

The risk of periprocedural complications after coronary angioplasty of bifurcation lesions appears to be related to the degree of atherosclerotic involvement of the side branch as it originates from the parent vessel. To accurately assess the risk of side branch occlusions and to avoid conflicting definitions of side branches and ostial stenoses, a classification system for bifurcation lesions has been proposed.

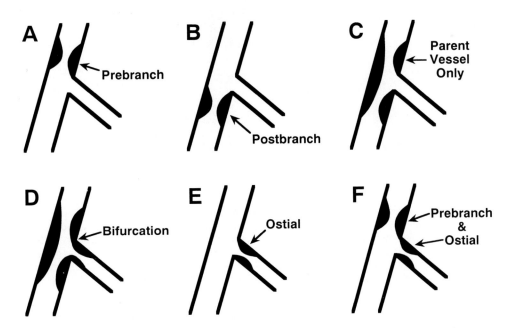

Figure 5–1
Schematic classification system for bifurcation stenoses. Type A: Prebranch stenosis not involving the ostium of the side branch. Type B: Postbranch stenosis of the parent vessel not involving the origin of the side branch. Type C: Stenosis encompassing the side branch but not involving the ostium. Type D: Stenosis involving the parent vessel and ostium of the side branch. Type E: Stenosis involving the ostium of the side branch only. Type F: Stenosis discretely involving the parent vessel and ostium of the side branch. Prior studies have suggested that patients with types D and F bifurcation stenoses (with atherosclerotic disease of both the side branch and the parent vessel) are at risk for complications during balloon angioplasty of the parent vessel. (Courtesy of Duke University Angiographic Core Laboratory, Duke University, Durham, NC.)

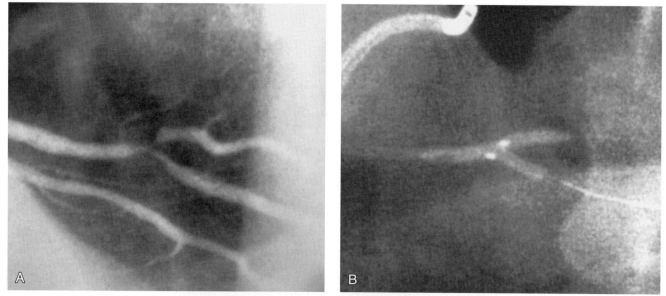

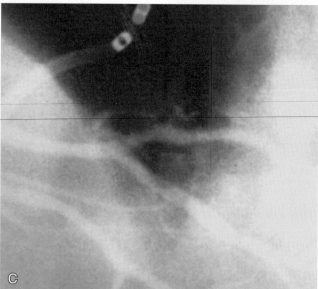

Figure 5–2

A type D bifurcation lesion involving the origin of the posterior descending branch and posterolateral segmental artery of the right coronary artery was demonstrated *(Panel A)*. Sequential balloon inflations in the posterior descending branch and posterolateral segmental arteries resulted in suboptimal alternating results in either artery suggestive of "plaque shifting" between the two branches. This phenomenon is also known as *snowplowing*, a term that conveys the balloon's effect on plaque at a bifurcation site, as illustrated in Figure 5–3. As a result, simultaneous or "kissing" balloon inflations were performed using 2.5-mm balloon dilatation catheters *(Panel B)*. After balloon deflation, <10% residual stenoses were obtained in both branches *(Panel C)*.

Type "D" Bifurcation Lesion

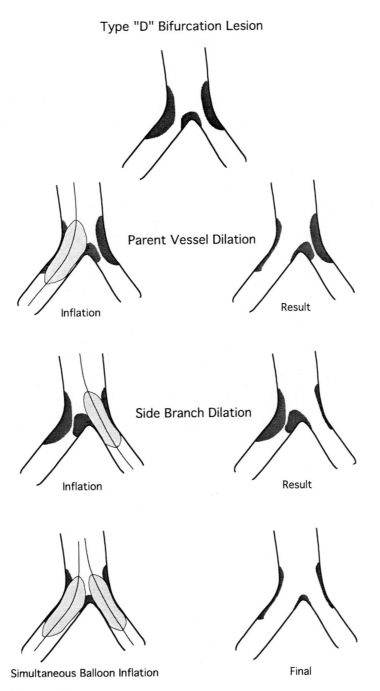

Parent Vessel Dilation

Inflation   Result

Side Branch Dilation

Inflation   Result

Simultaneous Balloon Inflation   Final

Figure 5–3
Schematic representation of "snowplowing" of atherosclerotic
plaque between the parent vessel and the side branch.
Simultaneous balloon inflations in the parent vessel and the side
branch may be effective in relieving both obstructions.

Side branches that are <1.5 mm in diameter are generally not protected using additional coronary guide wires;
lesion angulation, calcification, or severe ostial disease may
also make more difficult or preclude side branch protection
in vessels that are ≥1.5 mm in diameter.

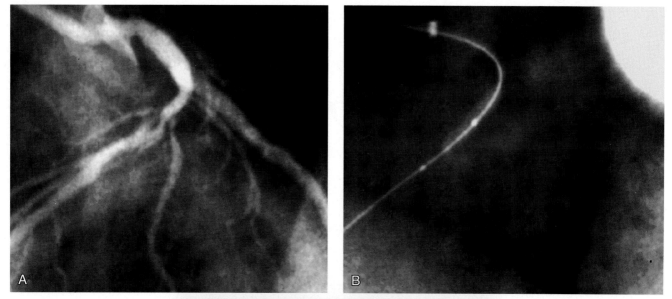

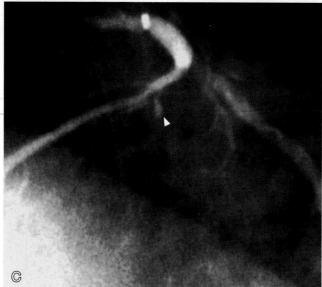

Figure 5–4
A type D bifurcation lesion of the left anterior descending artery and diagonal branch *(Panel A)* was treated with standard balloon angioplasty of the parent vessel without side branch protection *(Panel B)*. After a single balloon inflation, the diagonal branch became occluded *(arrow)* and could not be salvaged despite attempts to cross the occlusion with conventional coronary guide wires *(Panel C)*.

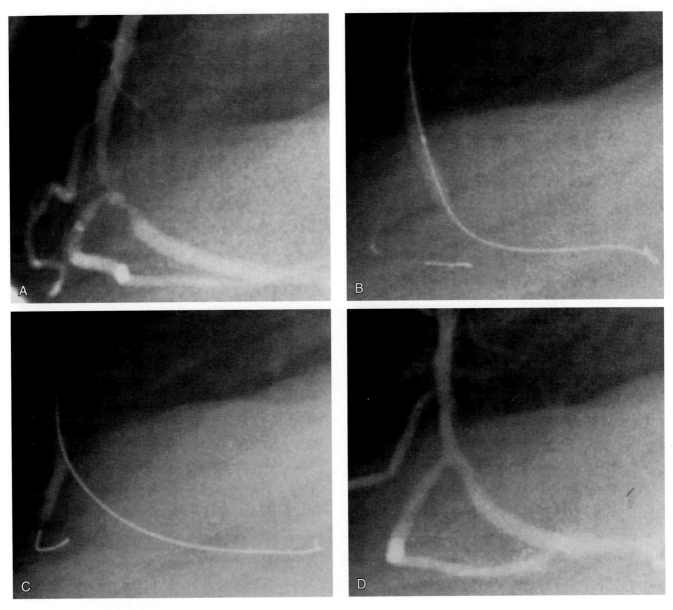

Figure 5–5
A type D bifurcation stenosis of the distal right coronary artery and acute marginal branch *(Panel A)*
was treated using guide wire protection of the side branch. A 3.0-mm balloon catheter was inflated in
the distal right coronary artery *(Panel B)*, resulting in transient loss of flow into the acute marginal
branch. A standard "over-the-wire" 2.5-mm balloon catheter could not be advanced across the acute
marginal branch lesion. With the exchange guide wire in place, a 2.5-mm "fixed-wire" balloon
catheter was advanced into the acute marginal branch, and the guide wire was removed. A 2.5-mm
balloon catheter was then inflated *(Panel C)*. A minimal degree of plaque shifting occurred, a 20%
residual stenosis was noted in the distal right coronary artery, and a 30% residual stenosis was
obtained in the acute marginal branch *(Panel D)*.

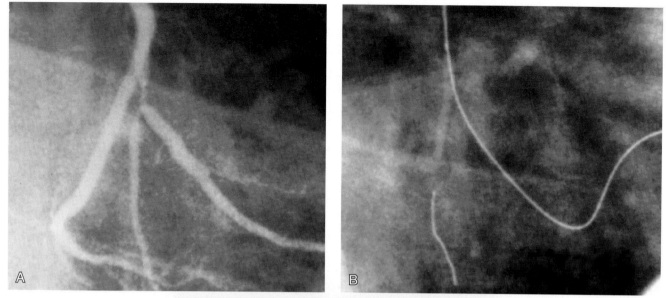

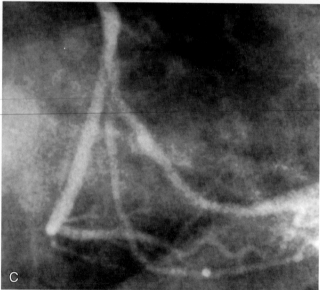

Figure 5–6

A type D bifurcation lesion of an obtuse marginal branch was treated with standard balloon angioplasty *(Panel A)*. Although the ostium of the superior branch of the obtuse marginal branch was only 50% stenosed, a guidewire was advanced across the lesion, and the side branch was protected. A 2.5-mm fixed-wire balloon catheter was inflated in the inferior branch of the obtuse marginal branch *(Panel B)*, resulting in a 20% residual stenosis *(Panel C)*. No evidence of compromise of the superior branch of the obtuse marginal branch was noted.

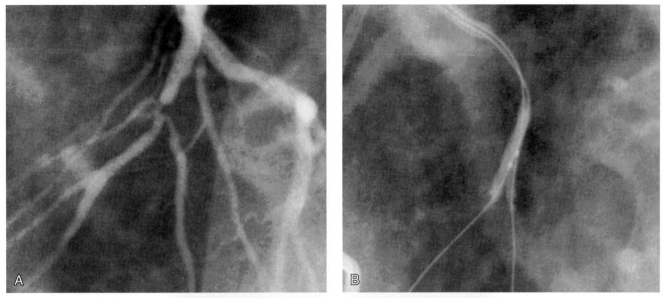

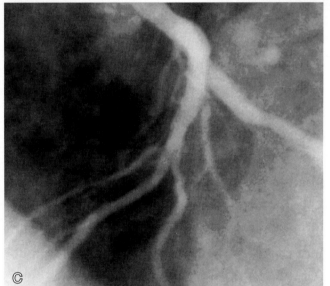

Figure 5–7
A type F bifurcation of the left anterior descending artery and of its diagonal branch *(Panel A)* was treated with standard balloon angioplasty. Radiopaque guide wires were placed within the left anterior descending artery and the diagonal branch, and sequential balloon inflations were performed in each vessel. After balloon inflation in the left anterior descending artery, occlusion of the diagonal branch developed. Plaque shifting resulted in a 40% residual stenosis within the left anterior descending artery after recanalization of the diagonal branch. Simultaneous balloon inflations *(Panel B)* resulted in <20% residual stenoses in both the left anterior descending and diagonal branches *(Panel C)*.

The significance of side branch occlusion after coronary angioplasty is related to the size of the branch vessel, the extent of myocardium it subserves, and the adequacy of the angiographic result in the parent vessel. Management of side branch occlusion has ranged from conservative observation of smaller side branch occlusions to emergency coronary bypass surgery for larger branch occlusions that result in significant myocardial ischemia.

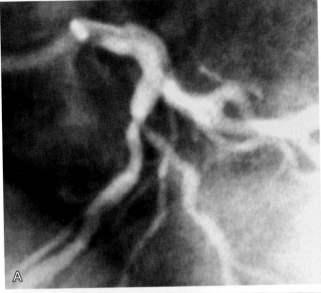

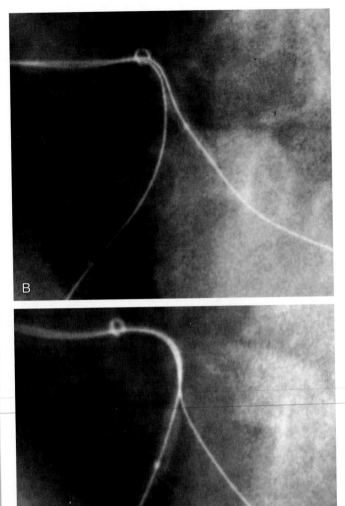

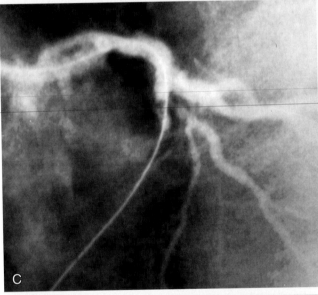

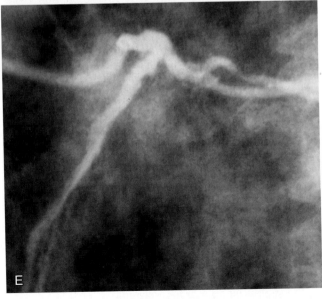

Figure 5–8

A type D bifurcation lesion of the left anterior descending artery and diagonal branch *(Panel A)* was approached with simultaneous wiring of both the parent and branch vessels using radiopaque guide wires. Balloon angioplasty of the diagonal branch was first performed using a 2.5-mm balloon catheter *(Panel B)*. After balloon deflation, total occlusion of the left anterior descending artery occurred; this was presumably due to dissection, superimposed thrombus, or both *(Panel C)*. Balloon dilatation of the left anterior descending artery with a 3.0-mm balloon dilatation catheter resulted in recanalization of the left anterior descending artery; however, occlusion of the diagonal branch developed *(Panel E)*. Additional attempts to restore anterograde perfusion in the diagonal branch were unsuccessful. Although the diagonal branch appeared to supply a large region of myocardium, the patient remained free of ischemic pain and did not demonstrate electrocardiographic changes; hence, an emergency coronary bypass operation was not performed. A prophylactic intra-aortic balloon pump was placed, and the patient developed an uncomplicated non–Q wave myocardial infarction.

Directional Atherectomy
of Bifurcation Lesions

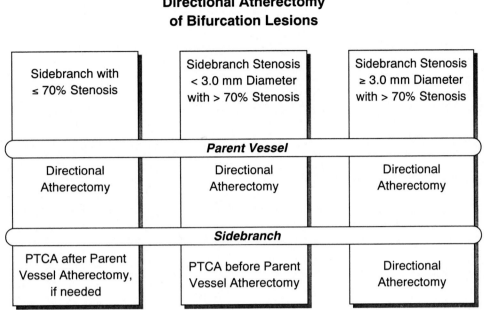

Figure 5–9
Directional atherectomy of bifurcation lesions.

Directional coronary atherectomy, which excises athero-sclerotic plaque, has been used in the treatment of patients with bifurcation lesions located in larger parent vessels (≥3.0 mm). Use of this modality potentially avoids the snowplowing effect noted after sequential balloon inflations within bifurcation lesions. Larger side branches (≥3.0 mm) allow the use of sequential directional atherectomy in both the parent vessel and the side branch (Figure 5–9). With this technique, guide wire protection of the side branch during initial parent vessel atherectomy is rarely required.

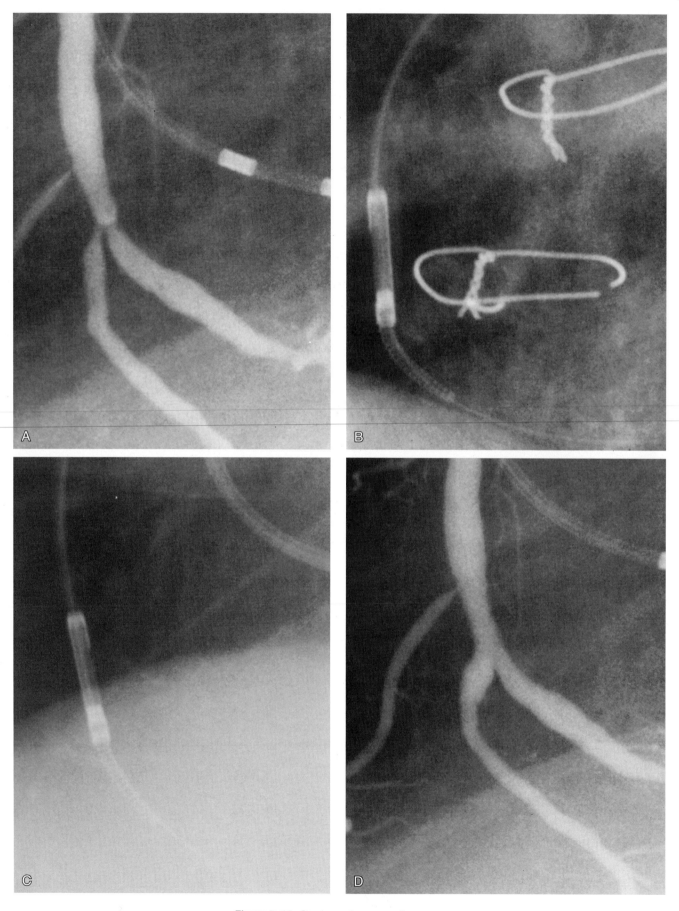

Figure 5–10. *See legend on opposite page*

Figure 5–10
A type D bifurcation stenosis involving the distal right coronary artery and acute marginal branch was noted *(Panel A)*. Directional coronary atherectomy using a 6-French device was performed in both the parent vessel and the side branch *(Panels B and C)*, resulting in 10% residual stenoses in each *(Panel D)*. (Reprinted from Altmann D, Popma J, Pichard A, et al. Impact of directional atherectomy on adjacent branch vessels. Am J Cardiol 1993; 72:351–354.)

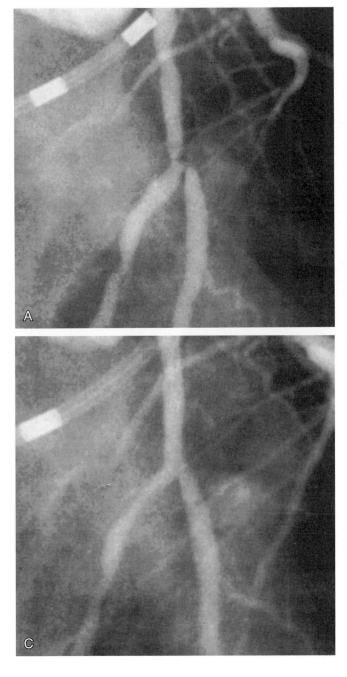

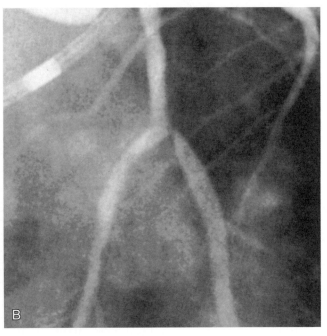

Figure 5–11
A type D bifurcation stenosis of the midportion of the left circumflex and obtuse marginal branch was selected for directional atherectomy *(Panel A)*. Atherectomy was first performed using a 6-French DVI EX device in the circumflex, resulting in a 20% residual stenosis *(Panel B)*. The 0.014-inch coronary guide wire was then repositioned into the obtuse marginal branch, and additional cuts were performed *(Panel C)*. A moderate degree of coronary vasoconstriction occurred in the left circumflex; this vasoconstriction responded to intracoronary nitroglycerin administration.

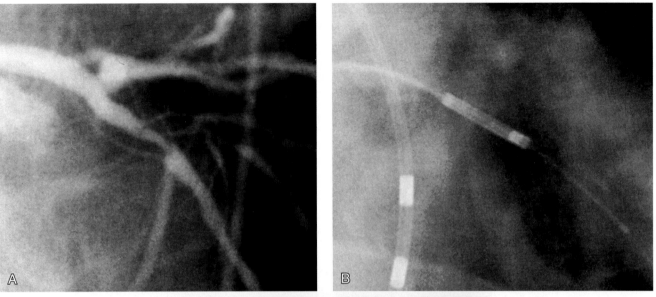

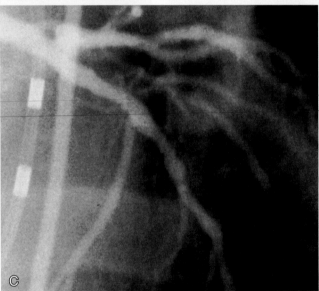

Figure 5–12
An eccentric bifurcation lesion of the midportion of the left anterior descending artery was demonstrated *(Panel A)*. The diagonal branch was <1.5 mm in diameter and had diffuse disease in its proximal segment. A 6-French atherectomy device was positioned across the lesion, and excisions were performed with avoidance of the origin of the diagonal branch *(Panel B)*. A 20% residual stenosis was obtained without further compromise of the side branch *(Panel C)*.

Selected calcified bifurcation stenoses may be treated with rotational atherectomy. Guide wire protection of the side branch is not possible with the use of this technique, and loss of side branches (especially with types D and F bifurcations) can occur after parent vessel treatment conse-quent to plaque shifting or vasospasm. In patients with high-risk bifurcation lesions, it may be advisable to dilate the side branch before performing rotational atherectomy within the parent vessel.

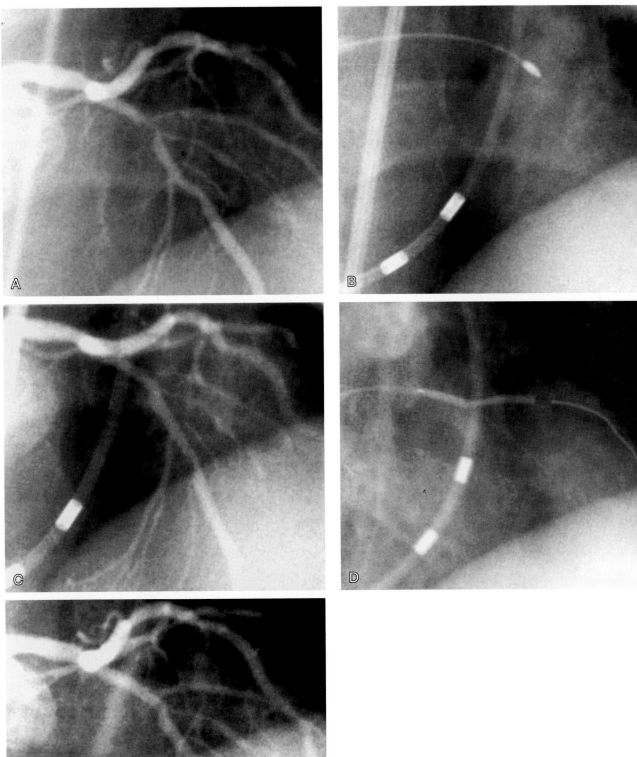

Figure 5–13
A calcified, eccentric stenosis of the midportion of the left anterior descending artery involved the origin of a diagonal branch *(Panel A)*. Rotational atherectomy was performed using 1.5- and 1.75-mm burrs *(Panel B)*. After two passes, diminished flow into the diagonal branch was noted *(Panel C)*. A 2.0-mm fixed-wire balloon catheter was advanced into the diagonal branch, and a single balloon inflation was performed *(Panel D)*. After balloon deflation, an excellent anatomic result in the parent and branch vessels was demonstrated *(Panel E)*.

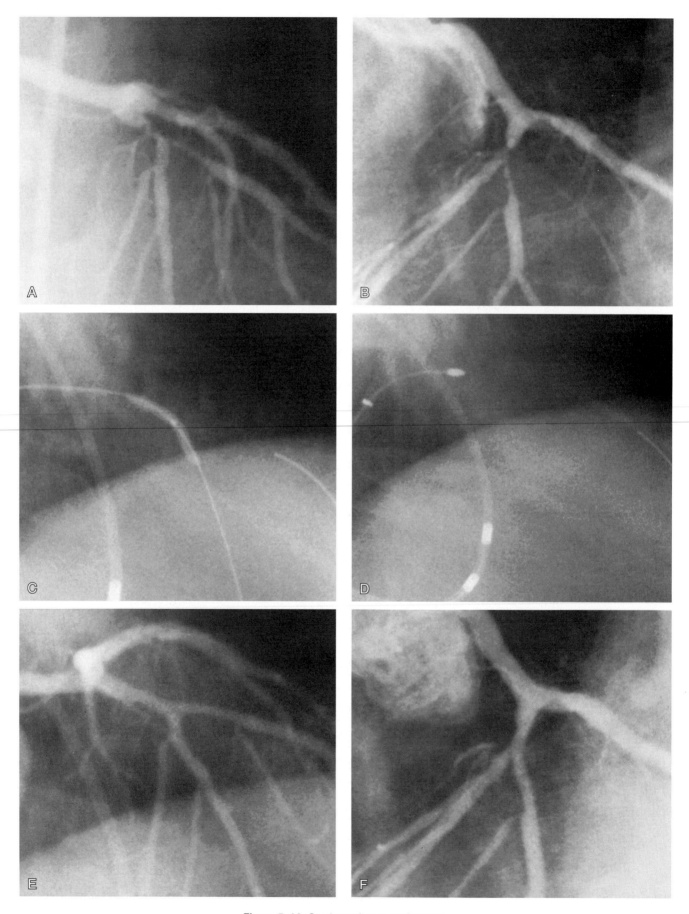

Figure 5–14. *See legend on opposite page*

Figure 5–14
A type F bifurcation stenosis of the left anterior descending artery and diagonal branch was noted in two projections *(Panels A and B)*. Moderate lesion calcium was noted fluoroscopically in the stenosis involving the diagonal branch. Coronary angioplasty was performed using a 2.5-mm balloon catheter in the left anterior descending artery *(Panel C)*. After balloon deflation, a <10% residual stenosis was demonstrated, and the guide wire in the left anterior descending coronary artery was removed. Rotational atherectomy of the diagonal branch was performed using 1.5- and 2.0-mm burrs *(Panel D)*. An excellent result was obtained in both projections *(Panel E and F)*.

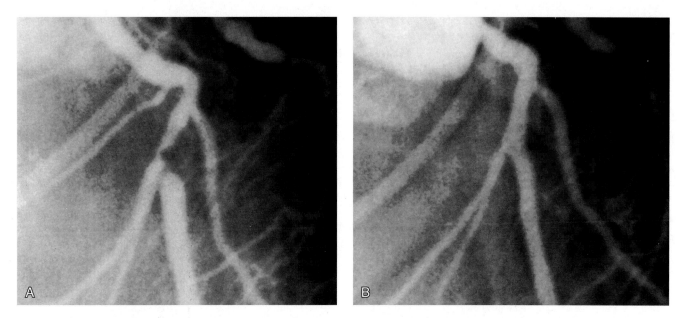

Figure 5–15
A calcified, eccentric, type F bifurcation lesion of the midportion of the left circumflex and large obtuse marginal branch *(Panel A)* was treated with rotational atherectomy of the latter. After adjunct balloon angioplasty using a 3.0-mm balloon catheter, a <10% residual stenosis was obtained *(Panel B)*.

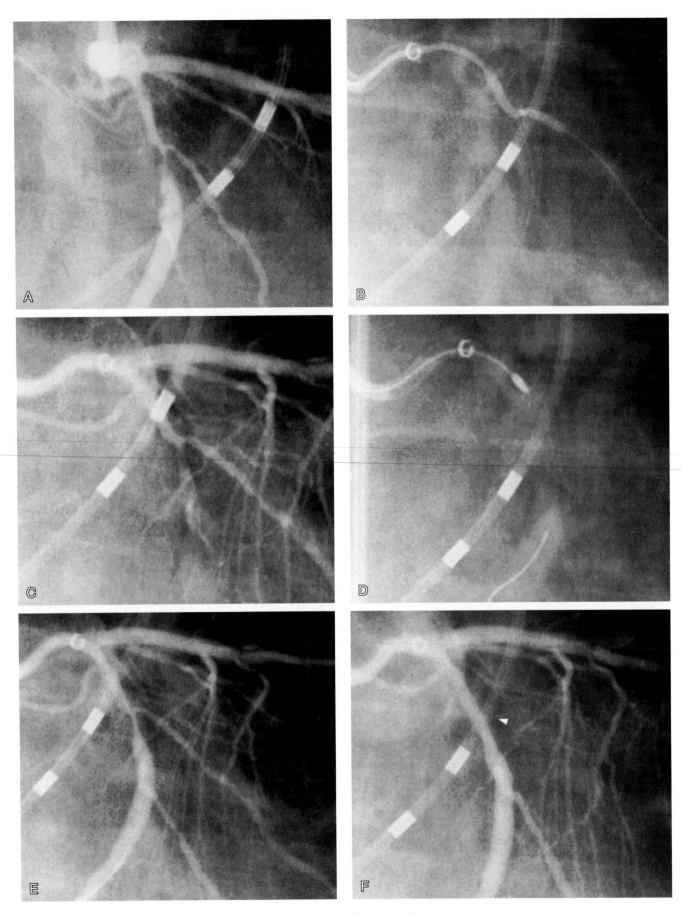

Figure 5–16. *See legend on opposite page*

Figure 5–16

A calcified bifurcation lesion of the proximal segment of the left circumflex *(Panel A)* was treated with a combination of balloon angioplasty and rotational atherectomy. Balloon angioplasty of a diseased first obtuse marginal branch was performed *(Panel B)*; this resulted in occlusion of the left circumflex *(Panel C)*. A 1.75-mm burr was advanced across the occluded segment in the left circumflex *(Panel D)* and yielded a small increase in the minimal lumen diameter *(Panel E)*. Adjunct balloon angioplasty using a 3.0-mm balloon dilatation catheter resulted in a 20% residual stenosis; however, the first obtuse marginal branch became occluded *(arrow, Panel F)*. Attempts to recanalize the obtuse marginal branch were unsuccessful.

SELECTED REFERENCES

Altmann D, Popma J, Pichard A, et al. Impact of directional atherectomy on adjacent branch vessels. Am J Cardiol 1993; 72:351–354.

Ciampricotti R, El Gamal M, van Gelder B, et al. Coronary angioplasty of bifurcational lesions without protection of large side branches. Cathet Cardiovasc Diagn 1992; 27:191–196.

den Heijer P, Bernink PJLM, van Dijk RB, et al. The kissing balloon technique with two over-the-wire balloon catheters through a single 8-French guiding catheter. Cathet Cardiovasc Diagn 1991; 23:47–49.

George B, Myler R, Stertzer S, et al. Balloon angioplasty of coronary bifurcation lesions: The kissing balloon technique. Cathet Cardiovasc Diagn 1986; 12:124–138.

Mansour M, Fishman R, Kuntz R, et al. Feasibility of directional atherectomy for the treatment of bifurcation lesions. Coron Artery Dis 1992; 3:761–765.

Meier B, Gruentzig A, King S III, et al. Risk of side branch occlusion during coronary angioplasty. Am J Cardiol 1984; 53:10–14.

Oesterle S, McAuley B, Buchbinder M, Simpson J. Angioplasty at coronary bifurcations: Single-guide, two-wire technique. Cathet Cardiovasc Diagn 1986; 12:57–63.

Renkin J, Wijns W, Hanet C, et al. Angioplasty of coronary bifurcation stenoses: Immediate and long-term results of the protecting branch technique. Cathet Cardiovasc Diagn 1991; 22:167–173.

Vetrovec G, Cowley M, Wolfgang T, Ducey K. Effects of percutaneous transluminal coronary angioplasty on lesion-associated branches. Am Heart J 1985; 109:921–925.

Weinstein J, Baim D, Sipperly M, et al. Salvage of branch vessels during bifurcation lesion angioplasty: Acute and long-term follow-up. Cathet Cardiovasc Diagn 1991; 22:1–6.

Saphenous Vein Graft Lesions

Coronary angioplasty provides an alternative to repeat coronary bypass surgery in selected patients with recurrent symptoms from aortocoronary saphenous vein graft (SVG) disease. Balloon angioplasty in this setting has been associated with high rates of procedural success (>85%) and relatively low rates of complications (<5%). In a recent review of 16 SVG angioplasty series comprising 1571 patients by de Feyter and associates, an overall procedural success rate of 88% was reported; complications were infrequent and included death (1%), myocardial infarction (4%), and the need for coronary bypass operation (2%). Overall procedural success rates were lower in patients with lesions of the proximal (86%) than in those with lesions in mid- (93%) and distal (90%) segments of the SVGs; angiographic evidence of recurrence was more frequently observed in patients with proximal lesions (58%) than in those

with mid- and distal segment lesions (52% and 28%, respectively). The risk of complications and restenosis may be higher in some patients, particularly those with aged grafts, grafts with degeneration (lumen irregularity or ectasia occluding ≥50% of the graft lumen), diffuse disease, intraluminal thrombus, or aorto-ostial lesion location.

New angioplasty devices have been used as an alternative or adjunct to balloon angioplasty for three general indications: (1) to improve the initial angiographic result, (2) to reduce complications associated with balloon angioplasty of degenerated or complex SVG lesions, and (3) to improve late angiographic outcome and reduce overall restenosis. To aid in the selection of balloon and new angiographic devices for the treatment of SVG lesions, an algorithm for device selection is proposed (Figure 6–1).

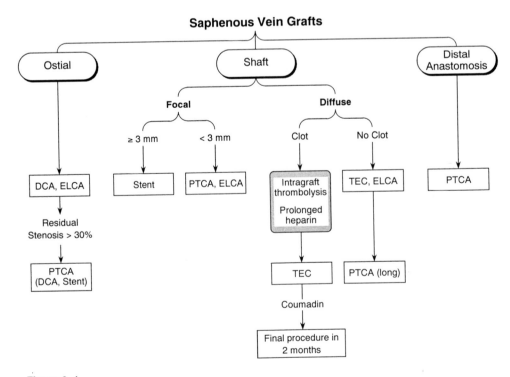

Figure 6–1
Algorithm for the treatment of SVG lesions.

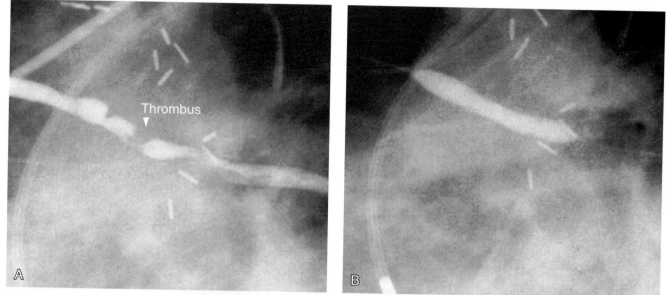

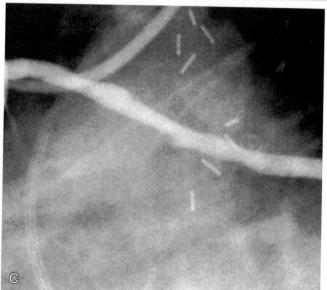

Figure 6–2
A highly eccentric, tubular lesion in the midsegment of the SVG to the obtuse marginal branch was incompletely opacified because of the severity of the stenosis and superimposition of thrombus *(Panel A)*. A 3.5-mm balloon was positioned across the lesion and inflated *(Panel B)*. Balloon expansion was incomplete at 8 atm, suggesting rigidity and fibrosis of the lesion. After balloon deflation, overall improvement of the lumen contour was observed, although some residual lumen irregularity was noted in the inferior aspect of the SVG *(Panel C)*. Nevertheless, brisk flow into the distal vessel was obtained without evidence of distal embolization. Despite the favorable initial angiographic results, the patient developed recurrent symptoms 3 months later, and repeat angiography demonstrated restenosis at the midbody dilatation site (not shown).

Standard balloon angioplasty should be considered as an alternative to repeat bypass operation in patients with focal (<10-mm) and tubular (10- to 20-mm) stenoses that involve the shaft portion and distal anastomosis of the SVG, particularly when smaller SVG size (<3.0 mm) or proximal vessel tortuosity precludes the use of a new angioplasty devices.

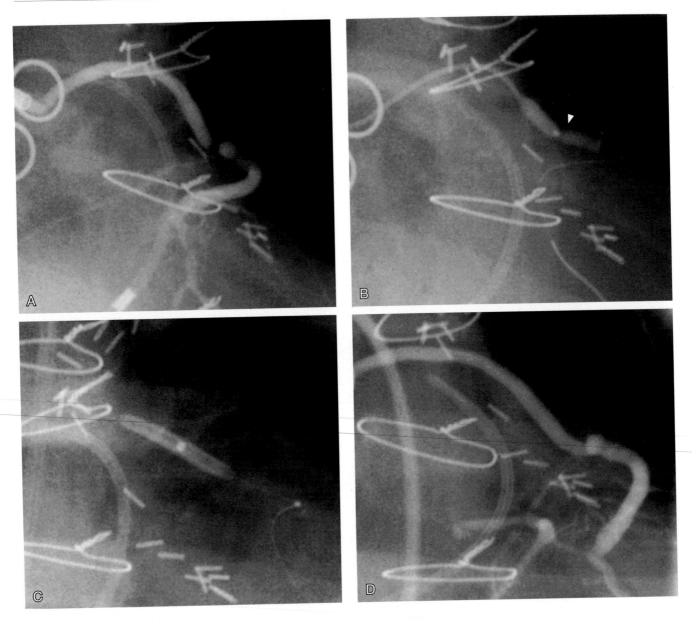

Figure 6–3
A severe lesion (>90% occlusion) at the side-to-side anastomotic segment of a sequential SVG to the diagonal and obtuse marginal branches was located in a region of severe angulation *(Panel A)*. A 3.0-mm balloon catheter was used to cross the lesion, and the balloon was inflated to 10 atm. Despite this relatively high pressure, a significant waist was noted *(arrow, Panel B)*. Importantly, the patient developed severe chest pain and elevation of the pulmonary artery pressure with each attempted balloon inflation. For this reason, a prolonged (10-minute) balloon inflation using a 3.0-mm perfusion balloon catheter was performed *(Panel C)*, and full balloon expansion was obtained after 5 minutes. An excellent (<10%) residual stenosis was obtained with brisk flow into the distal vessel *(Panel D)*.

Significant distal embolization may occur in 10% of lesions located within degenerated SVGs and is attributable to the friability of graft material and superimposed thrombus. Depending on the amount of material dislodged, clinical manifestation of distal embolization may range from transient reductions in anterograde coronary perfusion to abrupt closure, myocardial infarction, and death. Distal embolization is best treated with intragraft administration of nitroglycerin, 100 to 300 μg, or of verapamil, ≤1 mg in 100-μg increments, to alleviate microvascular spasm, or with intragraft administration of thrombolytic agents if thrombus at the lesion site is present. Often, the embolic episode resolves spontaneously with time. Occasionally, hemodynamic support using an intra-aortic balloon pump may be necessary.

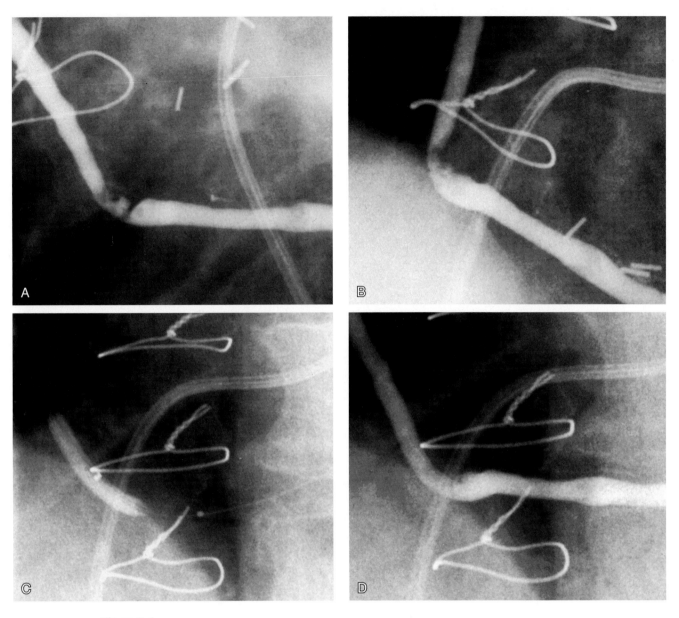

Figure 6–4
A filling defect was noted in this patient with an eccentric, ulcerated lesion in the distal portion of the SVG to the posterior descending artery *(Panel A)*. The proximal and midsegments of the graft had moderate lumen irregularities. After initial dilatation using a 3.0-mm balloon catheter, transient reduction of anterograde flow associated with chest pain was observed, and electrocardiographic evidence of inferior ischemia (consistent with distal embolization was demonstrated *(Panel B)*. Intragraft nitroglycerin, 200 μg, and verapamil, 100 μg, were administered; this improved anterograde flow and brought about resolution of the ischemia. A 3.5-mm perfusion balloon catheter was advanced across the residual lesion, and the balloon was inflated for 5 minutes *(Panel C)*. After final balloon deflation, a 20% residual stenosis was obtained *(Panel D)*.

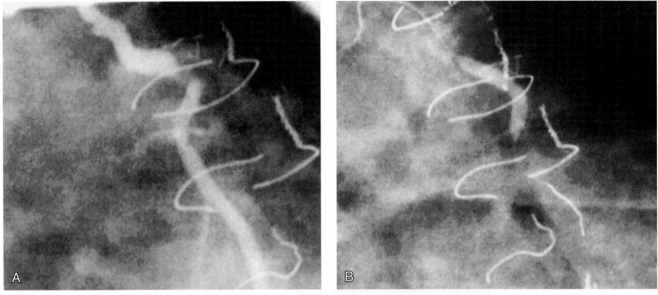

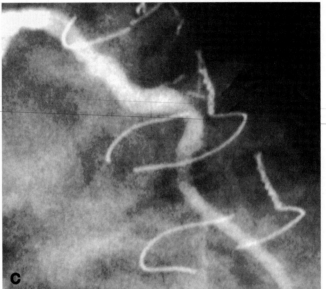

Figure 6–5
A highly angulated stenosis was demonstrated in this patient within the body of a mildly degenerated SVG to the left anterior descending artery *(Panel A)*. A 3.0-mm balloon dilatation catheter was advanced across the stenosis and inflated to 8 atm *(Panel B)*. After final balloon deflation, a 30% residual stenosis remained *(Panel C)*; the residual stenosis was in part due to the relative undersizing of the balloon catheter. Larger balloons were not used because of the risk of coronary dissection in this angulated lesion location.

Patients with aorto-ostial lesions may also be difficult to manage with standard balloon angioplasty as a result of the marked fibrosis, lesion rigidity, and enhanced elastic recoil that typically occurs in the aorta. Often, a suboptimal result is obtained when balloon methods alone are used, leading to late angiographic and clinical evidence of recurrence.

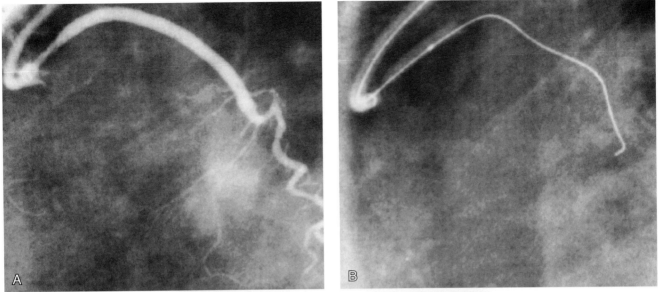

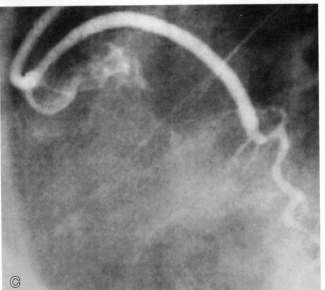

Figure 6–6
An ostial lesion of the nondegenerated SVG to the first diagonal branch *(Panel A)* was crossed with a
3.0-mm compliant balloon catheter. The guiding catheter was withdrawn into the aorta, and the
balloon was inflated across the origin of the SVG *(Panel B)*. Incomplete balloon expansion occurred
at nominal pressure, and the compliant balloon catheter was replaced with a 3.5-mm noncompliant
balloon catheter inflated to 16 atm (not shown). After balloon deflation, no evidence of dissection was
observed, but a 30% residual stenosis persisted *(Panel C)* likely because of lesion rigidity, excessive
plaque burden, and elastic recoil.

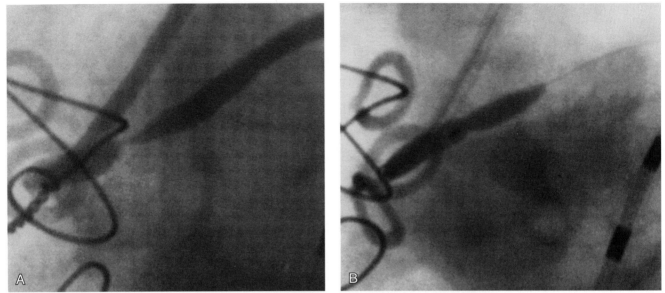

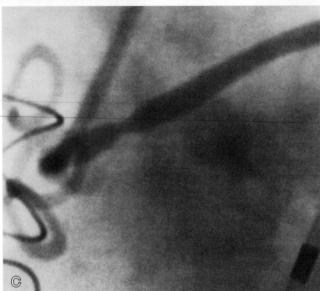

Figure 6–7
A concentric lesion involving the ostium and proximal segments of the SVG to the left anterior descending artery *(Panel A)* was treated with a 3.5-mm noncompliant balloon *(Panel B)*. Incomplete balloon expansion was noted at 18 atm. After balloon deflation, a moderate (40%) residual stenosis persisted *(Panel C)*, underscoring the marked rigidity of this lesion.

Standard balloon angioplasty of highly eccentric and "flaplike" lesions may result in a suboptimal angiographic outcome attributable to excessive elastic recoil within the segment. Occasionally, flaplike lesions occur in the region of a normal venous valve, making the distinction between normal vein graft anatomy and SVG pathology difficult.

In native coronary arteries, balloon-to-artery oversizing (>1.2:1) has been shown to result in the more frequent occurrence of coronary complications such as dissection and abrupt closure. Although SVGs may generally be more elastic than native coronary arteries, they are susceptible to similar angiographic complications if oversized angioplasty balloons are used.

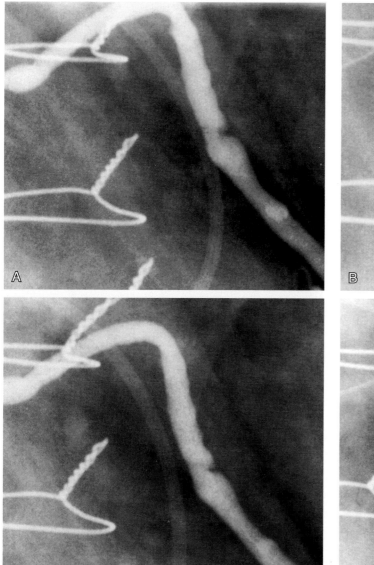

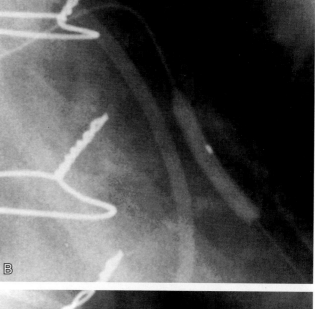

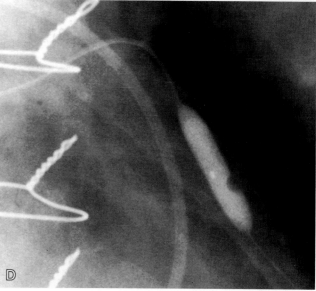

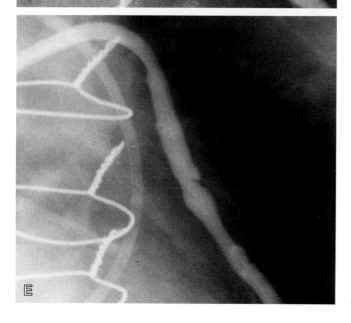

Figure 6–8
A flaplike lesion in the midbody of the SVG to the left anterior descending artery was demonstrated *(Panel A)*; mild luminal irregularities were noted throughout the artery's length. A 3.5-mm balloon dilatation catheter was positioned across the lesion and inflated to 6 atm, resulting in full balloon expansion *(Panel B)*. After balloon deflation, the flaplike lesion recoiled, and a 40% residual stenosis was obtained *(Panel C)*. To further improve the angiographic result by overstretching the segment, a 4.0-mm balloon was advanced across the lesion and inflated to 6 atm *(Panel D)*. After final balloon deflation, the intimal flap was again seen (30% residual stenosis) *(Panel E)*.

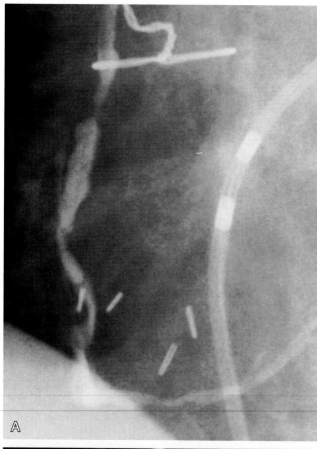

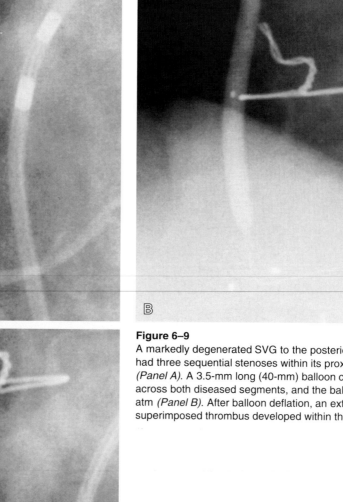

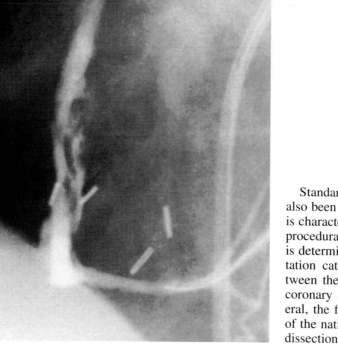

Figure 6–9

A markedly degenerated SVG to the posterior descending artery had three sequential stenoses within its proximal and midsegments *(Panel A)*. A 3.5-mm long (40-mm) balloon catheter was advanced across both diseased segments, and the balloon was inflated to 8 atm *(Panel B)*. After balloon deflation, an extensive dissection with superimposed thrombus developed within the graft *(Panel C)*.

Standard balloon angioplasty of anastomotic lesions has also been shown to have a high procedural success rate and is characterized by infrequent lesion recurrence. One major procedural difficulty associated with anastomotic dilatation is determination of the appropriate size of the balloon dilatation catheter. Often, a significant mismatch occurs between the reference diameters of the SVG and the native coronary artery just distal to the anastomotic site. In general, the final balloon size is selected based on the caliber of the native coronary artery. With this approach, coronary dissections can be minimized.

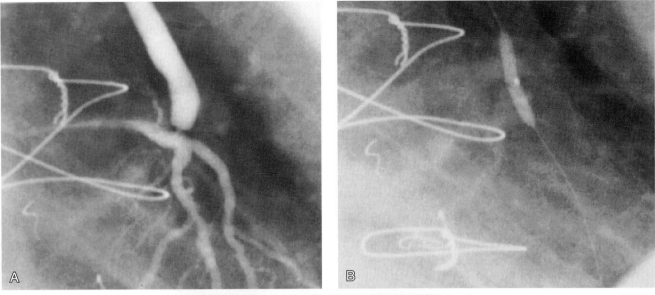

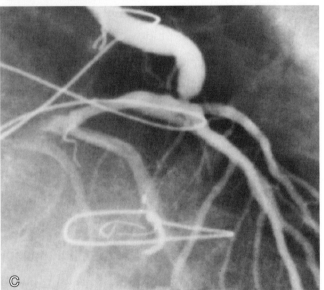

Figure 6–10

A severe stenosis (80%) of the anastomosis of the SVG to the left anterior descending artery was noted *(Panel A)*. A 3.0-mm balloon was advanced across the lesion and inflated to 8 atm; this resulted in full balloon expansion across the anastomotic site *(Panel B)*. Although the residual minimal lumen diameter at the anastomosis approximated that of the native vessel, the distal segment of the SVG appeared to have a residual stenosis *(Panel C)*.

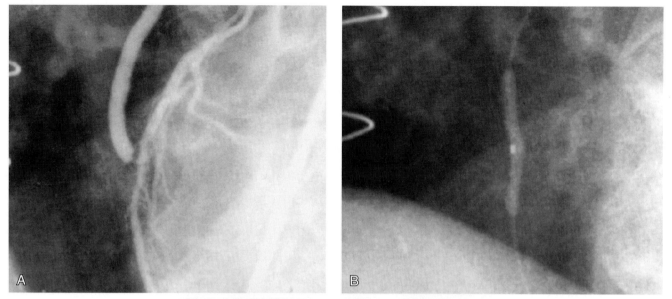

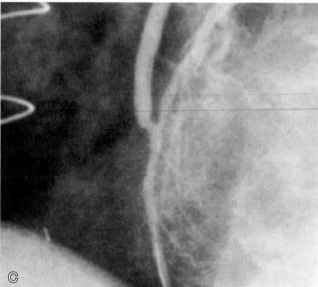

Figure 6–11
An anastomotic site stenosis of a nondegenerated SVG to the left anterior descending artery *(Panel A)* was treated with a 3.0-mm balloon catheter, which was selected to match the native artery's diameter *(Panel B)*. After final balloon deflation, the minimal lumen diameter was similar to that of the native artery, but a relative residual stenosis was demonstrated within the distal SVG segment *(Panel C)*.

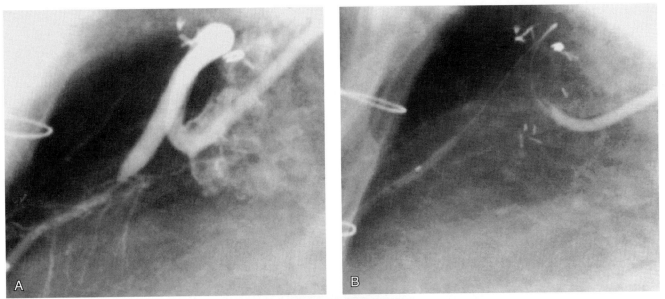

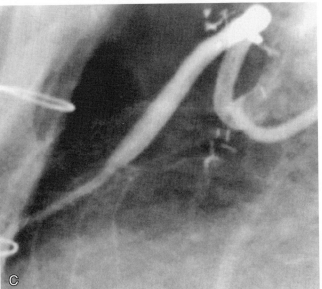

Figure 6–12
A concentric stenosis of the anastomosis of the SVG to the left anterior descending artery *(Panel A)* was treated with a 3.0-mm balloon catheter *(Panel B)*. After a prolonged (5-minute) balloon inflation, a 20% residual stenosis was obtained *(Panel C)*. No evidence of coronary dissection was observed.

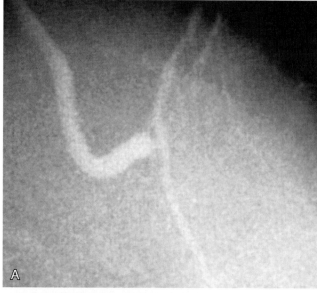

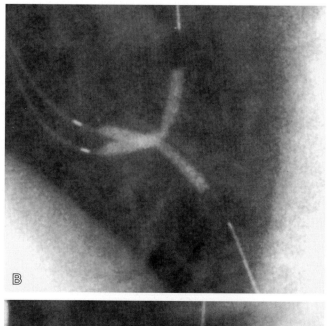

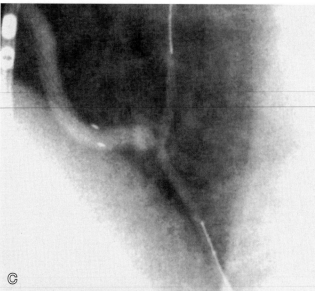

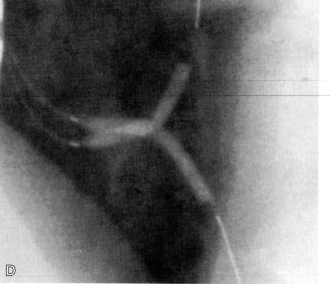

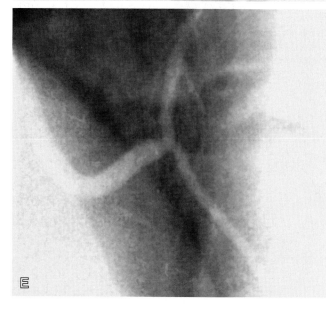

Figure 6–13
A restenotic lesion of the anastomosis of the SVG to the left
anterior descending artery was notable for marked elastic recoil
during the patient's prior balloon angioplasty procedure *(Panel A).*
Because of the marked discrepancy between the caliber of the
SVG and that of the native left anterior descending artery, a kissing
balloon inflation was performed with one 2.5-mm balloon catheter
directed retrograde and one 2.5-mm balloon catheter directed
anterograde within the left anterior descending artery *(Panel B).*
After initial balloon inflation, a 40% residual stenosis due to an
excessive amount of elastic recoil was noted *(Panel C).* The 2.5-
mm balloons were then exchanged for 3.0-mm balloons, and
another simultaneous balloon inflation was performed *(Panel D).*
After the final kissing balloon inflation, a 20% residual stenosis was
obtained *(Panel E).*

In patients who have undergone prior coronary bypass operations, coronary angioplasty can be performed within a native coronary vessel through the SVG conduit. This technique is particularly useful when proximal portions of the native vessels are occluded or have significant proximal tortuosity—factors that preclude an anterograde approach to the diseased segment.

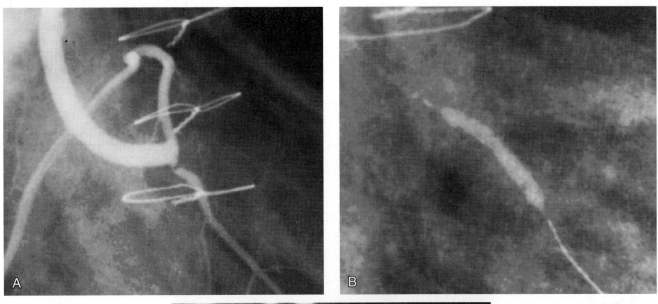

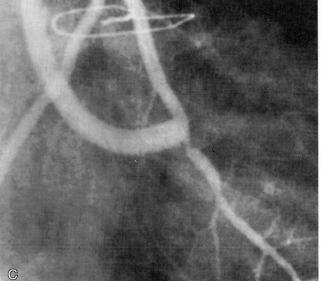

Figure 6–14
An eccentric stenosis was demonstrated just distal to the anastomosis of the nondegenerated SVG to the left anterior descending artery *(Panel A)*. A 3.0-mm fixed-wire balloon dilatation catheter was advanced through the SVG across the lesion and inflated to 8 atm *(Panel B)*. A moderate (30%) residual stenosis with intraluminal haziness was noted despite slight oversizing of the balloon catheter *(Panel C)*. The anterograde flow remained brisk, and no angiographic evidence of dissection was observed.

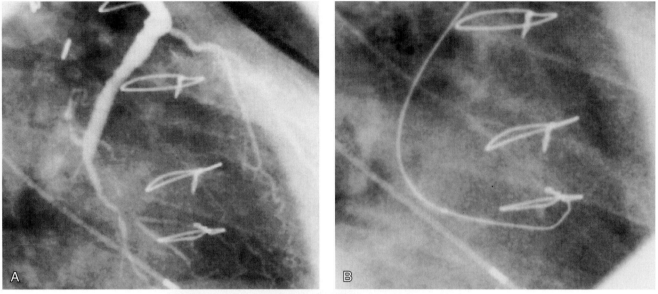

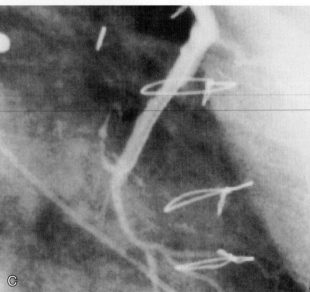

Figure 6–15
A complex bifurcation stenosis was noted in the native second obtuse marginal branch distal to the anastomosis of the sequential SVG to the first and second obtuse marginal branches *(Panel A)*. A 2.5-mm balloon catheter was advanced across the lesion *(Panel B)* and inflated to nominal pressures. After a single balloon inflation, no significant residual stenosis was seen *(Panel C)*.

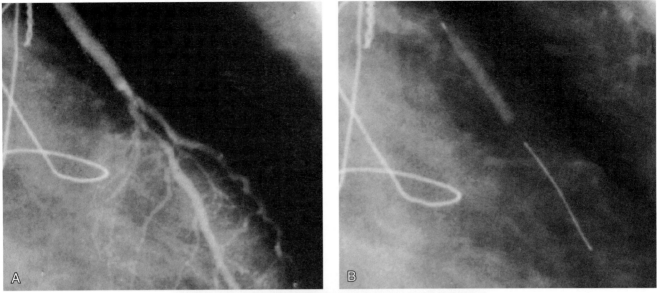

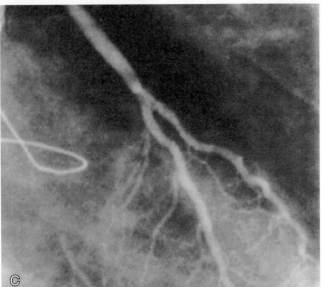

Figure 6–16
A tubular, eccentric stenosis in the midsegment of the left anterior descending artery *(Panel A)* was treated with a 3.0-mm fixed-wire balloon dilatation catheter. Complete balloon expansion was achieved at nominal pressures *(Panel B)*. After balloon deflation, a <10% residual stenosis was obtained *(Panel C)*.

Directional atherectomy has been useful as an alternative to standard balloon angioplasty in selected patients with SVG lesions. Most often, directional atherectomy is used alone or in combination with other techniques to provide improved initial angiographic results in SVG ostial lesions. By directly excising the fibrous plaque, directional atherec-tomy may render the segment more amenable to adjunct balloon angioplasty (if required to treat a residual stenosis). Directional atherectomy may also be useful in selected de novo lesions within the body of nondegenerated SVGs, especially focal lesions with severe eccentricity or flaplike appearance.

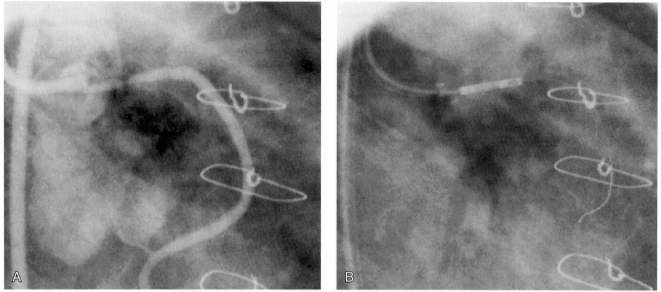

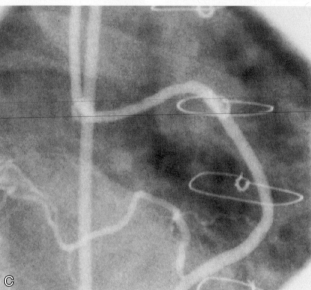

Figure 6–17
A discrete lesion in the proximal segment of an SVG to the obtuse marginal branch *(Panel A)* was crossed with a 7-French DVI EX atherectomy device *(Panel B)*. Circumferential excisions to a maximum of 30 psi were performed and resulted in the removal of approximately 20 mg of tissue. After directional atherectomy, no residual stenosis was identified within the SVG *(Panel C)*.

The technique of device ''synergy'' has been used by some to treat complex SVG lesions. For example, one device (a directional or extraction atherectomy device, or an excimer laser) may serve to initially ''debulk'' the lesion, potentially altering overall plaque compliance and reducing lesion rigidity, while a second device serves to further ''debulk'' the remaining plaque (directional atherectomy device) or scaffold the inner lumen surface (stenting). For a truly ''synergistic'' technique, the combination of devices must be more than additive; the ultimate goal of such an approach is to achieve the best final angiographic result more safely than would be possible with noncombined techniques.

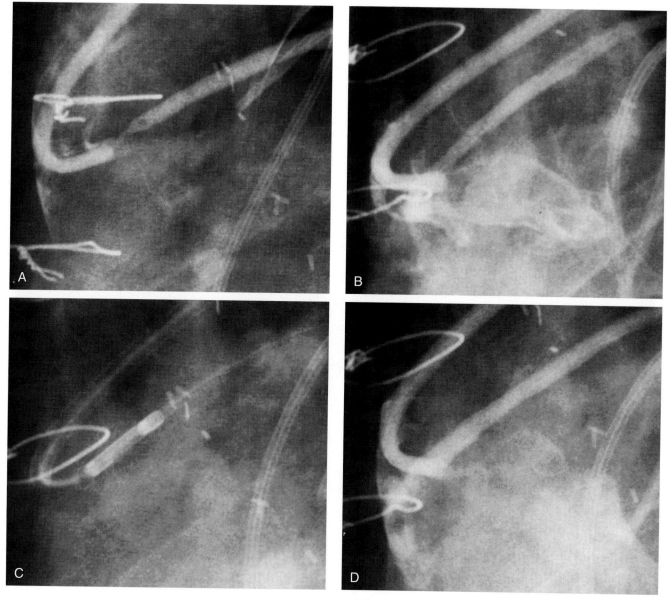

Figure 6–18

A filling defect was noted just beyond a restenotic lesion that involved the ostium of the SVG to the left anterior descending artery *(Panel A)*. A 2.2-mm excimer laser (308-nm) catheter was advanced across the ostial lesion in three sequential passes. After excimer laser angioplasty, marked improvement in stenosis severity was demonstrated *(Panel B)*. A 7-French DVI EX atherectomy device was advanced across the lesion, and circumferential cuts to a maximum of 30 psi were performed, yielding abundant tissue retrieval *(Panel C)*. Mild ectasia was demonstrated at the site of the original stenosis *(Panel D)*.

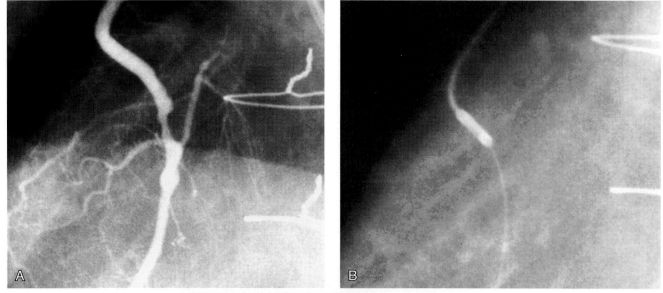

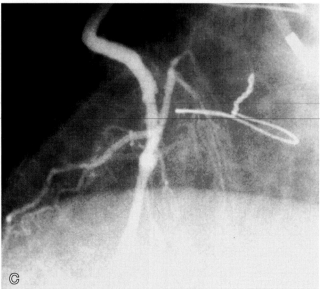

Figure 6–19
Standard balloon angioplasty of the eccentric stenosis in the distal segment of the nondegenerated SVG to the left anterior descending artery failed to significantly improve stenosis severity due to elastic recoil *(Panel A)*. As a result, a 7-French DVI EX atherectomy device was advanced across the lesion, and circumferential cuts were performed to a maximum pressure of 30 psi *(Panel B)*. A scant amount of fibrous tissue was retrieved; however, a marked improvement in the overall lumen contour was observed *(Panel C)*.

Directional atherectomy should be used with caution in patients with degenerated SVGs because of the propensity of the relatively stiff catheters to dislodge graft material in a vessel and predispose the graft to distal embolization. Of importance, this complication may also occur in nondegenerated SVGs because angiography frequently does not reliably identify the presence or absence of friable material.

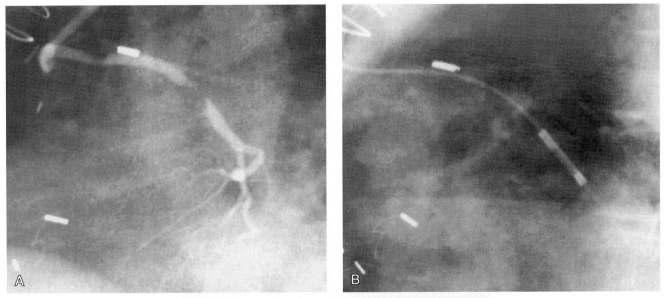

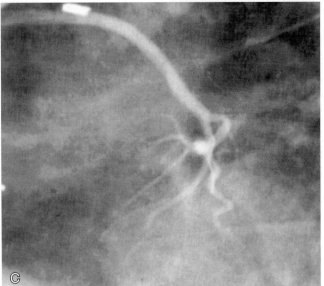

Figure 6–20
Two sequential lesions within a nondegenerated SVG to the first diagonal branch *(Panel A)* were
treated with a 6-French DVI SCA atherectomy device. Circumferential cuts were made within the
proximal and midsegments *(Panel B)*. Although marked improvement in the graft contour was
achieved and a minimal residual stenosis was demonstrated *(Panel C)*, no tissue was removed from
the nose cone. Immediately after withdrawal of the device, the patient developed chest pain and
demonstrated anterior ST segment elevation consistent with distal microembolization.

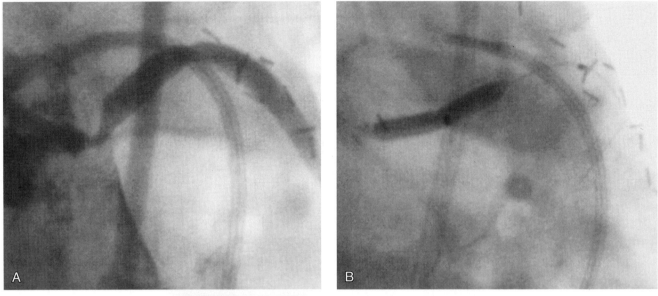

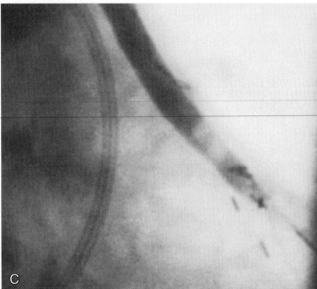

Figure 6–21
An eccentric lesion of the ostium of a degenerated SVG to the left anterior descending artery *(Panel A)* was treated with a 7-French DVI EX atherectomy device inflated to a maximum of 30 psi. Because of a 30% residual stenosis, adjunct balloon dilatation was performed *(Panel B)*. After balloon deflation, the patient developed marked anterior ST segment elevation, and angiography demonstrated large, intraluminal filling defects *(Panel C)* consistent with distal embolization. Despite the use of intragraft administration of urokinase and nitroglycerin, the patient experienced a Q wave myocardial infarction.

Although rotational atherectomy has been reserved by protocol for native coronary arteries, it has been used on a compassionate basis in selected patients with recalcitrant SVG lesions, that is, fibrous, undilatable lesions or recurrent restenotic lesions in nondegenerated SVGs.

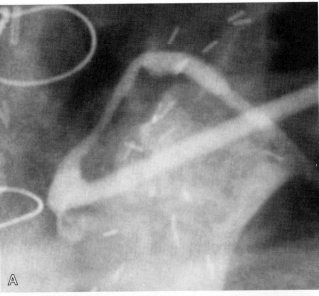

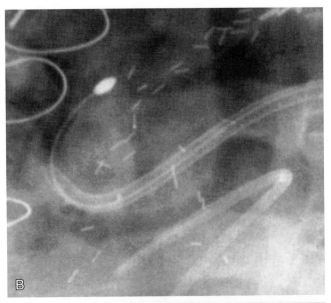

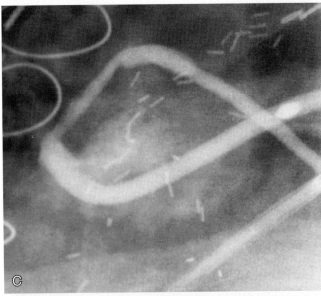

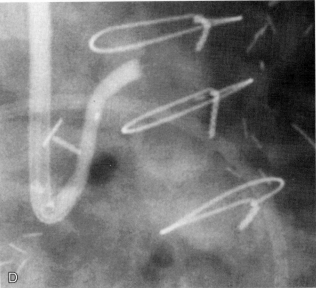

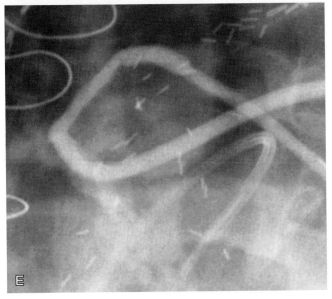

Figure 6–22
A diffuse, restenotic lesion in the proximal segment of the SVG to the left anterior descending artery had undergone multiple prior coronary interventions with balloon angioplasty, directional atherectomy, and excimer laser angioplasty *(Panel A)*. On account of the presence of extensive fibrosis within the lesion, rotational atherectomy was performed using 1.5- and 2.0-mm burrs *(Panel B)*. A 40% residual stenosis *(Panel C)* was treated with a 3.0-mm balloon catheter; this resulted in near complete balloon expansion *(Panel D)*. After final balloon deflation, a 20% residual stenosis was obtained *(Panel E)*.

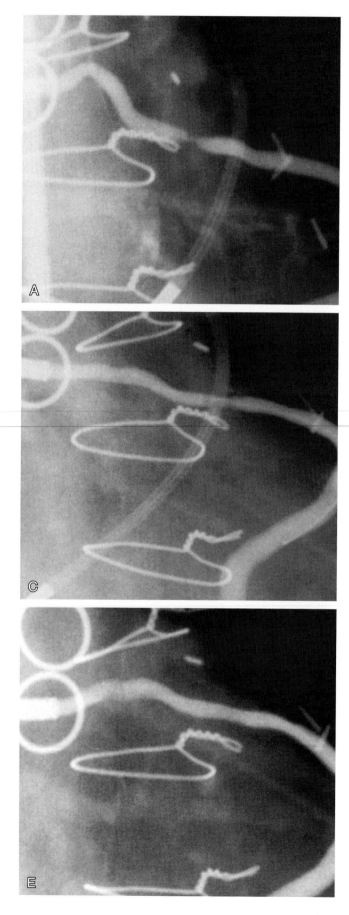

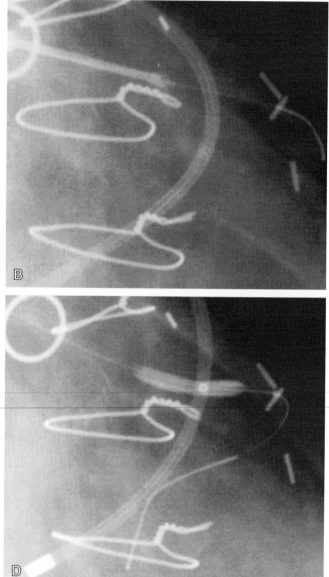

Transluminal extraction atherectomy has also been shown to be a useful treatment modality for patients with SVG disease; it may be particularly advantageous in those SVGs with degeneration or superimposed thrombus. After macroshavings of atherosclerotic plaque are mechanically cut, particles are removed through the catheter by continuous vacuum suction. With removal of the particulate debris, the potential for the development of distal embolization may be reduced.

Figure 6–23

The concentric stenosis in the midsegment of the SVG to the obtuse marginal branch *(Panel A)* was treated with a 2.5-mm transluminal extraction atherectomy device *(Panel B)*. Multiple passes across the treatment site resulted in a marked improvement in the stenosis severity *(Panel C)*. Adjunct balloon dilatation *(Panel D)* was used to smooth the arterial contour, and an excellent residual stenosis (<10%) was obtained *(Panel E)*.

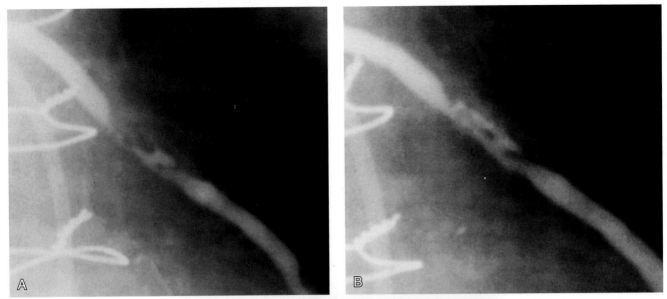

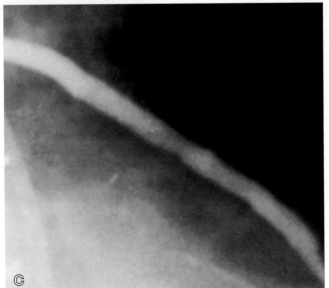

Figure 6–24
An eccentric, ulcerated stenosis of the midsegment of the SVG to the left anterior descending artery *(Panel A)* was treated with a 2.5-mm extraction atherectomy catheter (not shown). After the initial passes, a localized linear dissection occurred *(Panel B)*. Adjunct balloon dilatation was performed with a 3.0-mm balloon dilatation catheter, "tacking up" the dissection flap *(Panel C)*.

The use of tubular slotted stents to treat degenerated and nondegenerated SVG lesions may be a beneficial alternative to standard balloon angioplasty. Intragraft stenting has several potential advantages over atherectomy and balloon angioplasty in SVG disease. First, the stainless steel filaments of the stent provide a scaffold upon which the friable contents of the SVG can be buttressed against the graft wall, preventing distal embolization and intimal flaps from creating turbulent anterograde flow. Second, inflation times for predilatation and postdilatation and for stent deployment may be shorter than with standard balloon angioplasty, reducing the duration of ischemia during SVG angioplasty. Finally, a very low residual diameter stenosis (0–10%) can often be predictably achieved with intragraft stenting; this low diameter stenosis has the potential to favorably influence the late angiographic outcome and to reduce clinical lesion recurrences.

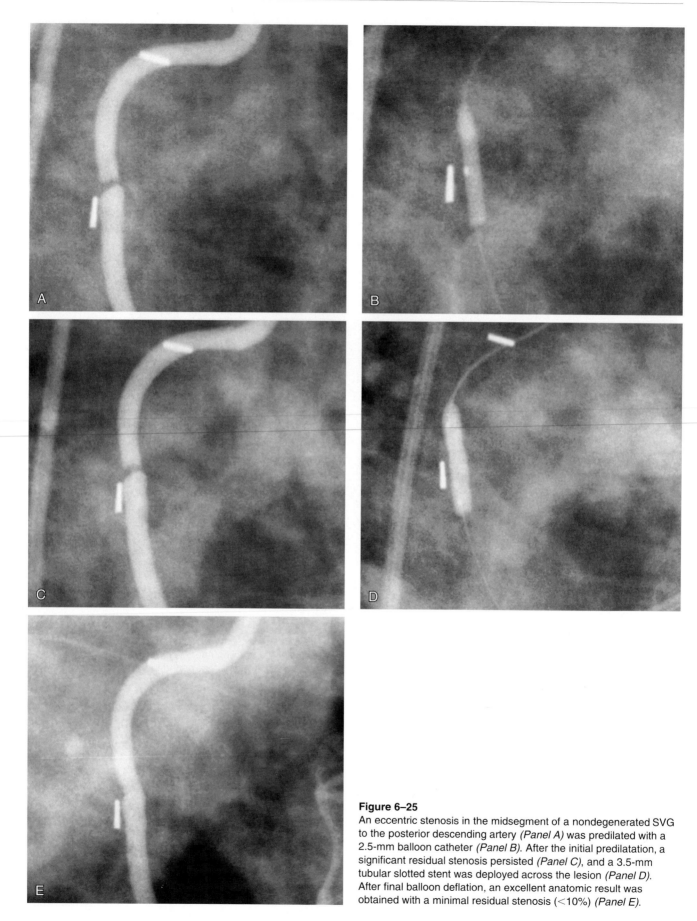

Figure 6–25

An eccentric stenosis in the midsegment of a nondegenerated SVG to the posterior descending artery *(Panel A)* was predilated with a 2.5-mm balloon catheter *(Panel B)*. After the initial predilatation, a significant residual stenosis persisted *(Panel C)*, and a 3.5-mm tubular slotted stent was deployed across the lesion *(Panel D)*. After final balloon deflation, an excellent anatomic result was obtained with a minimal residual stenosis (<10%) *(Panel E)*.

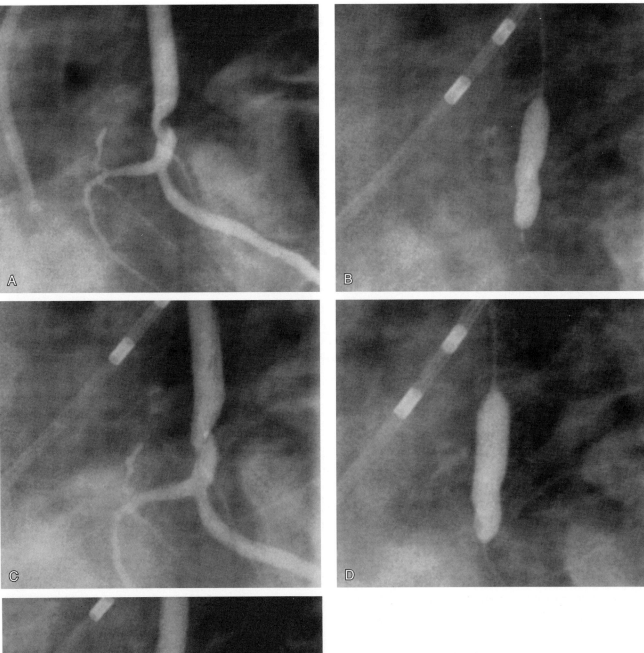

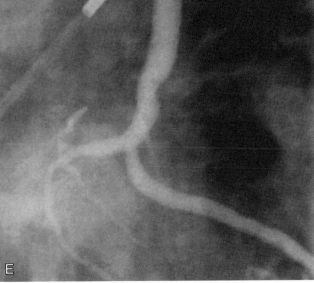

Figure 6–26

An eccentric lesion in the distal segment of the SVG to the obtuse marginal branch *(Panel A)* was unsuccessfully treated with standard balloon angioplasty because of incessant elastic recoil. A 3.5-mm tubular slotted stent was advanced with a balloon catheter across the lesion, and the balloon was inflated to 6 atm *(Panel B)*. An improvement in the residual lumen contour was achieved, but a 30% residual stenosis persisted *(Panel C)*. As a result, a 4.0-mm balloon catheter was inflated to 8 atm *(Panel D)*, resulting in a <20% residual stenosis *(Panel E)*.

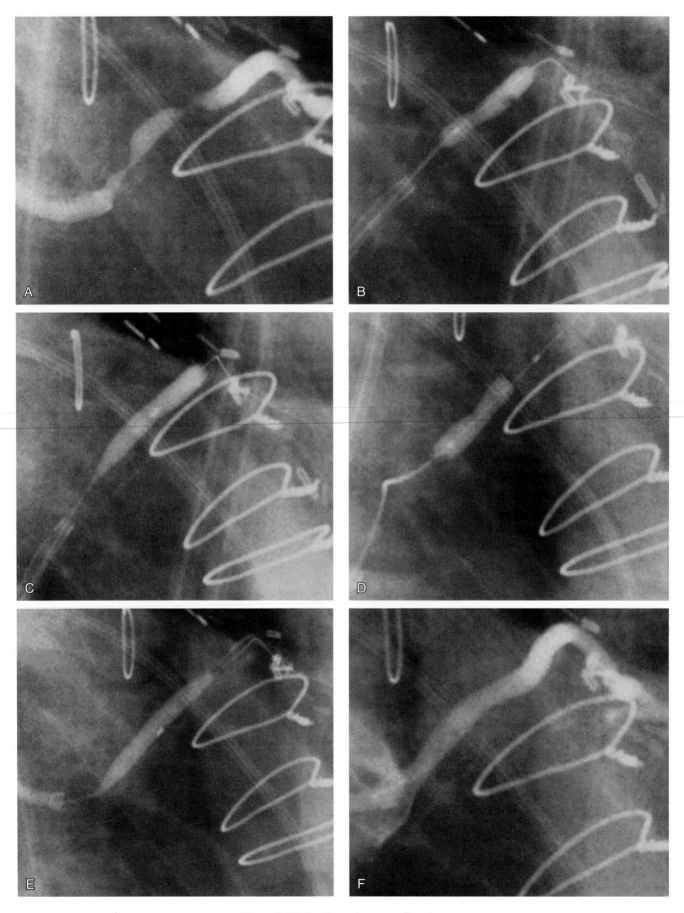

Figure 6–27. *See legend on opposite page*

Figure 6–27
Sequential lesions in the ostium and proximal segments of the SVG to the diagonal branch recurred in this patient 3 months after directional atherectomy *(Panel A)*. Intravascular ultrasound was used to quantitate the length of the diseased segments (12 mm and 14 mm for the ostial and proximal lesions, respectively) and to determine the distance between the two lesions (7 mm) in anticipation of intragraft stenting. Since sequential stents could be placed without overlap, a 3.0-mm tubular slotted stent was deployed in the proximal segment, which had been predilated with a 2.5-mm balloon catheter *(Panel B)*. Note the lesion rigidity and incomplete stent expansion with initial dilatation. A 3.0-mm noncompliant balloon catheter was then inflated to 12 atm, resulting in full balloon expansion *(Panel C)*. A 3.0-mm Palmaz-Schatz stent was then positioned across the ostial lesion, and the balloon inflated to nominal pressure. Incomplete stent expansion again occurred *(Panel D)*. A 3.0-mm noncompliant balloon was again inflated to 12 atm *(Panel E)*. After final balloon inflation, an excellent angiographic result was obtained, and no residual stenosis was demonstrated *(Panel F)*. Intravascular ultrasound demonstrated full stent strut apposition to the wall of the graft.

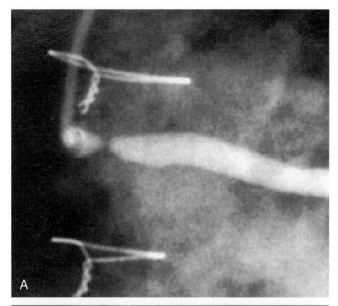

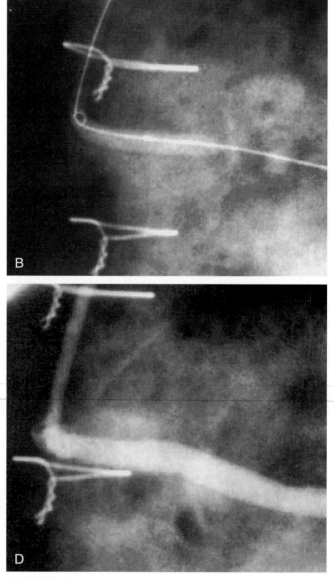

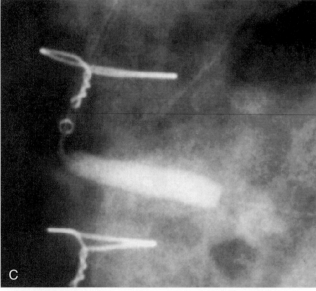

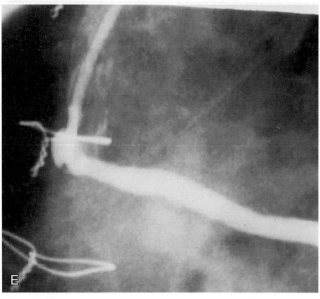

Figure 6–28

A concentric stenosis of the ostium of the SVG to the obtuse marginal branch *(Panel A)* recurred in this patient despite two prior treatment attempts with standard balloon angioplasty. A 3.5-mm tubular slotted stent was deployed across the stenosis after predilatation with a 2.5-mm balloon catheter *(Panel B)*. To maximize the final lumen dimensions, a 4.0-mm balloon was inflated across the lesion with the guiding catheter withdrawn to allow full balloon inflation across the ostium *(Panel C)*. An excellent final angiographic result was obtained *(Panel D)*, and this result was maintained at angiographic follow-up 6 months later *(Panel E)*.

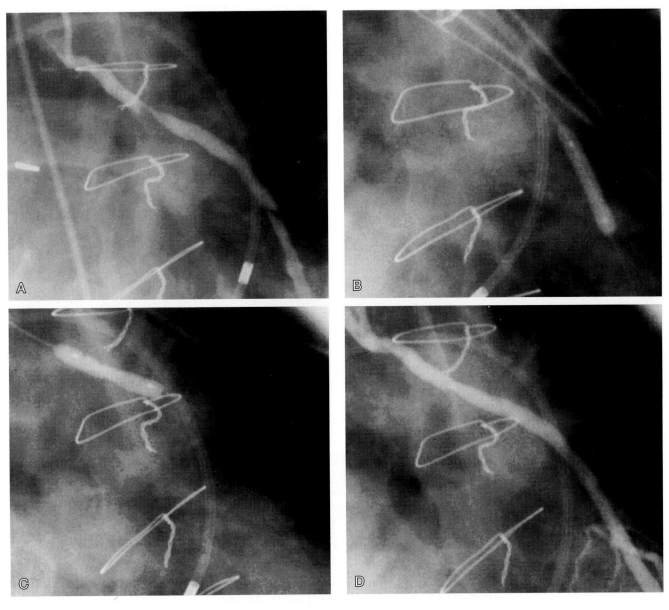

Figure 6–29
Sequential stenoses in a degenerated segment of the SVG to the left anterior descending artery
(Panel A) were noted. After predilatation with a 2.5-mm balloon catheter, sequential 3.5-mm tubular
slotted stents were deployed across the distal *(Panel B)* and proximal *(Panel C)* segments of the
graft. Adjunct dilatation was performed using a 3.5-mm balloon at both the distal and proximal sites,
resulting in an excellent angiographic result and no evidence of distal embolization or dissection
(Panel D).

The larger ''biliary'' tubular slotted stent, alone or in combination with another new device, has also been used to treat complex SVG disease. Moreover, by partially ''de-bulking'' the fibrous cap and fibrocellular atherosclerotic plaque before stenting, a more favorable angiographic result may be obtained.

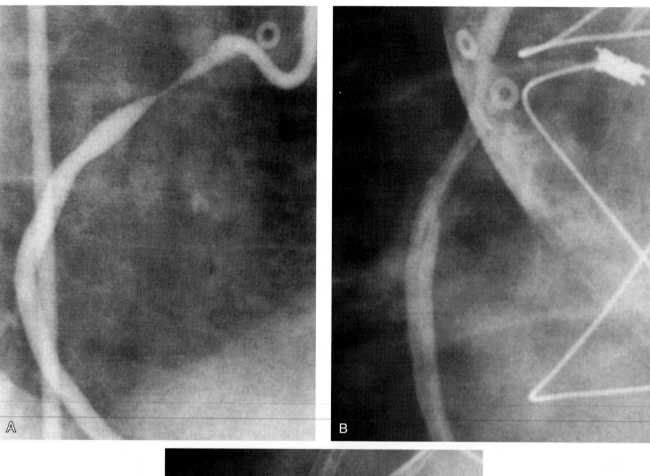

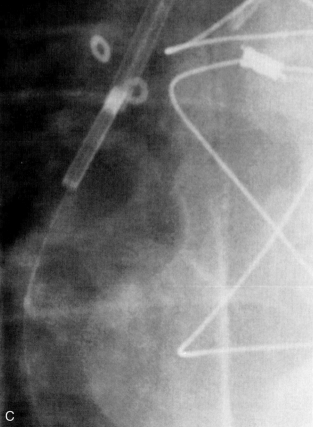

Figure 6–30. See legend on opposite page

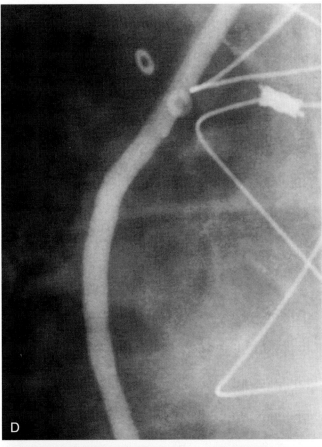

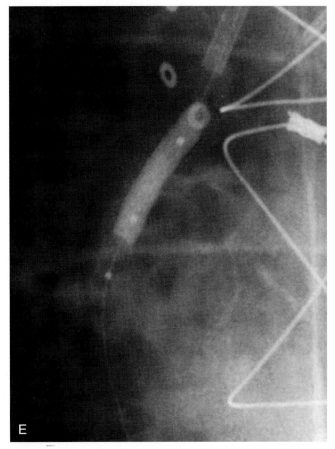

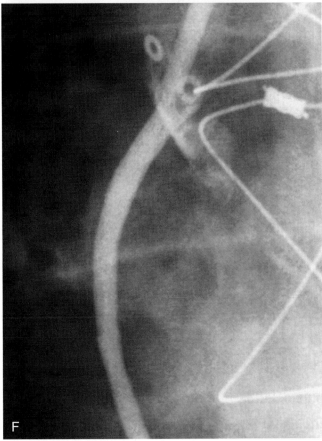

Figure 6–30
An eccentric lesion of the ostium of the SVG to the distal right coronary artery *(Panel A)* was predilated with a 2.5-mm balloon catheter but incomplete balloon expansion occurred (not shown). As a result, a 60% residual stenosis was obtained after initial predilatation *(Panel B)*. To partially debulk the rigid lesion, a 7-French DVI EX atherectomy device was advanced across the lesion, and circumferential cuts were performed *(Panel C)*. A moderate amount of fibrous tissue was retrieved, and a 10% residual stenosis was obtained *(Panel D)*. A 4.0-mm Palmaz-Schatz 204 stent was positioned with a balloon catheter across the ostial stenosis, and the balloon was inflated to 6 atm *(Panel E)*. After final balloon inflation, an excellent angiographic result was achieved *(Panel F)*.

Although the goal of intragraft stent implantation is to obtain a minimal residual diameter stenosis (<10%), over-dilatation may predispose a patient to complications (e.g., dissection and perforation) similar to those for balloon angioplasty of native and SVG lesions.

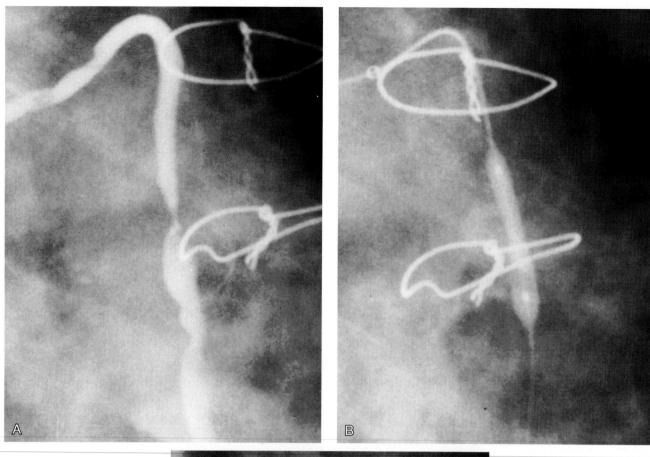
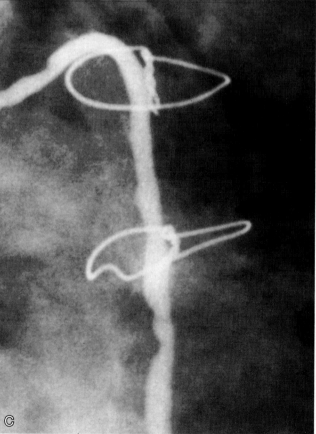

Figure 6–31. *See legend on opposite page*

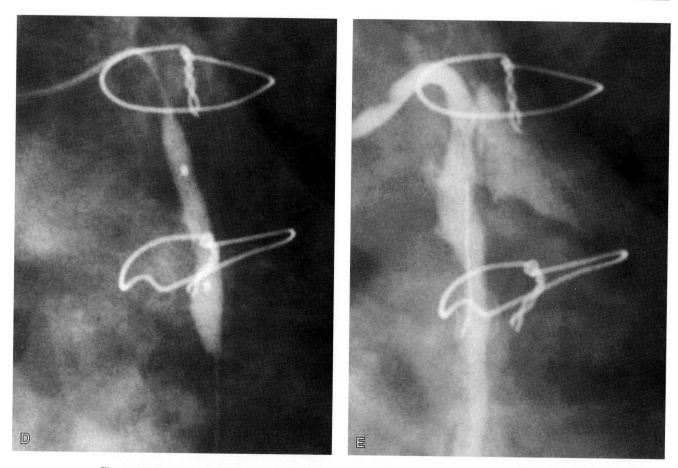

Figure 6–31
Sequential lesions in the midbody of the SVG to the obtuse marginal branch *(Panel A)* were treated with a 3.5-mm tubular slotted stent *(Panel B)*. Stent deployment was notable for incomplete balloon expansion owing to lesion rigidity. A 40% residual stenosis in the midportion of the SVG *(Panel C)* was treated with a second balloon inflation at higher inflation pressures *(Panel D)*. As a result of segment overexpansion, a localized SVG perforation occurred *(Panel E)*.

Photoablation of atherosclerotic plaque using concentric or directional excimer laser angioplasty catheters has also been used with encouraging initial results in patients with degenerated and nondegenerated SVG lesions. Due to the undersizing of the largest available excimer laser catheter (2.2 mm), balloon dilatation or stent implantation is required in the vast majority of patients (>90%).

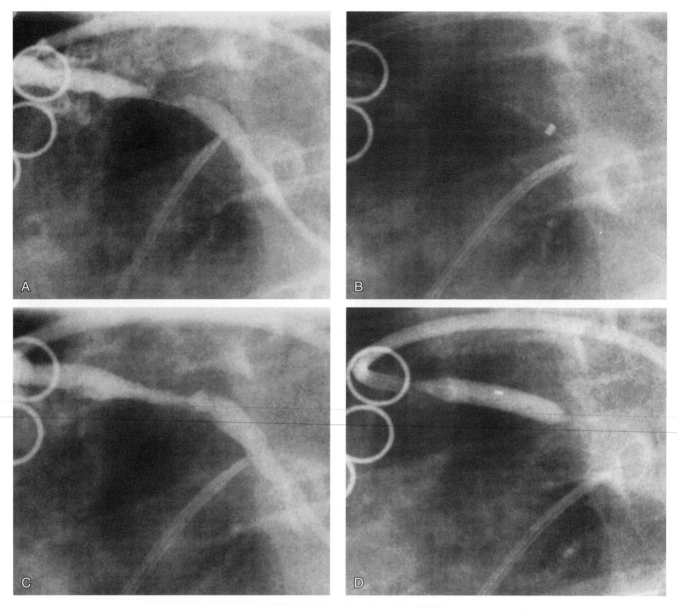

Figure 6–32. *See legend on opposite page*

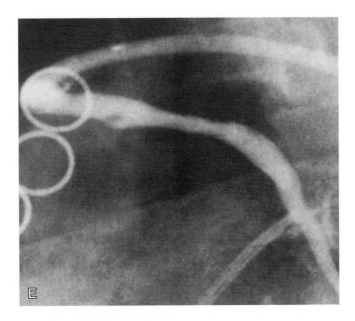

Figure 6–32
An eccentric stenosis in the midsegment of a degenerated SVG to the left anterior descending artery *(Panel A)* was treated with multiple passes of a 2.2-mm excimer laser catheter *(Panel B)*. After initial photoablation, a 50% residual stenosis was obtained *(Panel C)*. Adjunct balloon angioplasty was performed with a 3.5-mm balloon catheter *(Panel D)*, resulting in a 40% residual stenosis. Because of the severe degeneration of the SVG and elastic recoil of the lesion, no further dilatations with balloon angioplasty were performed *(Panel E)*.

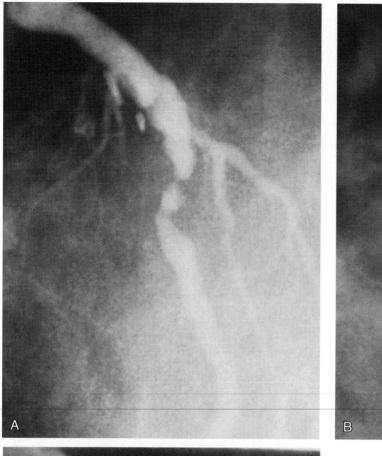

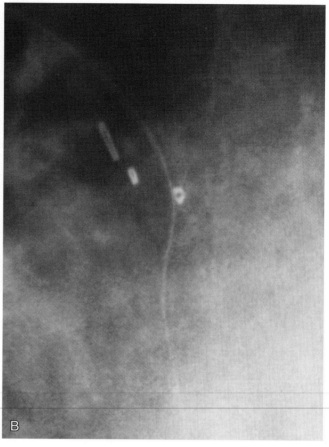

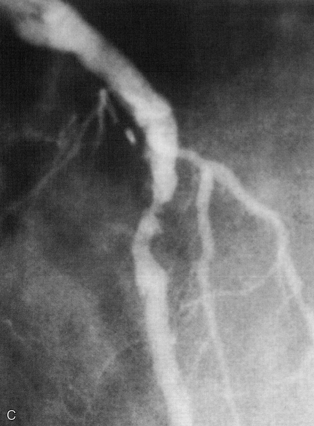

Figure 6–33

A complex, eccentric lesion in the sequential limb of the SVG to the diagonal branch and left anterior descending arteries *(Panel A)* was treated with a 1.8-mm directional excimer laser catheter *(Panel B)*. After the initial pass, a 40% residual stenosis was obtained with brisk anterograde flow into the graft *(Panel C)*. Adjunct balloon dilatation was performed using a 3.5-mm balloon catheter *(Panel D)*, resulting in a residual stenosis of <10% *(Panel E)*.

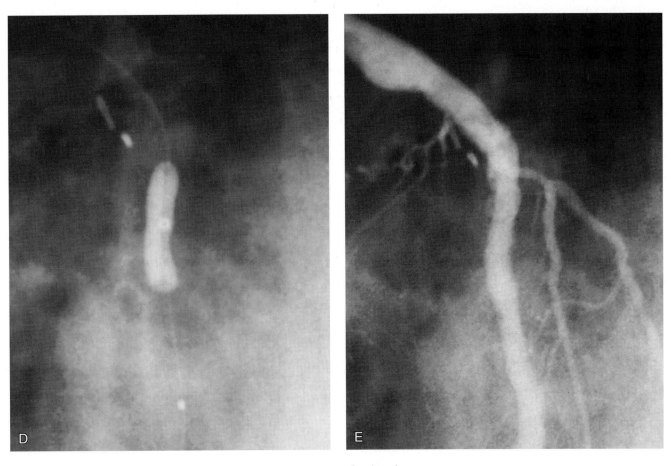

Figure 6–33. *Continued*

SELECTED REFERENCES

Aueron F, Gruentzig A. Distal embolization of a coronary artery bypass graft atheroma during percutaneous transluminal coronary angioplasty. Am J Cardiol 1984; 53:953–954.

Block P, Cowley M, Kaltenbach M, et al. Percutaneous angioplasty of stenoses of bypass grafts or of bypass graft anastomotic sites. Am J Cardiol 1984; 53:666–668.

Cooper I, Ineson N, Demirtas E, et al. Role of angioplasty in patients with previous coronary artery bypass surgery. Cathet Cardiovasc Diagn 1989; 16:81–86.

Corbelli J, Franco I, Hollman J, et al. Percutaneous transluminal coronary angioplasty after previous coronary artery bypass surgery. Am J Cardiol 1985; 56:398–403.

Cote G, Myler R, Stertzer S, et al. Percutaneous transluminal angioplasty of stenotic coronary artery bypass grafts: 5 years' experience. J Am Coll Cardiol 1987; 9:8–17.

de Feyter P, Van Suylen R, de Jaegere P, et al. Balloon angioplasty for the treatment of lesions in saphenous vein bypass grafts. J Am Coll Cardiol 1993; 21:1539–1549.

de Scheerder I, Strauss B, de Feyter P, et al. Stenting of venous bypass grafts: A new treatment modality for patients who are poor candidates for reintervention. Am Heart J 1992; 123:1046–1054.

Dorros G, Lewin R, Mathiak L, et al. Percutaneous transluminal coronary angioplasty in patients with two or more previous coronary artery bypass grafting operations. Am J Cardiol 1988; 61:1243–1247.

Ernst S, van der Feltz T, Ascoop C, et al. Percutaneous transluminal coronary angioplasty in patients with prior coronary artery bypass grafting. J Thorac Cardiovasc Surg 1987; 93:268–275.

Kaufmann U, Garratt K, Vlietstra R, Holmes D. Transluminal atherectomy of saphenous vein aortocoronary bypass grafts. Am J Cardiol 1990; 65:1430–1433.

Platko W, Hollman J, Whitlow P, Franco I. Percutaneous transluminal angioplasty of saphenous vein graft stenosis: Long-term follow-up. J Am Coll Cardiol 1989; 14:1645–1650.

Plokker H. Meester B, Serruys P. The Dutch experience in percutaneous transluminal angioplasty of narrowed saphenous vein grafts used for aortocoronary bypass. Am J Cardiol 1991; 67:361–366.

Pomerantz R, Kuntz R, Carrozza J, et al. Acute and long-term outcome of narrowed saphenous venous grafts treated by endoluminal stenting and directional atherectomy. Am J Cardiol 1992; 70:161–167.

Reeves F, Bonan R, Cote G, et al. Long-term angiographic follow-up after angioplasty of venous coronary bypass grafts. Am Heart J 1991; 122:620–627.

Trono R, Sutton C, Hollman J, et al. Multiple myocardial infarctions associated with atheromatous emboli after PTCA of saphenous vein grafts. Cleve Clin J Med 1989; 56:581–584.

Internal Mammary Artery Angioplasty

In patients undergoing coronary artery bypass grafting, the left and right internal mammary arteries are the conduits of choice over saphenous vein grafts because of these arteries' low incidence of atherosclerotic involvement. On occasion, however, these grafts develop obstructive lesions at the anastomotic site into the native coronary artery or, less often, within the body of the internal mammary artery. Although they frequently pose a technical challenge, these obstructive lesions can be approached with balloon angioplasty, which results in symptomatic relief and precludes repeat bypass operation. The internal mammary arteries are sensitive to mechanical trauma, and care must be taken to avoid injury to the origin of the internal mammary artery. Coaxial guiding catheter alignment into the internal mammary artery is essential to provide adequate support for advancement of the angioplasty equipment through the often tortuous vessel (Figure 7–1).

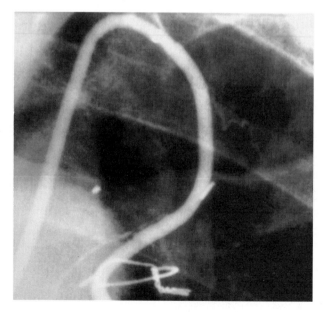

Figure 7–1
Coaxial alignment of the internal mammary guiding catheter in the left internal mammary artery.

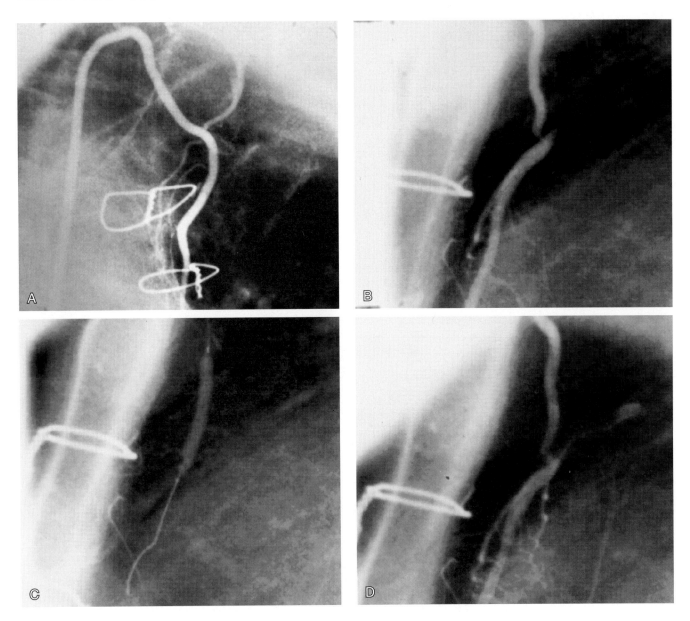

Figure 7–2
Acceptable guiding catheter alignment was obtained at the origin of the left internal mammary artery
into the left anterior descending artery *(Panel A)*. A severe stenosis (>90%) at the anastomotic site
was noted *(Panel B)*; thus, a 3.0-mm fixed-wire balloon catheter was advanced across the stenosis,
and the balloon inflated to 6 atm *(Panel C)*. After final balloon deflation, a 40% residual stenosis was
obtained with a moderate degree of residual intraluminal haziness *(Panel D)*.

Anastomotic lesions of the left internal mammary artery
are most often treated with balloon angioplasty. These lesions are sometimes rigid, requiring high balloon inflation
pressures for complete balloon expansion. Elastic recoil
may also limit the final angiographic result.

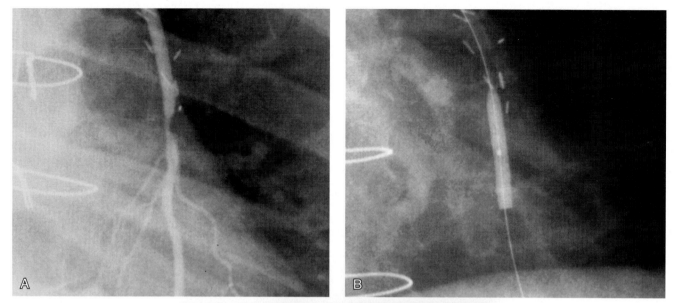

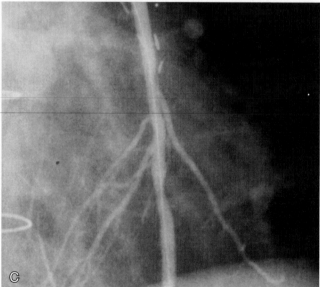

Figure 7–3
An eccentric lesion of the anastomosis of the left internal mammary artery into the left anterior descending artery *(Panel A)* was treated with a 2.5-mm balloon catheter *(Panel B)*. Full balloon expansion was achieved, and an excellent angiographic result was obtained *(Panel C)*.

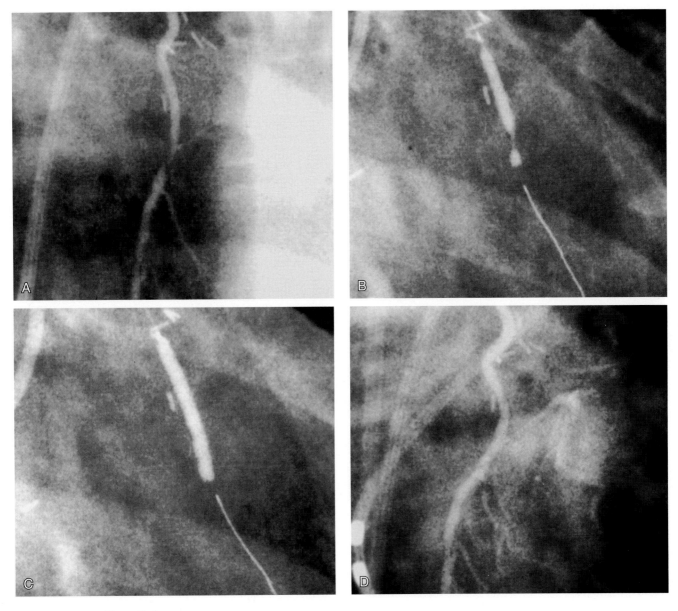

Figure 7–4

A concentric stenosis involving the anastomotic site of the left internal mammary artery into the left anterior descending artery *(Panel A)* was dilated with a 2.5-mm balloon catheter *(Panel B)*. At 8 atm, a residual waist was demonstrated. After inflation of the balloon to a maximum of 12 atm, the waist was relieved *(Panel C)*, and a 20% residual stenosis was achieved *(Panel D)*.

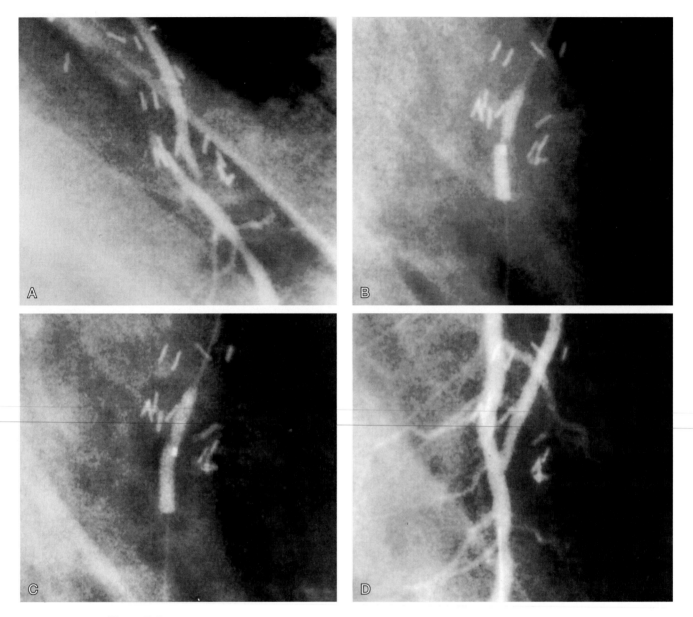

Figure 7–5
An anastomotic lesion of the left internal mammary artery into the left anterior descending artery was
treated with a 2.5-mm balloon catheter *(Panel A).* At 4 atm, a waist was demonstrated *(Panel B);*
complete balloon expansion occurred at 8 atm *(Panel C).* After a 5-minute inflation, a residual
stenosis of <10% was obtained *(Panel D).*

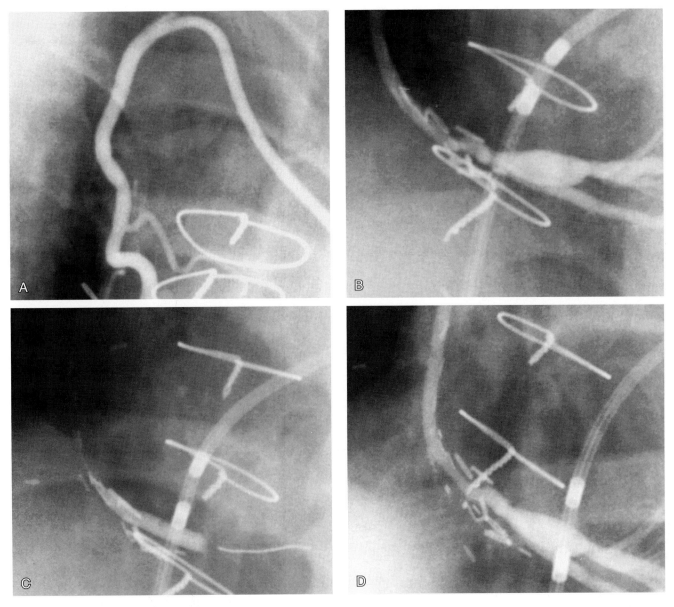

Figure 7–6
Coaxial alignment into the right internal mammary artery was achieved with an 8-French internal mammary artery guiding catheter *(Panel A)*. An anastomotic stenosis of the right internal mammary artery into the distal right coronary artery *(Panel B)* was treated with a 3.0-mm fixed-wire balloon catheter *(Panel C)*. After a 3-minute balloon inflation, a 30% residual stenosis persisted *(Panel D)*.

Coronary angioplasty of native coronary lesions can also be performed through the left or right internal mammary arteries in a manner similar to that for the treatment of native lesions via saphenous vein grafts.

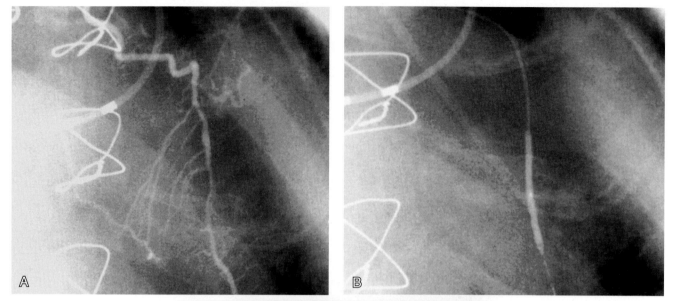

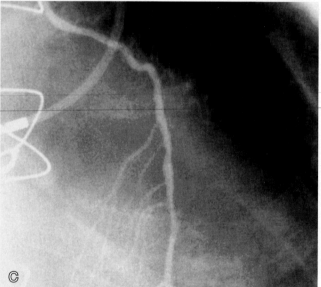

Figure 7–7
Diffuse obstructive disease was demonstrated in the midportion of the native left anterior descending artery distal to the anastomosis of the left internal mammary artery. The internal mammary artery was very tortuous but was crossed with a 0.010-inch wire. A 2.5-mm balloon catheter was advanced across the left anterior descending artery, and the balloon was inflated to 6 atm *(Panel B)*, resulting in a 30% residual stenosis within the native left anterior descending artery *(Panel C)*.

The internal mammary arteries are susceptible to vasospasm with mechanical trauma. This vasospasm generally responds to the intra-arterial administration of nitroglycerin.

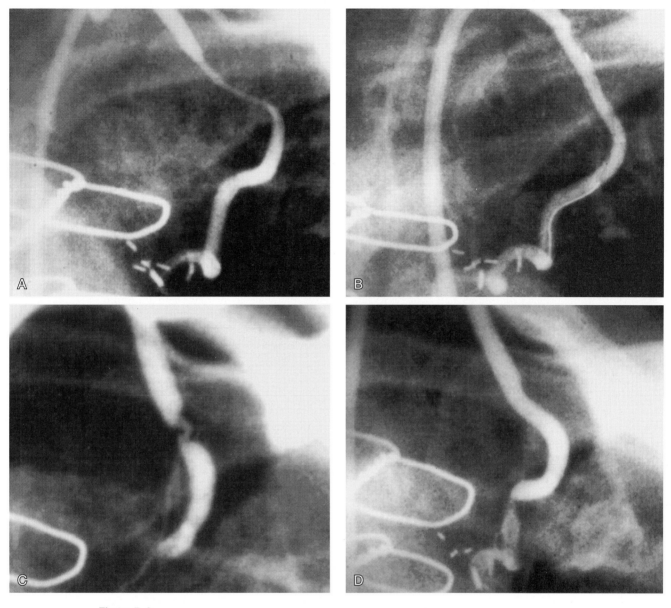

Figure 7–8
A tubular narrowing of the proximal segment of the left internal mammary artery *(Panel A)* developed on passage of the guide wire into the distal portion of the left internal mammary artery. Intra-arterial nitroglycerin, 200 μg, was administered, and the arterial spasm resolved *(Panel B)*. Similarly, a focal narrowing of the distal segment of the left internal mammary artery developed during angioplasty *(Panel C)* and responded to intra-arterial nitroglycerin administration *(Panel D)*.

SELECTED REFERENCES

Bell M, Holmes D. Percutaneous transluminal angioplasty of internal mammary artery grafts. J Invasive Cardiol 1989; 1:239–245.

Crean P, Mathieson P, Rickards A. Transluminal angioplasty of a stenosis of an internal mammary artery graft. Br Heart J 1986; 56:473–475.

Dimas A, Arora R, Whitlow P, et al. Percutaneous transluminal angioplasty involving internal mammary artery grafts. Am Heart J 1991; 122:423–429.

Kereiakes D, George B, Stertzer S, Myler R. Percutaneous transluminal angioplasty of left internal mammary artery grafts. Am J Cardiol 1985; 55:1215–1216.

Pinkerton C, Slack J, Orr C, VanTassel J. Percutaneous transluminal angioplasty involving internal mammary artery bypass grafts: A femoral approach. Cathet Cardiovasc Diagn 1987; 13:414–418.

Popma J, Cooke R, Leon M, et al. Immediate procedural and long-term clinical results of internal mammary artery angioplasty. Am J Cardiol 1992; 69:1237–1239.

Shimshak T, Giorgi L, Johnson W, et al. Application of percutaneous transluminal coronary angioplasty to the internal mammary artery graft. J Am Coll Cardiol 1988; 12:1205–1214.

Singh S. Coronary angioplasty of internal mammary artery graft. Am J Med 1987; 82:361–362.

Steffenino G, Meier B, Finci L, et al. Percutaneous transluminal angioplasty of right and left internal mammary artery grafts. Chest 1990; 90:849–851.

Thrombus-Containing Lesions

Angiographic evidence of thrombus is generally manifested by the appearance of discrete, intraluminal filling defects adjacent to or connected to the arterial surface. The presence of intracoronary thrombus has been associated with higher, although somewhat variable, rates of ischemic complications after coronary angioplasty (range: 6–73%); these rates are generally attributable to the occurrence of abrupt closure and distal embolization. The presence of thrombus on angiography suggests that the underlying plaque morphology is unstable, potentially consequent to recent ulceration and exposure of the subintimal connective tissue elements to platelets and thrombin. Notably, small amounts of localized thrombus can be treated with standard balloon angioplasty with a low risk for distal embolization or other significant sequelae.

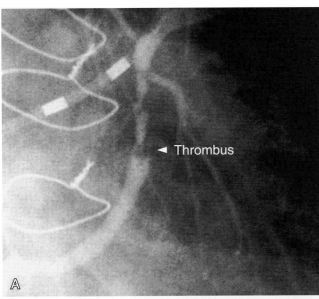

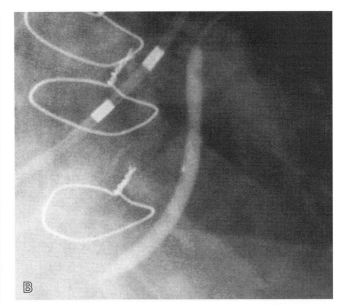

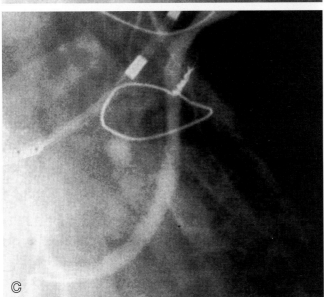

Figure 8–1
A sequential saphenous vein graft (SVG) to the obtuse marginal and posterior descending branches of this patient had discrete intragraft filling defects within its lumen *(Panel A)*. A 3.0-mm long (40-mm) balloon was used to dilate the entire midsegment of the SVG *(Panel B)*. After two inflations, no residual thrombus was visualized, and an excellent angiographic result was obtained *(Panel C)*.

Larger amounts of coronary thrombus should be approached with caution when standard balloon methods are used. Aggressive anticoagulation with intravenous heparin and oral aspirin, possibly combined with thrombolytic administration, is generally recommended for 1–5 days prior to attempted coronary angioplasty of large thrombus-containing lesions. Use of new IIb/IIIa platelet integrin antagonists or direct thrombin inhibitors are also promising treatments for such lesions.

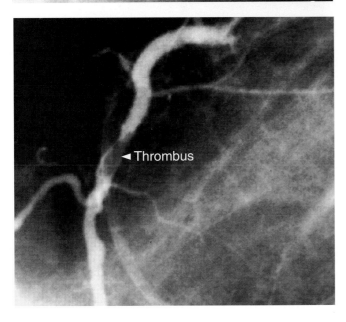

Figure 8–2
A large intraluminal filling defect was present in this patient who presented with unstable angina, which was manifested by a recent acceleration of symptoms, pain at rest, and transient ST segment depression in the inferior leads. The identification of thrombus in this setting suggests recent plaque ulceration and high risk for complications with coronary angioplasty.

On occasion, thrombus superimposed on a minimal atherosclerotic lesion appears angiographically identical to an obstructive, flow-limiting stenosis.

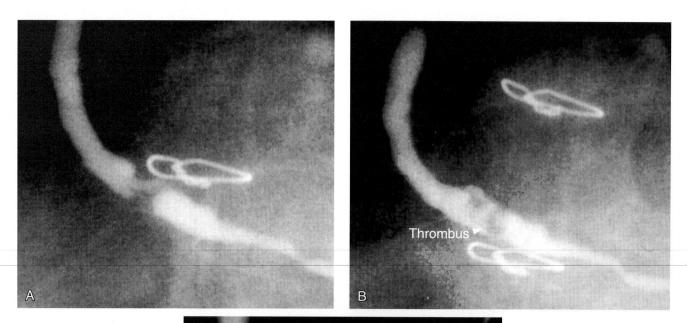

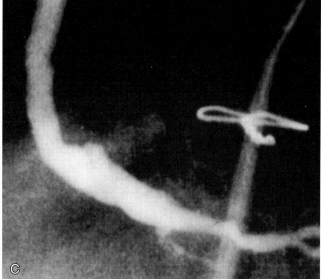

Figure 8–3

A concentric stenosis in the distal portion of the SVG to the right coronary artery was treated with 500,000 U of urokinase prior to planned coronary angioplasty *(Panel A)*. After 40 minutes, dissolution of the thrombus was demonstrated *(Panel B)*. A continuous infusion of intravenous urokinase, 75,000 U/h, was given for 24 hours. Repeat angiography 24 hours later demonstrated near complete resolution of the apparent stenosis *(Panel C)*, suggesting that the entire lesion was secondary to the superimposition of intragraft thrombus. (Reprinted from Cospito P, Popma J, Satler L, et al. Prolonged intravenous urokinase infusion: An alternative pharmacologic approach in the treatment of thrombus-containing saphenous vein graft stenoses. Cathet Cardiovasc Diagn 1992; 26:291–294, with permission.)

Patients with acute myocardial infarction who fail to reperfuse after the administration of thrombolytic therapy may have coronary thrombi—potentially due to platelet-platelet aggregation and fibrin cross-linking at the site of excess thrombus burden—that preclude the use of mechanical methods of arterial recanalization.

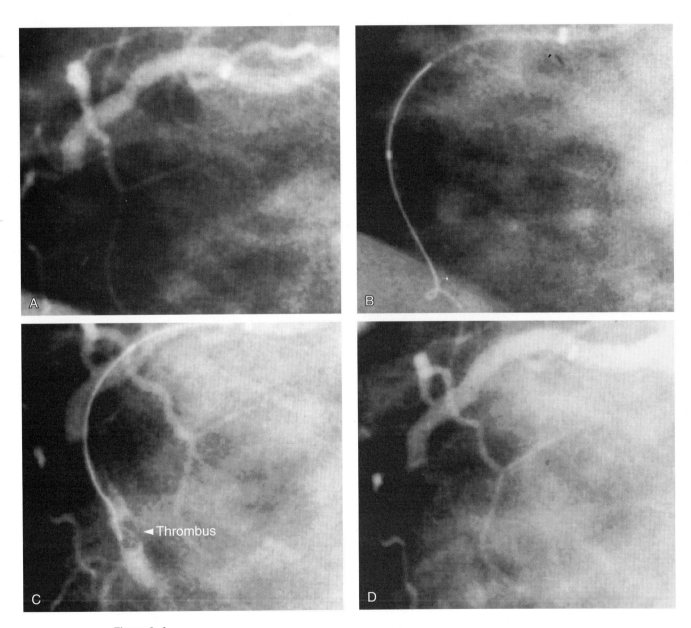

Figure 8–4
Thrombosis of the midsegment of the right coronary artery resulted in an acute inferior wall myocardial infarction in this patient 12 hours prior to presentation. Tissue plasminogen activator, 100 mg, was administered over 3 hours; 4 hours after the administration of the thrombolytic agent, symptoms and inferior ST segment elevation persisted. Emergency coronary angiography was performed and demonstrated a total occlusion of the midsegment of the right coronary artery *(Panel A)*. Standard balloon angioplasty was attempted using a 3.0-mm balloon catheter *(Panel B)*. Although faint anterograde flow was demonstrated *(Panel C)*, a marked amount of intracoronary thrombus remained. Total coronary occlusion occurred 10 minutes after the final balloon inflation *(Panel D)*.

New angioplasty devices (e.g., directional atherectomy devices) may be used in thrombus-containing lesions, provided that the thrombus burden is not excessive. In a multicenter series of 400 patients undergoing directional atherectomy, complex thrombus-containing lesions were associated with favorable procedural outcome (Ellis et al., 1991). Procedural success was obtained in all 30 lesions that contained intracoronary thrombus, and no episodes of

abrupt closure were noted. Importantly, late abrupt closure may occur more frequently in vessels with thrombus-containing lesions, despite good initial angiographic results. This emphasizes the need for postprocedural heparin administration (for 48–72 hours), possibly combined with chronic oral anticoagulation therapy with warfarin (1–3 months).

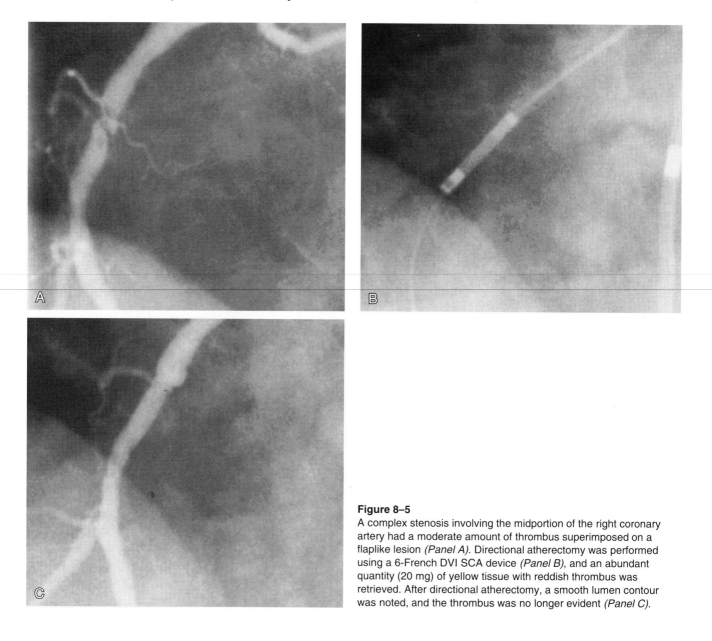

Figure 8–5

A complex stenosis involving the midportion of the right coronary artery had a moderate amount of thrombus superimposed on a flaplike lesion *(Panel A)*. Directional atherectomy was performed using a 6-French DVI SCA device *(Panel B)*, and an abundant quantity (20 mg) of yellow tissue with reddish thrombus was retrieved. After directional atherectomy, a smooth lumen contour was noted, and the thrombus was no longer evident *(Panel C)*.

Figure 8–6

A recent total occlusion of the midsegment of the right coronary artery *(Panel A)* was treated with excimer laser angioplasty using a 1.3-mm catheter *(Panel B)*. After the initial photoablation, the vessel was recanalized; however, a significant amount of "grapelike" filling defects were noted in the midportion of the right coronary artery *(Panel C)*. Prolonged inflation with a 3.5-mm balloon dilatation catheter was performed *(Panel D)*, but the irregular, thrombus-containing lesion in the midportion of the right coronary artery persisted *(Panel E)*. Directional atherectomy was then performed using a 7-French DVI EX device (not shown), and circumferential cuts were made. After final excision, a marked improvement in the lumen contour was observed, and no angiographic evidence of residual thrombus was present *(Panel F)*.

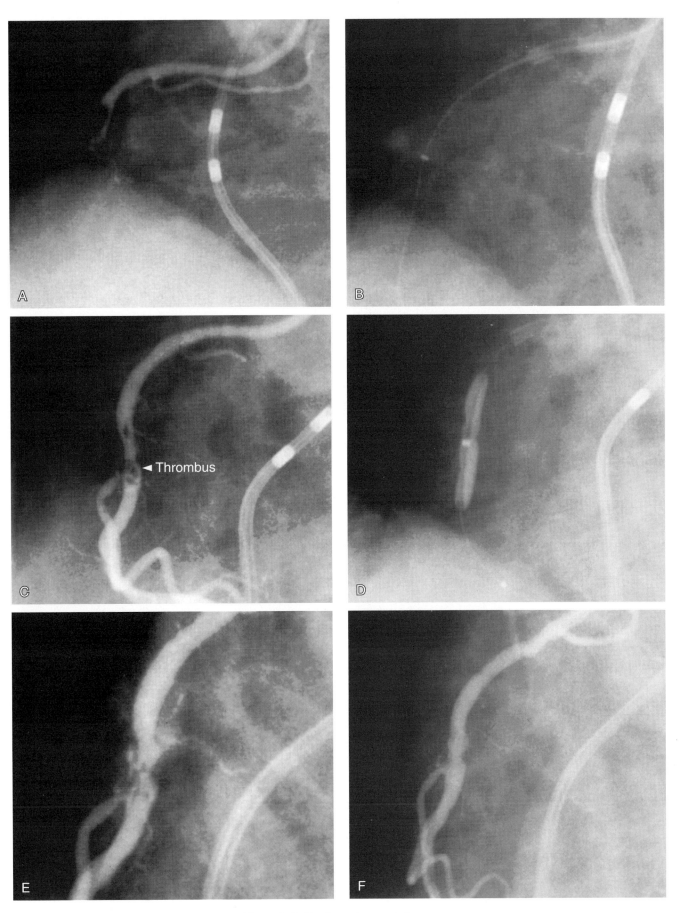

Figure 8–6. *See legend on opposite page*

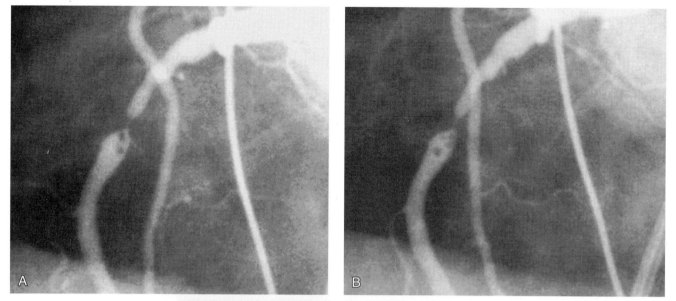

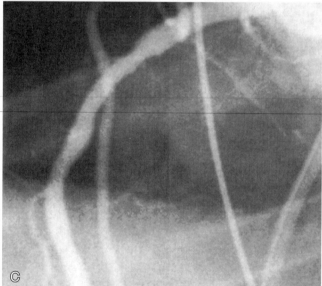

Figure 8–7
A concentric stenosis in the midportion of the right coronary artery had circumferential pedunculated filling defects adherent to the vessel wall just distal to the stenosis *(Panels A and B)*. Directional atherectomy was performed using a 7-French DVI EX device (not shown), and an excellent angiographic result was obtained without evidence of dissection or reduction in anterograde flow *(Panel C)*

Transluminal extraction atherectomy has also been specifically targeted for the management of thrombus-containing lesions, particularly those located in SVGs.

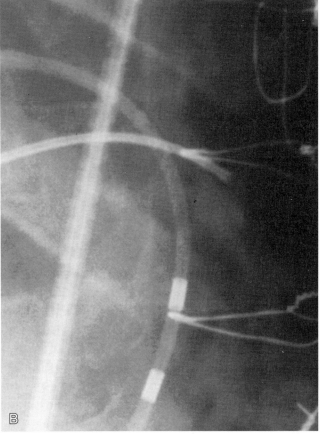

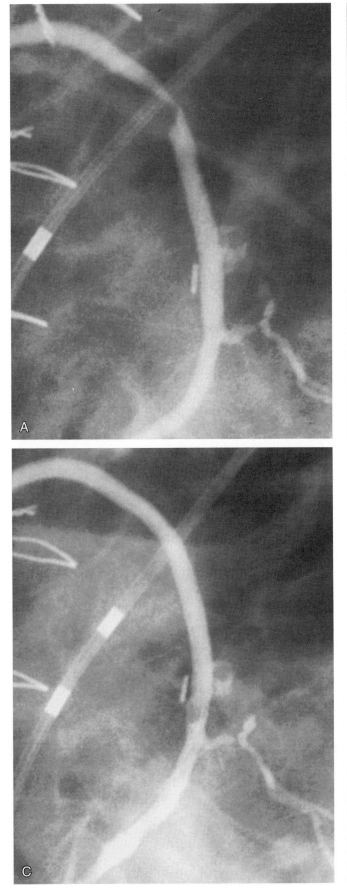

Figure 8–8

An eccentric stenosis in the midportion of the sequential SVG to the obtuse marginal branches *(Panel A)* was treated with a 2.5-mm transluminal extraction catheter (TEC) device *(Panel B)*. After 8 passes across the lesion, a 40% residual stenosis was obtained (not shown). Adjunct balloon dilatation was performed with a 3.5-mm balloon catheter, yielding an excellent angiographic result and normal flow of the distal segment. Either streaming or a possible filling defect was noted distal to the original lesion *(Panel C)*.

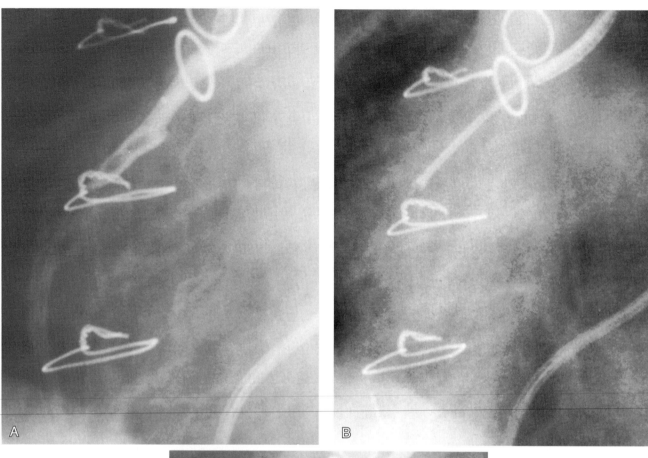

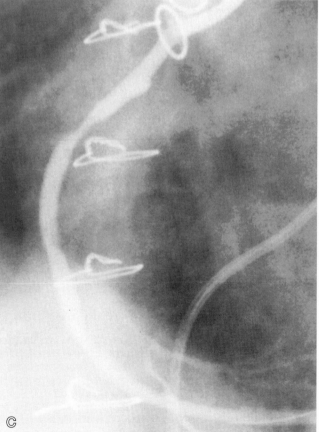

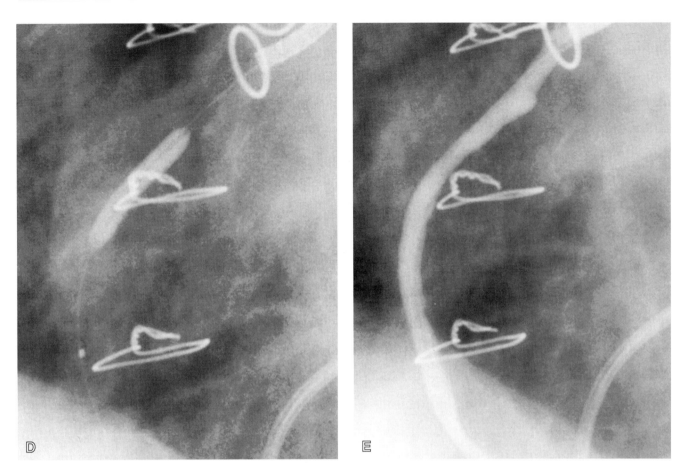

Figure 8–9
The SVG to the distal right coronary artery was totally occluded in its proximal portion *(Panel A)*. A large intragraft thrombus was noted. A 2.5-mm TEC device was advanced across the segment of total occlusion, and multiple passes were performed *(Panel B)*. After initial extraction atherectomy, anterograde SVG flow was re-established, and no evidence of distal embolization was observed *(Panel C)*. Because of the presence of a 40% residual stenosis, adjunct balloon dilatation was performed with a 3.5-mm balloon catheter *(Panel D)*. After final balloon inflation, a smooth lumen contour was demonstrated with rapid flow into the distal right coronary artery *(Panel E)*.

Despite the utility of the TEC device in the removal of thrombus, distal embolization in lesions that contain an excess amount of thrombus remains a concern. Distal embolization occurs most often after adjunct balloon dilatation consequent to dislodgment of the friable thrombotic or graft material.

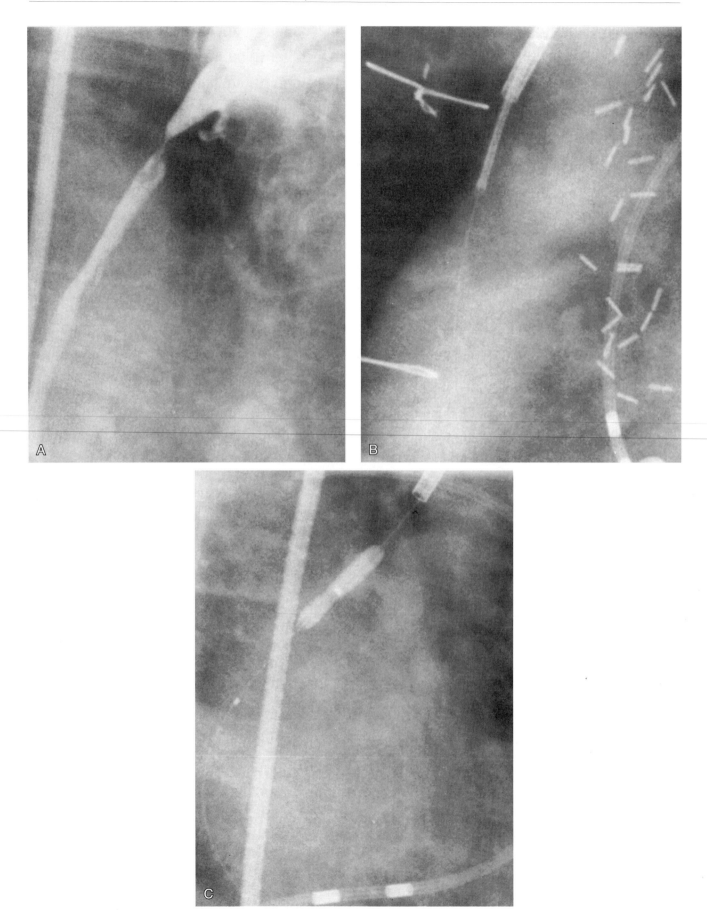

Figure 8–10. *See legend on opposite page*

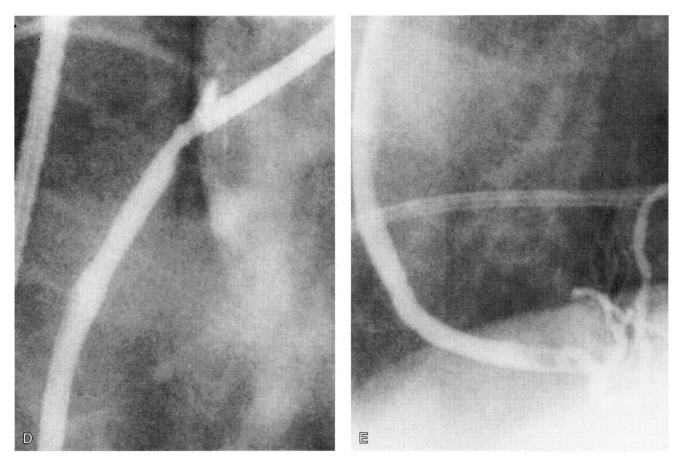

Figure 8–10
A thrombus-containing lesion in the proximal segment of a SVG to the posterior descending artery *(Panel A)* was treated with a 2.3-mm TEC device *(Panel B)*. Because of a 50% residual stenosis (not shown), a 3.5-mm balloon catheter was advanced across the residual stenosis, and a single balloon inflation was performed *(Panel C)*. After dilatation, flow was delayed into the distal portion of the graft despite an acceptable angiographic result *(Panel D)*. An intraluminal filling defect consistent with an embolus was noted in the distal portion of the SVG *(Panel E)*.

In selected patients with degenerated and friable SVGs in whom the risk of distal embolization is high, planned staging of the SVG angioplasty has been tried. Transluminal extraction atherectomy may first be used to remove the superficial plaque debris and thrombus. Because distal embolization often occurs after adjunct balloon angioplasty to treat a suboptimal initial result, the residual stenosis may not be treated with adjunct dilatation during the initial procedure. Instead, the patients undergo systemic anticoagulation therapy with coumadin for 6 weeks. After this period, definitive coronary angioplasty using balloons or intragraft stenting can be performed.

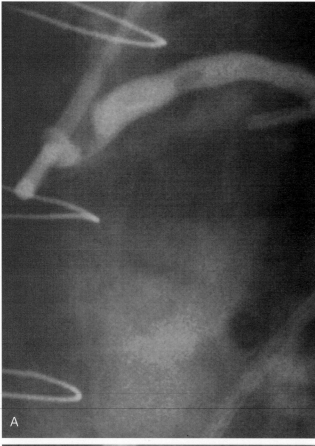

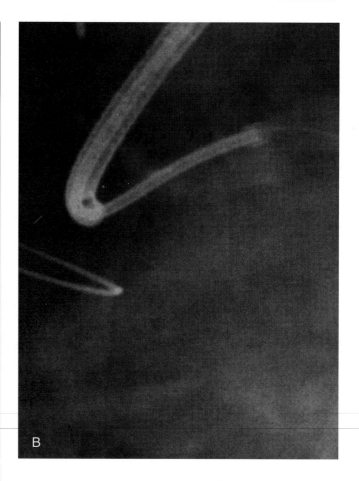

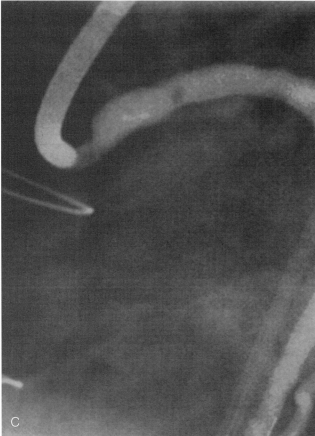

Figure 8–11

An eccentric stenosis of the ostium of the SVG to the left anterior descending artery *(Panel A)* was treated with a 2.5-mm TEC device *(Panel B)*. After six sequential passes, a progressive improvement in the severity of the stenosis was observed *(Panel C)*. Although a significant residual stenosis (60%) and an intraluminal filling defect remained, the lesion was not treated further with adjunct balloon dilatation because of concerns about possible distal embolization. As an alternative, the patient was treated with oral coumadin and returned 6 weeks later for definitive intragraft stent placement; this approach allowed sufficient time for the degenerated SVG to heal.

SELECTED REFERENCES

Arora R, Platko W, Bhadwar K, Simpfendorfer C. Role of intracoronary thrombus in acute complications during percutaneous transluminal coronary angioplasty. Cathet Cardiovasc Diagn 1989; 16:226–229.

Deligonul U, Gabliani G, Caralis D, et al. Percutaneous transluminal coronary angioplasty in patients with intracoronary thrombus. Am J Cardiol 1988; 62:474–476.

Ellis S, DeCesare N, Pinkerton C, et al. Relation of stenosis morphology and clinical presentation to the procedural results of directional coronary atherectomy. Circulation 1991; 84:644–653.

Ellis S, Roubin G, King S III, et al. Angiographic and clinical predictors of acute closure after native vessel coronary angioplasty. Circulation 1988; 77:372–379.

Ellis S, Topol E, Gallison L, et al. Predictors of success for coronary angioplasty performed for acute myocardial infarction. J Am Coll Cardiol 1988; 12:1407–1415.

Goudreau E, DiSciascio G, Vetrovec G, et al. Intracoronary urokinase as an adjunct to percutaneous transluminal coronary angioplasty in patients with complex coronary narrowings or angioplasty-induced complications. Am J Cardiol 1992; 69:57–62.

Kern M, Deligonul U, Presant S, Vandormael M. Resolution of intraluminal thrombus with augmentation of heparin during percutaneous transluminal coronary angioplasty. Am J Cardiol 1986; 58:852–853.

Mabin T, Holmes D, Smith H, et al. Intracoronary thrombus: Role in coronary occlusion complicating percutaneous transluminal coronary angioplasty. J Am Coll Cardiol 1985; 5:198–202.

MacDonald R, Feldman R, Conti C, Pepine C. Thromboembolic complications of coronary angioplasty. Am J Cardiol 1984; 54:916–917.

Mooney M, Mooney J, Goldenberg I, et al. Percutaneous transluminal coronary angioplasty in the setting of large intracoronary thrombi. Am J Cardiol 1990; 65:427–431.

Myler R, Shaw R, Stertzer S, et al. Lesion morphology and coronary angioplasty: Current experience and analysis. J Am Coll Cardiol 1992; 19:1641–1652.

Popma J, Leon M, Mintz G, et al. Results of coronary angioplasty using the transluminal extraction catheter. Am J Cardiol 1992; 70:1526–1532.

Savage M, Goldberg S, Hirschfeld J, et al. Clinical and angiographic determinants of primary coronary angioplasty success. J Am Coll Cardiol 1991; 17:22–28.

Sugrue D, Holmes D, Smith H, et al. Coronary artery thrombus as a risk factor for acute vessel occlusion during percutaneous transluminal coronary angioplasty: Improving results. Br Heart J 1986; 56:62–66.

CHAPTER 9

Long Lesions

Lesions of excessive length (≥10 mm) have been associated with reduced procedural success rates, particularly when segments are diffusely diseased (≥20 mm). The suboptimal procedural success rates may be related to the more extensive plaque burden seen in longer lesions, which renders some regions of the lesion less responsive to balloon dilatation. Notably, using contemporary angioplasty techniques (overlapping, extended balloon inflations) and long balloons (30–40 mm), some practitioners have reported procedural success rates of >90%, provided that the entire length of a vessel is not involved.

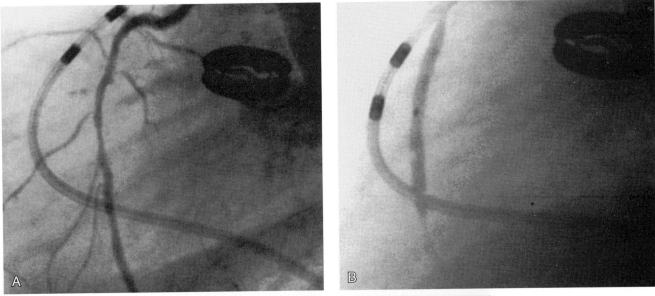

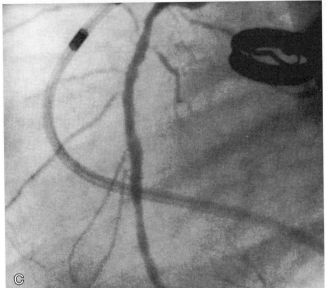

Figure 9–1
A diffusely diseased segment of the proximal portion and midportion of the right coronary artery
(Panel A) was treated with two inflations using a 3.0-mm long (40-mm) balloon catheter *(Panel B)*.
After the final balloon inflation, an improvement in lumen contour was obtained *(Panel C)*.

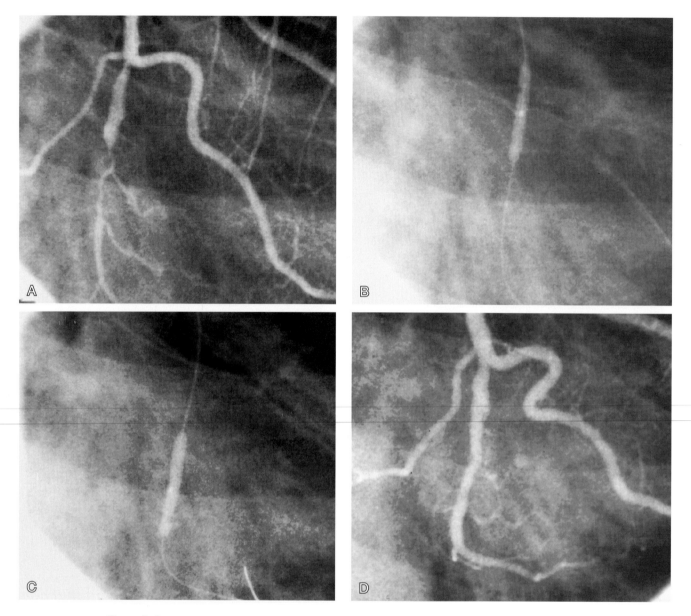

Figure 9–2
A tubular (18-mm) lesion *(Panel A)* was treated with standard balloon angioplasty using overlapping
2.5-mm balloon inflations in the midsegment *(Panel B)* and distal segment *(Panel C)* of the left
circumflex artery. After final balloon inflation, an excellent anatomic result was obtained, with a <10%
residual stenosis *(Panel D)*.

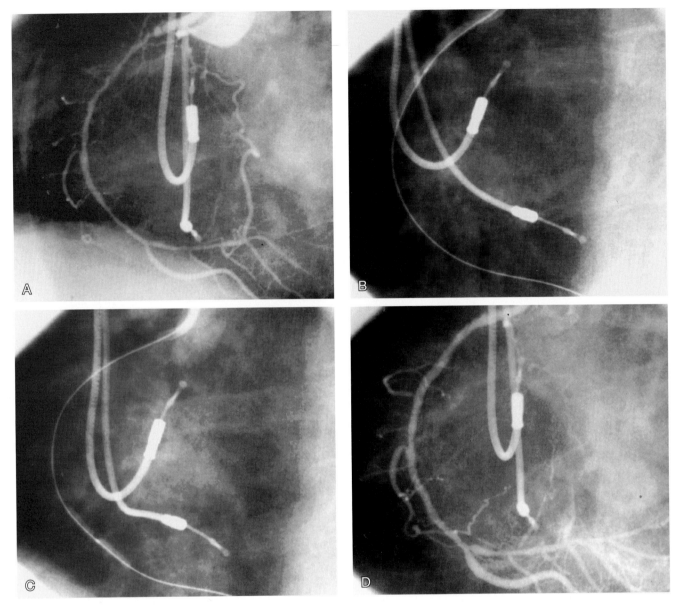

Figure 9–3
The right coronary artery of this patient was diffusely diseased in its proximal, medial, and distal segments *(Panel A)*. A 2.5-mm long (30-mm) balloon was inflated in the proximal and midsegments of the right coronary artery *(Panel B)*. After balloon deflation, the 2.5-mm long balloon could not be advanced across the distal stenosis. It was exchanged for a 2.5-mm standard-length balloon, which was inflated in the distal right coronary artery *(Panel C)*. After sequential inflations along the entire segment of the right coronary artery and following intracoronary infusion of nitroglycerin, 200 μg, a <20% residual stenosis was obtained *(Panel D)*.

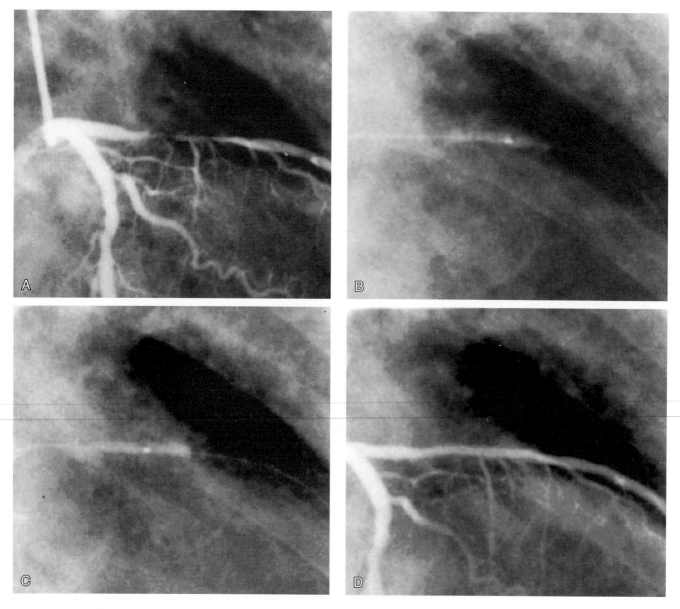

Figure 9–4
A tubular, eccentric lesion of the left anterior descending artery *(Panel A)* was treated with sequential balloon inflations in the proximal segment *(Panel B)* and midsegment *(Panel C)*. After final balloon inflation, a smooth lumen contour was obtained, with a <20% residual stenosis *(Panel D)*.

New angioplasty devices may be useful in long lesions owing to their ability to "debulk" the atherosclerotic plaque. A smaller postprocedural lumen diameter has been demonstrated in long (≥10 mm) as opposed to discrete (<10 mm) lesions after directional atherectomy by Popma and coworkers; this may account for the higher restenosis rates after directional atherectomy in long lesions. Rotational coronary atherectomy has also been used in diffusely diseased lesions, especially if lesion-associated calcium is present. Stand-alone rotational atherectomy of long lesions (≥10 mm) has a 70% procedural success rate, a 15% to 19% incidence of non–Q wave myocardial infarction, and a 75% angiographic restenosis rate. As a result, adjunct balloon dilatation is often performed after rotational atherectomy to maximize the lumen diameter. This results in an overall procedural success rate of >90%.

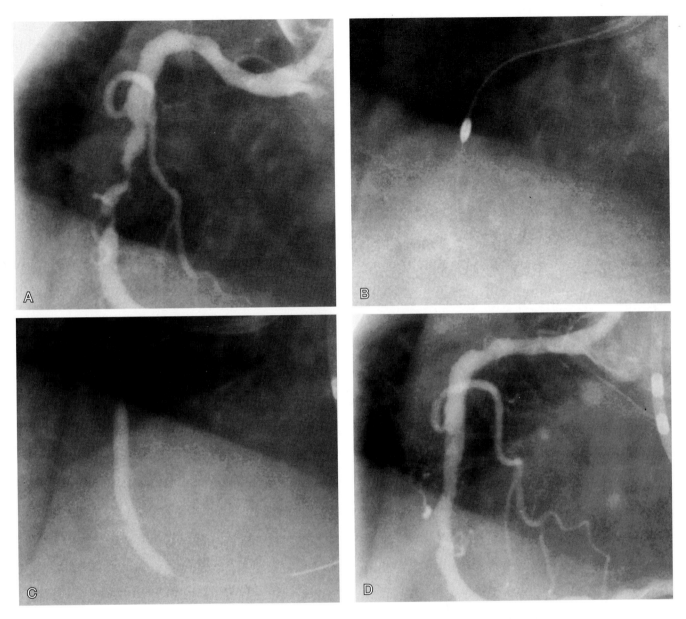

Figure 9–5
A calcified, tubular lesion in the midportion of the right coronary artery *(Panel A)* was treated with 1.5-
and 2.0-mm burrs *(Panel B)*. After eight passes with each burr, a 40% residual stenosis was obtained
(not shown), and a 3.0-mm long balloon was inflated in the distal and proximal segments of the lesion
(Panel C). After final balloon inflation, a smooth arterial lumen was obtained, with a 20% residual
stenosis *(Panel D)*.

Excimer laser ablation is another method of reducing the
overall plaque burden in long lesions and may be particularly useful in diffusely diseased or totally occluded segments.

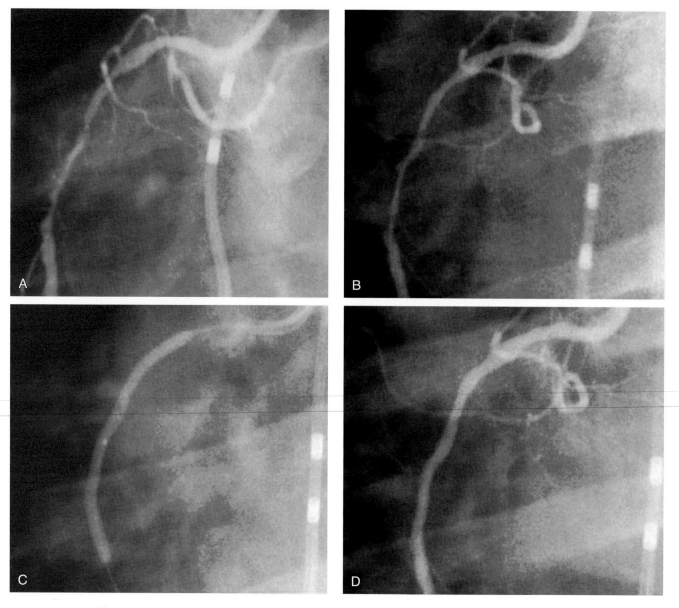

Figure 9–6
Diffusely diseased segments of the proximal and medial right coronary artery *(Panel A)* were treated with a 1.3-mm excimer laser (308-nm) catheter (not shown). After a single pass, a persistent narrowing of the vessel was evident *(Panel B)*. Adjunct balloon angioplasty using a 2.5-mm long (40-mm) balloon was performed *(Panel C)*, and a minimal (<20%) diameter stenosis was identified *(Panel D)*.

SELECTED REFERENCES

Bredlau C, Roubin G, Leimgruber P, et al. In-hospital morbidity and mortality in patients undergoing elective coronary angioplasty. Circulation 1985; 72:1044–1052.

Ellis S, Topol E, Gallison L, et al. Predictors of success for coronary angioplasty performed for acute myocardial infarction. J Am Coll Cardiol 1988; 12:1407–1415.

Goudreau E, DiSciascio G, Kelly K, et al. Coronary angioplasty of diffuse coronary artery disease. Am Heart J 1991; 121:12–19.

Meier B, Gruentzig A, Hollman J, et al. Does length or eccentricity of coronary stenoses influence the outcome of transluminal dilatation? Circulation 1983; 1983:497–499.

Myler R, Shaw R, Stertzer S, et al. Lesion morphology and coronary angioplasty: Current experience and analysis. J Am Coll Cardiol 1992; 19:1641–1652.

Popma J, DeCesare N, Ellis S, et al. Clinical, angiographic and procedural correlates of quantitative coronary dimensions after directional coronary atherectomy. J Am Coll Cardiol 1991; 18:1183–1189.

Savage M, Goldberg S, Hirschfeld J, et al. Clinical and angiographic determinants of primary coronary angioplasty success. J Am Coll Cardiol 1991; 17:22–28.

Teirstein P, Warth D, Haq N, et al. High speed rotational coronary atherectomy for patients with diffuse coronary artery disease. J Am Coll Cardiol 1991; 18:1694–1701.

CHAPTER 10

Proximal Vessel Tortuosity

With reductions in profile and improved trackability of contemporary angioplasty balloons, enhanced guiding catheter support, and the availability of transitionless coronary guide wires, lesions that were not accessible with standard balloon methods are now effectively treated with percutaneous angioplasty techniques. Both fixed-wire and over-the-wire systems have been advocated to treat lesions located distal to proximally tortuous vessels. Despite the improvements in angioplasty equipment, some lesions are still not amenable to standard angioplasty.

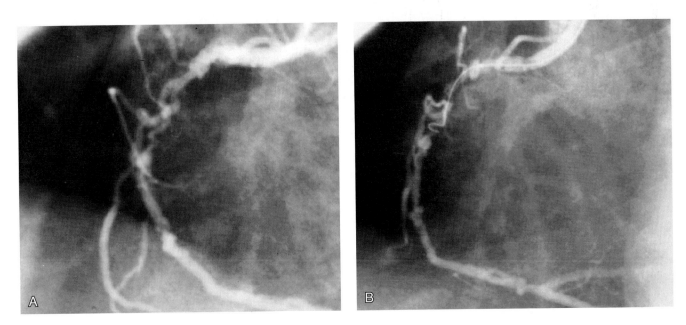

Figure 10–1
A severe (90%) stenosis of the midsegment of the right coronary artery was located distal to a segment of severe tortuosity due principally to asymmetric proximal plaque accumulation *(Panel A)*. Despite the use of a variety of floppy, intermediate, and standard guide wires and of sufficient guiding catheter backup, the lesion could not be crossed *(Panel B)*.

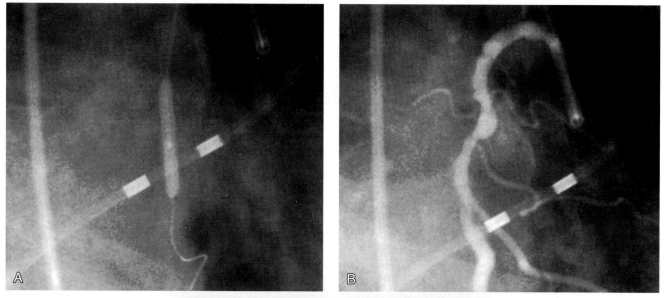

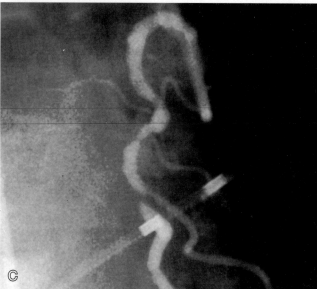

Figure 10–2

A concentric stenosis in the midportion of the right coronary artery just after the origin of a right ventricular marginal branch was located distal to a region of proximal tortuosity *(Panel A)*. A 2.5-mm balloon catheter was advanced across the lesion, and the balloon was inflated; this resulted in marked straightening of the vessel *(Panel B)*. After balloon deflation, mild intraluminal haziness was noted, but an acceptable angiographic result was obtained *(Panel C)*.

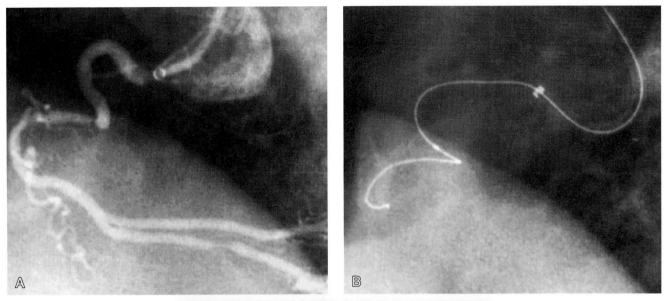

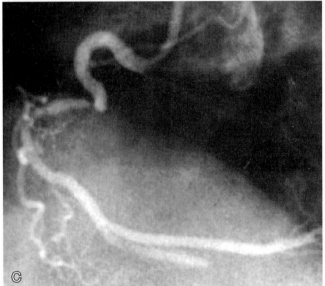

Figure 10–3
An angulated lesion was noted in the midportion of the right coronary artery just distal to a shepherd's crook origin. *(Panel A).* Although a wire could be positioned across the stenosis, the balloon catheter could not be advanced across the lesion *(Panel B)* because of inadequate guiding catheter support. The procedure was unsuccessful *(Panel C)* and was terminated after closure of the posterolateral branch resulting from distal wire dissection.

On occasion, the guiding catheter can be carefully used to provide sufficient intracoronary support to traverse segments of severe tortuosity.

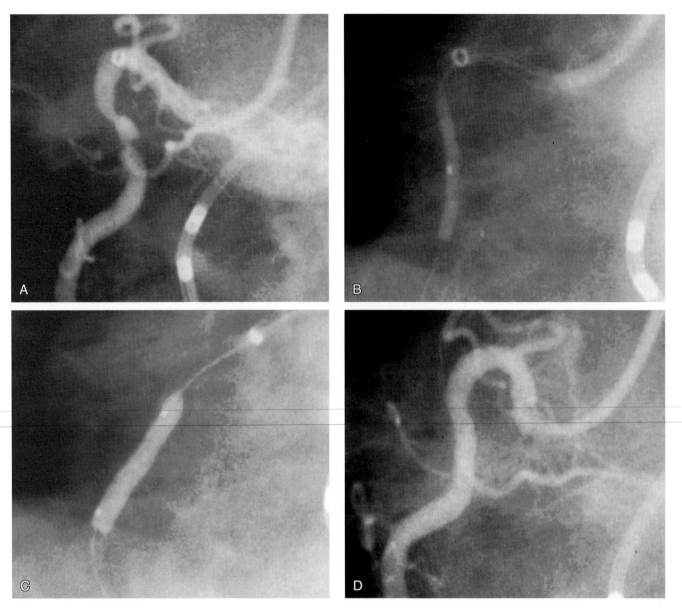

Figure 10–4

An eccentric, restenotic lesion located just distal to a severe shepherd's crook takeoff of the right coronary artery *(Panel A)* was predilated with a 2.5-mm balloon catheter *(Panel B)*. With the use of a left Amplatz guiding catheter for support, a 3.0-mm tubular slotted Palmaz-Schatz stent was deployed across the stenosis *(Panel C)*. This resulted in a residual stenosis of <10% *(Panel D)*.

Left Mainstem Lesions

O'Keefe and colleagues described the use of coronary angioplasty of the left main coronary artery in three specific clinical settings. In the first, left main coronary angioplasty is used for catastrophic left main thrombosis in the setting of acute myocardial infarction. Emergency recanalization of the left main coronary artery through the use of percutaneous methods may restore anterograde perfusion into the left coronary artery and re-establish hemodynamic stability, allowing patient transfer for more definitive coronary bypass operation.

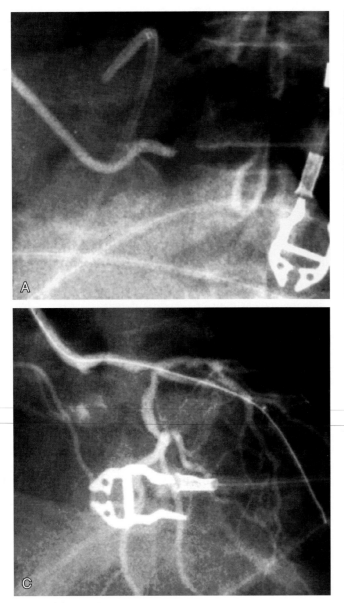

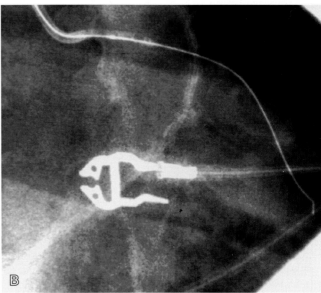

Figure 11–1

Acute thrombotic occlusion of the left main coronary artery resulted in profound anterior and posterior myocardial ischemia and hemodynamic collapse. With intra-aortic balloon pump support, immediate angiography demonstrated a total occlusion of the distal portion of the left main coronary artery *(Panel A)*. A coronary guide wire was used to recanalize the left coronary artery, and a 3.0-mm balloon catheter was quickly advanced across the lesion and its balloon inflated for 15 seconds *(Panel B)*. After balloon deflation, anterograde flow was restored into the left coronary artery *(Panel C)*. Although a significant residual stenosis remained, hemodynamic stability was re-established, and the patient was transferred for emergency coronary bypass surgery.

In the second setting, coronary angioplasty of the left main coronary artery is performed in patients in whom coronary bypass operation is not a therapeutic option because of underlying comorbid disease. Given the limited mortality and morbidity associated with coronary bypass surgery in this setting and the high rates of symptom recurrence after coronary angioplasty of the left main coronary artery, the latter therapy is appropriate for relatively few patients and should be considered only palliative.

When coronary angioplasty is performed in the unprotected left main coronary artery, several factors should be considered. First, whenever possible, hemodynamic and myocardial support should be provided with intra-aortic balloon counterpulsation, coronary sinus retroperfusion, or percutaneous cardiopulmonary support; however, the advantages and disadvantages of each of these approaches in patients with left main coronary disease have not been defined. Second, careful planning should be undertaken to ensure that the ischemic time is minimized; perfusion balloon catheters may be useful in this setting. Finally, suboptimal results may be obtained after coronary angioplasty of the left main coronary artery, and the balance of symptom recurrence must be carefully weighed against the potential risk of complications (e.g., coronary dissection) if oversized balloons are used.

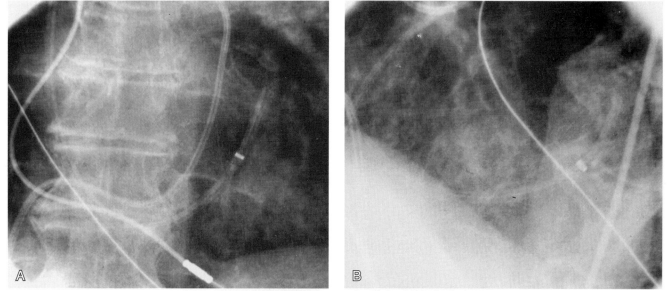

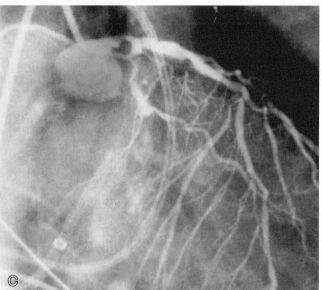

Figure 11–2
A prior attempt at coronary arteriography in this patient resulted in hemodynamic collapse and cardiac arrest prior to adequate definition of the coronary anatomy. To provide myocardial perfusion during diagnostic arteriography and potentially "high-risk" angioplasty, an 8.5-French coronary sinus retroperfusion catheter was advanced to the coronary sinus from the right internal jugular vein *(Panel A)*. Positioning of the coronary retroperfusion catheter was confirmed with contrast injections *(Panel B)*. Diagnostic arteriography demonstrated an eccentric stenosis of the left main coronary artery *(Panel C)*. Because of the extreme risk associated with coronary angioplasty in this setting, the patient was referred for coronary bypass operation.

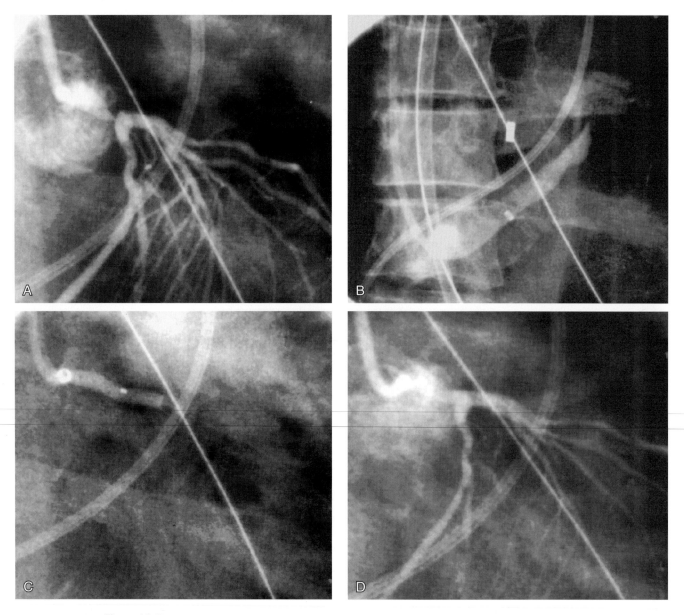

Figure 11–3
An eccentric stenosis was demonstrated in this patient in the distal segment of the left main coronary artery *(Panel A)*. Because of the patient's advanced age and underlying malignancy, coronary bypass surgery was not considered. To support myocardial perfusion during coronary angioplasty, coronary sinus retroperfusion was performed prior to the procedure. An 8.5-French retroperfusion catheter was advanced from the right internal jugular vein to the coronary sinus, and its position was confirmed with contrast injection *(Panel B)*. A 3.0-mm balloon was then inflated for 30 seconds across the distal left main stenosis *(Panel C)*. After balloon deflation, a 10% residual stenosis was obtained *(Panel D)*. The patient demonstrated no evidence of ischemia during left main coronary artery dilatation.

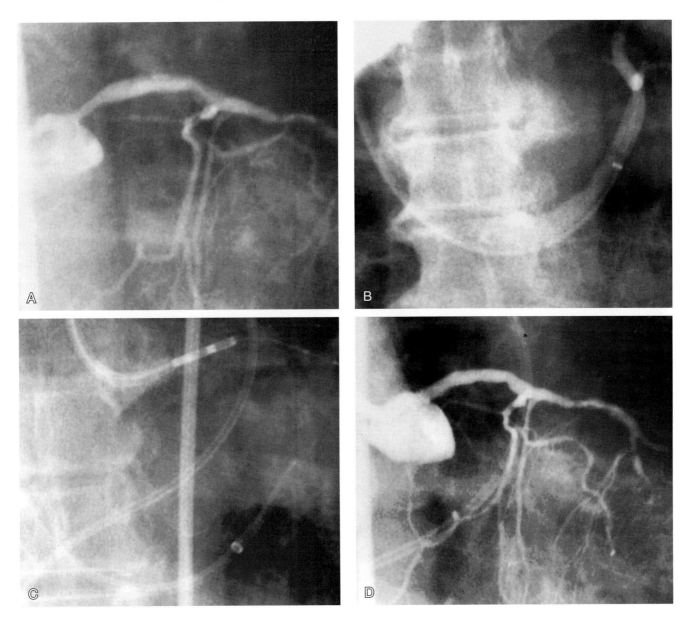

Figure 11–4
A concentric stenosis involving the ostium and proximal segments of the left main coronary artery
was demonstrated *(Panel A)*. Because of contraindications to coronary bypass surgery, supported
directional atherectomy was performed with coronary sinus retroperfusion positioned from the right
internal jugular vein. The position of the 8.5-French retroperfusion catheter within the coronary sinus
was confirmed with contrast injection *(Panel B)*. Circumferential cuts were performed with a 6-French
DVI SCA atherectomy device inflated to a maximum pressure of 40 psi *(Panel C)*. After directional
atherectomy, a <10% residual stenosis was obtained *(Panel D)*.

The third and most common setting is coronary angioplasty of the "protected" left main coronary artery. Patients
who have undergone prior coronary bypass surgery and
have one or more patent grafts to the left coronary artery
are generally considered at "low risk" for coronary angioplasty. However, because of the calcification and excess
plaque burden in this region, standard balloon angioplasty
may be limited by a suboptimal initial result and the frequent late recurrence of symptoms.

As an alternative to balloon angioplasty, directional coronary atherectomy may be useful in treating noncalcified
lesions that involve the left main coronary artery because
of its ability to remove large amounts of plaque; this technique may be particularly useful in vessels with bulky,
eccentric lesions that are difficult to dilate using standard
balloon methods.

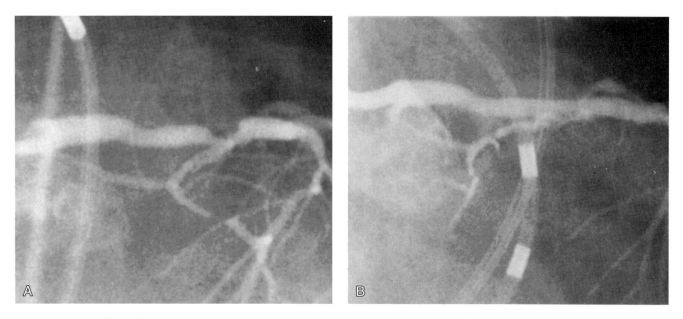

Figure 11–5
An eccentric stenosis in the distal aspect of the long left main coronary artery *(Panel A)* was treated with directional atherectomy using a 7-French DVI SCA device (not shown). After eight circumferential cuts, a <10% residual stenosis and a smooth lumen contour were obtained *(Panel B).*

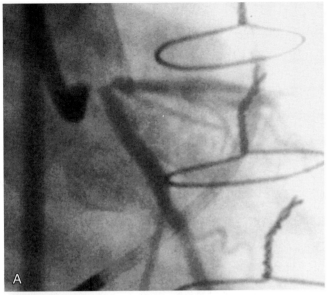

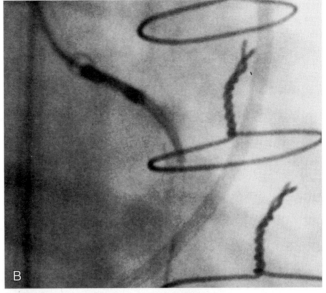

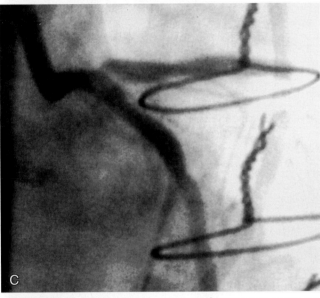

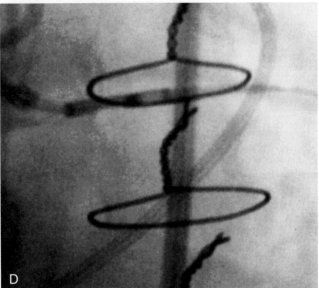

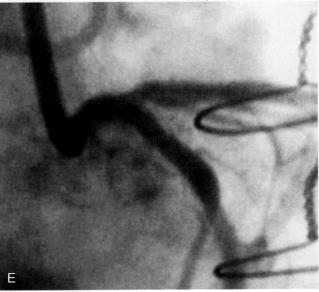

Figure 11–6
A noncalcified, ostial stenosis of the left main coronary artery
(Panel A) was treated with directional atherectomy. The 7-French
DVI EX catheter was first advanced into the native left circumflex
artery, and circumferential cuts of the distal left main coronary
artery were performed using a maximum pressure of 30 psi *(Panel
B)*. This resulted in a minimal residual stenosis in the left main
artery and the ostium of the left circumflex artery *(Panel C)*. The 7-
French DVI EX catheter was then repositioned in the left anterior
descending artery, and circumferential cuts were performed *(Panel
D)*. After final atherectomy, an excellent angiographic result was
obtained *(Panel E)*.

Rotational atherectomy has been used in calcified lesions that involve the left main coronary artery because of its ability to selectively ablate fibrocalcific plaque. Relative undersizing of the largest burr available for coronary use (2.5 mm) often requires that adjunct balloon dilatation or directional atherectomy be performed to maximize the final lumen dimensions.

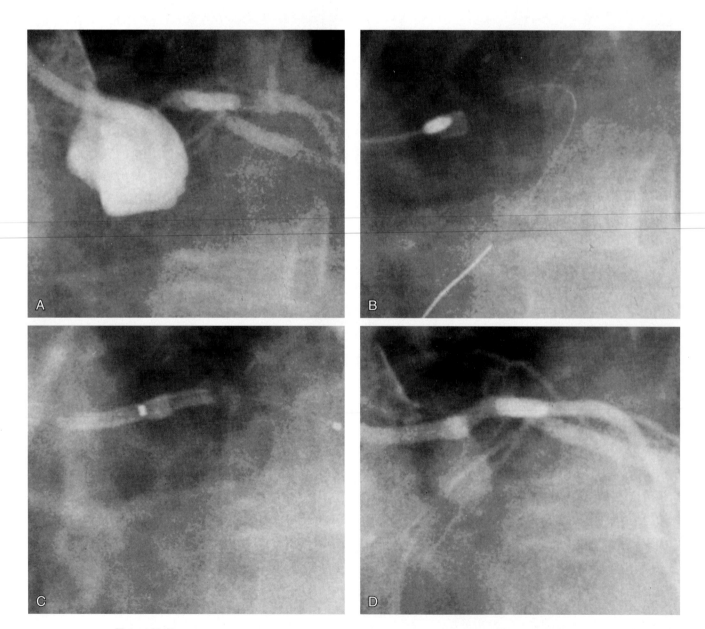

Figure 11–7
The ostial stenosis of the left main coronary artery had fluoroscopic evidence of severe calcification *(Panel A)*. Sequential rotational atherectomy using 1.75-, 2.25-, and 2.5-mm burrs *(Panel B)* resulted in improvement of the stenosis, but a 50% residual narrowing persisted. As a result, a prolonged balloon inflation was performed with a 3.5-mm balloon catheter *(Panel C)*; this resulted in an excellent angiographic result *(Panel D)*.

Extraction atherectomy may also be used in left main coronary lesions that contain a significant degree of thrombus. Continuous vacuum suction extracts the macroparticulate debris from the diseased segment, potentially reducing the risk of distal embolization.

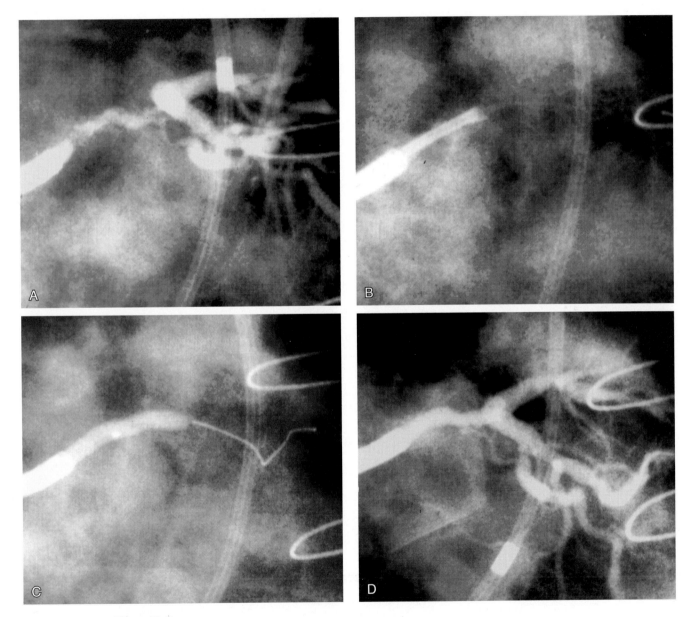

Figure 11–8
A thrombus-containing lesion involving the entire extent of the left main coronary artery *(Panel A)* was treated with six passes of a 6.5-French transluminal extraction catheter device. After extraction atherectomy, the lumen was improved, but a 50% residual stenosis remained (not shown). To maximize the final angiographic result, adjunct balloon dilatation was performed with a 3.5-mm balloon catheter *(Panel C)*; this resulted in a residual stenosis of <10% and no evidence of angiographic thrombus.

SELECTED REFERENCES

Eldar M, Schulhoff N, Herz I, et al. Results of percutaneous transluminal angioplasty of the left main coronary artery. Am J Cardiol 1991; 68:255–256.

Hamad N, Pichard A, Schwartz M, et al. Use of infusion catheter in acute left main coronary arterial occlusion. Am J Cardiol 1987; 60:191–192.

Kern M. Approach to the patient with left main coronary artery stenosis. Cathet Cardiovasc Diagn 1989; 18:181–182.

Lotan C, Milgalter E, Gotsman M. Dissection of the left main coronary artery: A complication of PTCA to the anterior descending artery. Clin Cardiol 1988; 11:120–121.

Muller D, Ellis S, Topol E. Atherectomy of the left main coronary artery with percutaneous cardiopulmonary bypass support. Am J Cardiol 1989; 64:114–116.

O'Keefe J, Hartzler G, Rutherford B, et al. Left main coronary angioplasty: Early and late results of 127 acute and elective procedures. Am J Cardiol 1989; 64:144–147.

Slack J, Pinkerton C, VanTassel J, Orr C. Left main coronary artery dissection during percutaneous transluminal coronary angioplasty. Cathet Cardiovasc Diagn 1986; 12:255–260.

Tommaso C, Vogel J, Vogel R. Coronary angioplasty in high-risk patients with left main coronary stenosis: Results from the National Registry of Elective Supported Angioplasty. Cathet Cardiovasc Diagn 1992; 25:169–173.

Vogel J, Ruiz C, Jahnke E, et al. Percutaneous (nonsurgical) supported angioplasty in unprotected left main disease and severe left ventricular dysfunction. Clin Cardiol 1989; 12:297–300.

Complications of Coronary Intervention: Diagnosis and Management

Pathologic studies have demonstrated that coronary angioplasty exerts its beneficial effect by stretching the normal artery and splitting the atherosclerotic plaque. Disruption of the normal coronary architecture may result in contrast extravasation into the media and adventitia and in protrusion of the atherosclerotic plaque and intimal flaps into the arterial lumen; these events are manifest angiographically as intraluminal haziness and coronary dissection. Often, the coronary dissection originates at the junction of the atherosclerotic plaque and the adjacent normal vessel.

Due to the marked heterogeneity of the postprocedural angiographic result, the National Heart, Lung and Blood Institute's (NHLBI) *Percutaneous Transluminal Coronary Angioplasty Registry* has proposed a classification system that characterizes coronary dissections according to morphologic subtype and their effect on distal coronary perfusion (Table 12–1). This classification system has proven useful in the standardization of the reporting of coronary dissection after balloon and new device angioplasty.

Although a variety of angiographic predictors for complications (including coronary dissections) have been identified, the predictive value of any specific clinical or morphologic feature is low, thus rendering risk assessment for coronary dissection in any specific patient or lesion subtype difficult.

Table 12–1 National Heart, Lung and Blood Institute Dissection Classification

Type	Definition
A	A small, radiolucent area that remains within the coronary lumen during contrast injection with minimal or no persistence of contrast after the dye has cleared
B	A parallel tract or double-lumen radiodense area that appears within the coronary lumen during contrast injection with minimal or no persistence after the contrast has cleared
C	A small amount of contrast persists outside the coronary lumen after the dye has cleared with or without a radiolucent area within the lumen during the contrast injection
D	A spiral type of luminal filling defect during the contrast injection which appears to be a complete occlusion not associated with delay in anterograde flow
E	A persistent, new intraluminal filling defect that appears during contrast injection associated with a delay in anterograde flow
F	A dissection with complete occlusion of the coronary lumen

(From Dorros G, Spring DA. Healing of coronary intimal dissection after percutaneous transluminal angioplasty. Am J Cardiol 1980; 45:423.)

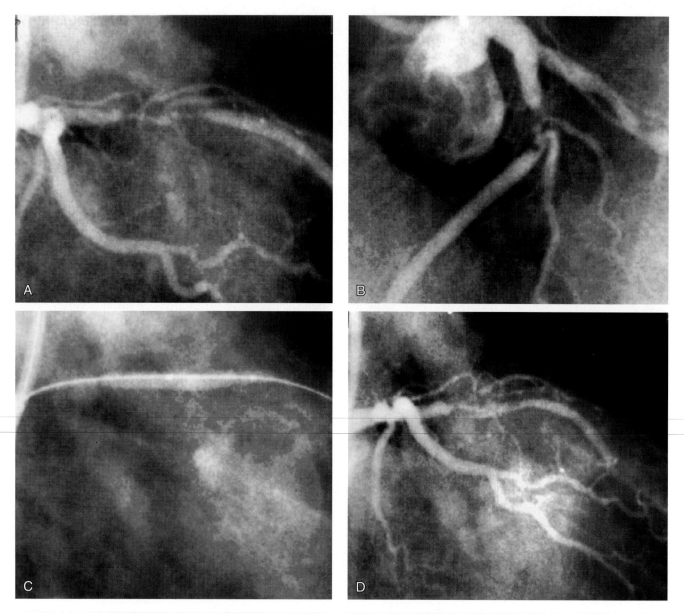

Figure 12–1
Visualization of this stenosis in the proximal segment of the left anterior descending artery demonstrated several features associated with increased risk for ischemic complications during coronary angioplasty. The unforeshortened right anterior oblique projection *(Panel A)* demonstrated the excess lesion length (18 mm). Lesion irregularity, eccentricity, and bifurcation location were noted in the left anterior oblique projection *(Panel B)*. Despite the presence of increased risk, standard balloon angioplasty (without side branch protection) was performed *(Panel C)*. After the initial balloon inflation, a spiral dissection developed that was associated with compromised anterograde perfusion *(Panel D)*. Emergency coronary bypass surgery was performed.

Coronary dissections may also develop after balloon angioplasty of seemingly "low-risk" type A lesions.

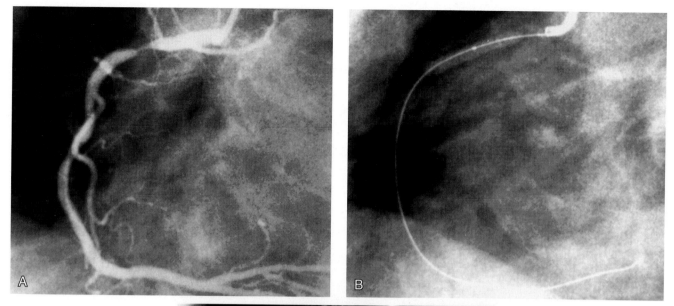

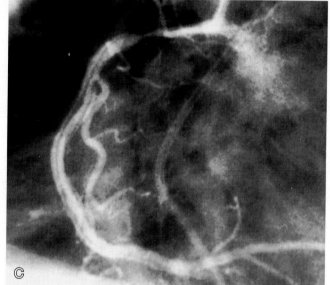

Figure 12–2
A type A stenosis (according to the American College of Cardiology/American Heart Association Classification) of the proximal segment of the right coronary artery *(Panel A)* was treated with standard balloon angioplasty *(Panel B)*. After the initial balloon inflation, a long spiral dissection developed that extended through the entire length of the vessel *(Panel C)*. Emergency coronary bypass surgery was performed.

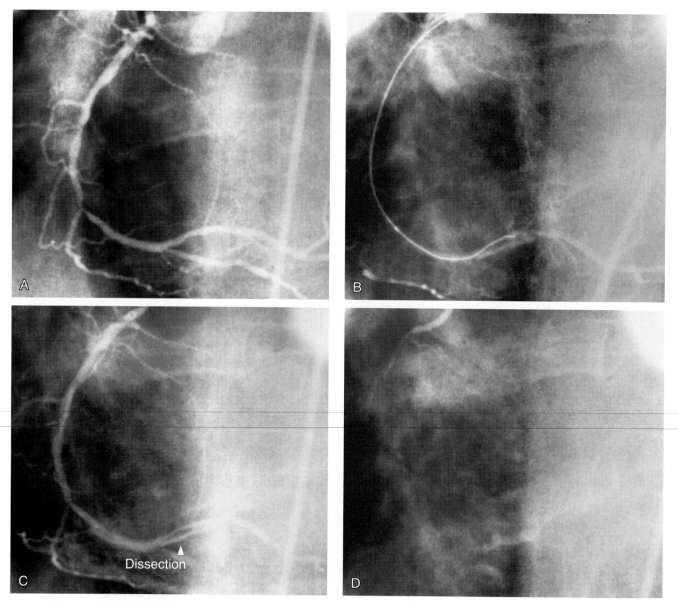

Figure 12–3
An eccentric stenosis in the distal portion of the right coronary artery was approached with standard balloon angioplasty *(Panel A)*. As the right ventricular marginal side branch did not appear to be involved in the stenosis, guide wire protection of the side branch was not performed. Dilatation was undertaken with the use of a 2.5-mm balloon catheter *(Panel B)*. A propagating spiral dissection developed from the proximal segment of the right coronary artery to the posterolateral branches of the right coronary artery *(Panel C)*, eventually resulting in total occlusion (NHLBI type F) *(Panel D)*.

The immediate prognostic significance of a coronary dissection is dependent on (1) the length of the dissection, (2) associated staining of contrast medium within the vessel wall, and (3) the effect on distal coronary perfusion.

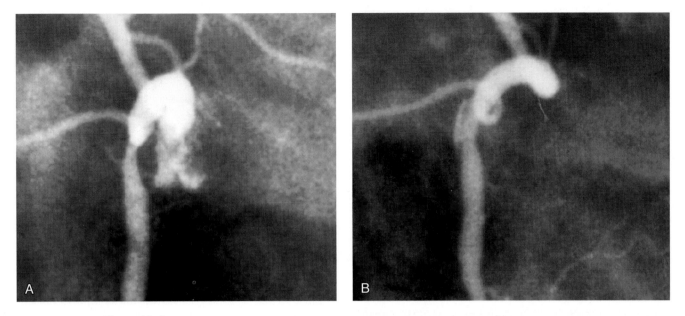

Figure 12–4
This eccentric stenosis in the proximal segment of the right coronary artery *(Panel A)* was dilated with a 3.0-mm balloon catheter. After the first balloon inflation, a localized 5-mm dissection (NHLBI type C) developed at the angioplasty site *(Panel B)*. No significant compromise of anterograde coronary perfusion was observed, and the patient was subsequently discharged without clinical sequelae.

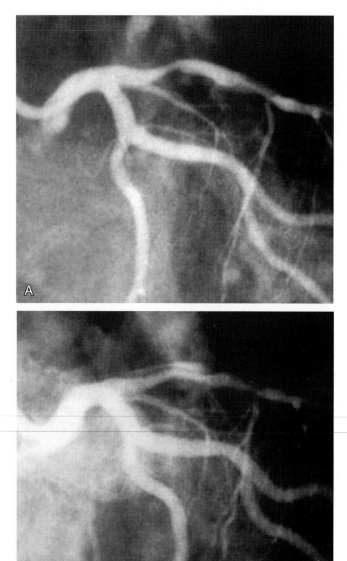

Figure 12–5

A tubular, eccentric lesion in the proximal portion of the left anterior descending artery was treated with standard balloon angioplasty *(Panel A)*. A 3.0-mm balloon was inflated to nominal (6 atm) pressure *(Panel B)*. A localized dissection was noted after initial balloon inflation. With subsequent balloon inflations, including ones using a 3.5-mm perfusion balloon, the dissection propagated proximally and was eventually associated with compromised anterograde perfusion (NHLBI type E) *(Panel C)*. In response to the patient's persistent chest pain and to electrocardiographic evidence of transmural myocardial ischemia, emergency coronary bypass surgery was performed.

Guiding catheter engagement of the left or right coronary arteries may also result in catheter-induced coronary dissection, particularly when the left main or right coronary ostia have focal atherosclerotic disease.

Figure 12–6

An eccentric stenosis of the midportion of the left circumflex was treated with standard balloon angioplasty *(Panel A)*. To provide additional backup support, the Judkins left-4 guiding catheter was advanced forward within the left main coronary artery *(Panels B and C)*. After balloon deflation, a dissection was noted in the proximal segment of the left anterior descending artery *(Panel D)*, presumably due to guiding catheter damage. The dissection became progressively more severe *(Panel E)* and eventually resulted in total occlusion of the left anterior descending artery *(Panel F)*. Emergency coronary bypass surgery was performed.

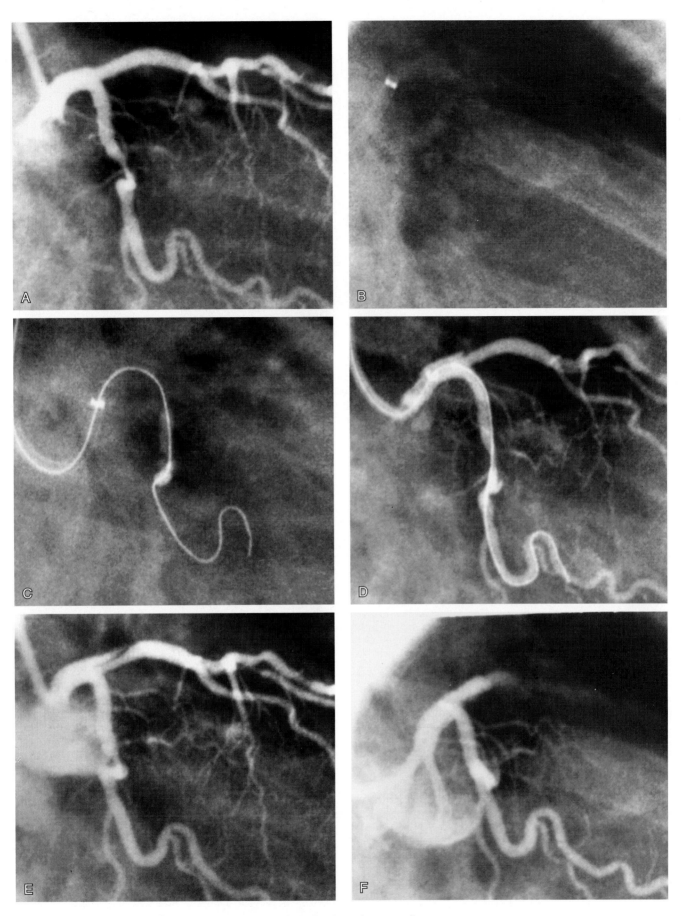

Figure 12–6. *See legend on opposite page*

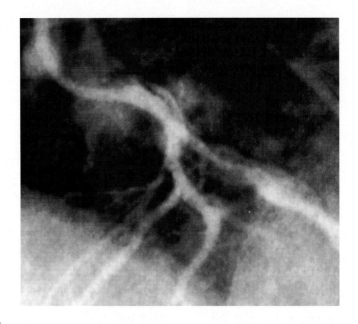

Figure 12–7
Directional coronary atherectomy was the planned treatment for the eccentric stenosis seen in the midportion of the left circumflex coronary artery. Following insertion of the 11-French guiding catheter into the left main coronary artery, a severe dissection of the left main coronary artery occurred. Although the patient was hemodynamically stable and no evidence of compromised perfusion was observed, coronary bypass surgery was performed.

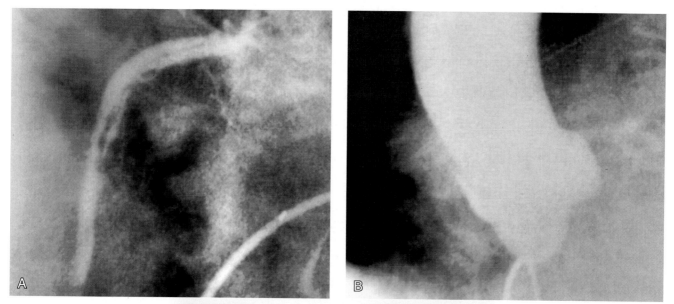

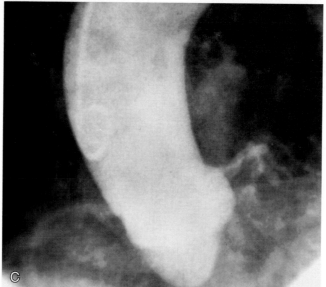

Figure 12–8

Direct coronary angioplasty was attempted in this patient with an acute inferior wall myocardial infarction. Coronary angiography demonstrated a total occlusion of the midportion of the right coronary artery. Guiding catheter insertion into the right coronary artery resulted in a spiral dissection (NHLBI type D) *(Panel A)*. The guiding catheter dissection also involved the ascending aorta *(Panel B)*. Because of relative contraindications to surgery, emergency repair of the ascending arch was not pursued. Recurrent symptoms developed 10 years later, and repeat aortography demonstrated repair and remodeling of the ascending aorta *(Panel C)*. Selective angiographic views of the right coronary artery demonstrated persistent patency.

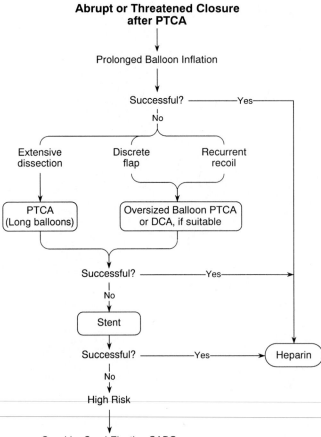

**Abrupt or Threatened Closure
after PTCA**

↓

Prolonged Balloon Inflation

↓

Successful? ————Yes————

No

Extensive   Discrete   Recurrent
dissection   flap   recoil

↓

PTCA   Oversized Balloon PTCA
(Long balloons)   or DCA, if suitable

↓

Successful? ————Yes————→

No

↓

Stent

↓

Successful? ————Yes————→ Heparin

No

↓

High Risk

↓

Consider Semi-Elective CABG

Figure 12–9
Algorithm for the management of abrupt or threatened closure
following percutaneous transluminal coronary angioplasty.

Depending on the severity of the dissection, the degree of ongoing ischemia, and the extent of jeopardized myocardium, a variety of treatment methods can be applied, ranging from careful observation with intravenous anticoagulation therapy to intracoronary stenting to emergency coronary bypass surgery (Fig. 12–9). In the absence of sustained compromise of distal coronary perfusion, localized coronary dissections can be initially managed with prolonged (5- to 15-minute) balloon inflations. In this circumstance, balloons are generally "upsized" by 0.5 mm, and low-pressure inflations are performed in an effort to compress the dissection flap and to seal the site of localized intramural contrast extravasation. Perfusion balloons may be used if significant ischemia results from prolonged balloon inflation. Alternative mechanical devices are also used to treat coronary dissections. Localized dissections and intramural flaps can be resected with directional atherectomy, whereas more extensive dissections can be treated with intracoronary stents.

Prolonged inflations using a perfusion balloon may be useful in the treatment of localized coronary dissections.

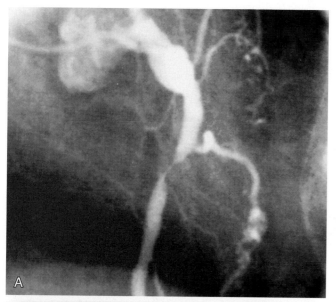

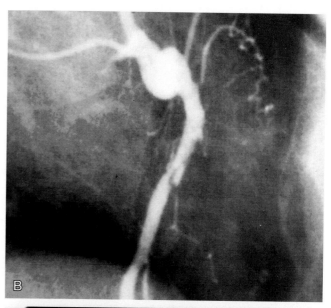

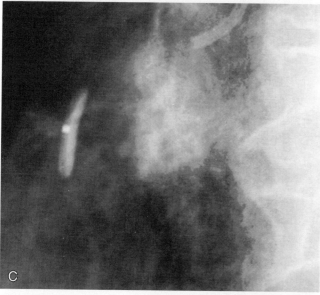

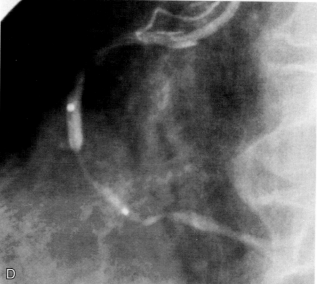

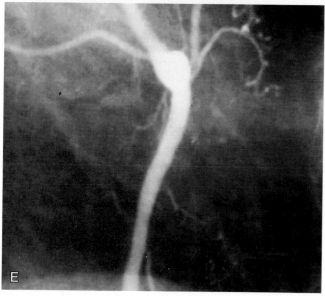

Figure 12–10

The eccentric stenosis located in the midportion of the right coronary artery of this patient *(Panel A)* was treated with a standard 3.0-mm balloon dilatation catheter. After initial balloon inflation, a 4.0-mm localized dissection (NHLBI type C) developed at the treatment site *(Panel B)*. A 3.5-mm perfusion balloon catheter was advanced across the dissection and inflated to 4 atm *(Panel C)*. Contrast medium injection with the balloon inflated demonstrated excellent anterograde perfusion *(Panel D)*. After a 10-minute inflation, the dissection was compressed, resulting in normal anterograde perfusion and no residual stenosis or lumen irregularity *(Panel E)*.

Coronary angioplasty performed in the peri-infarction period has been associated with an increased risk for procedural complications, which are most often attributable to thrombotic occlusions or the development of coronary dissection.

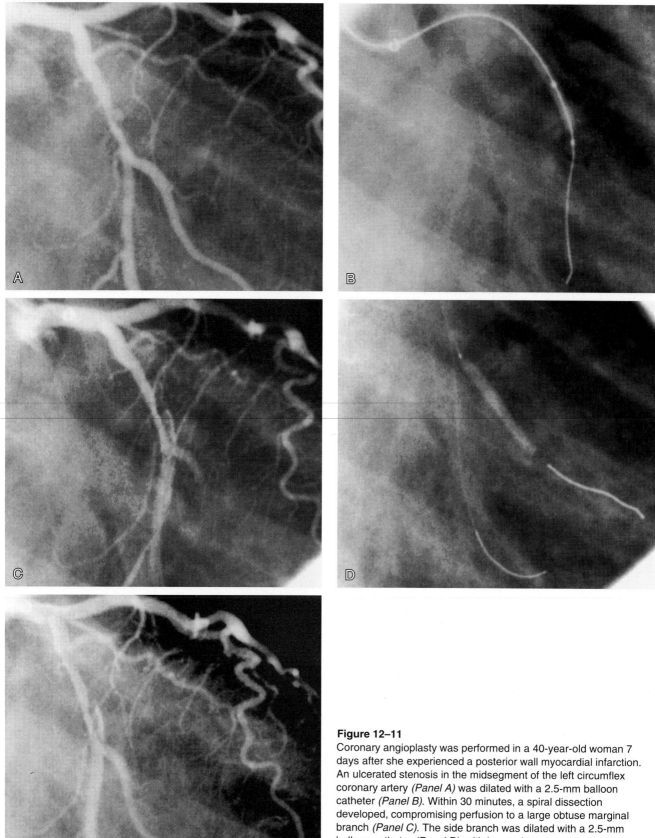

Figure 12–11

Coronary angioplasty was performed in a 40-year-old woman 7 days after she experienced a posterior wall myocardial infarction. An ulcerated stenosis in the midsegment of the left circumflex coronary artery *(Panel A)* was dilated with a 2.5-mm balloon catheter *(Panel B)*. Within 30 minutes, a spiral dissection developed, compromising perfusion to a large obtuse marginal branch *(Panel C)*. The side branch was dilated with a 2.5-mm balloon catheter *(Panel D)*, with incomplete restoration of anterograde perfusion to the obtuse marginal branch *(Panel E)*. Because of the recent myocardial infarction and the patient's single-vessel coronary artery disease, no further therapy was undertaken.

In the absence of an acute ischemic complication (e.g., abrupt closure), the late angiographic outcome after localized coronary dissection is often favorable.

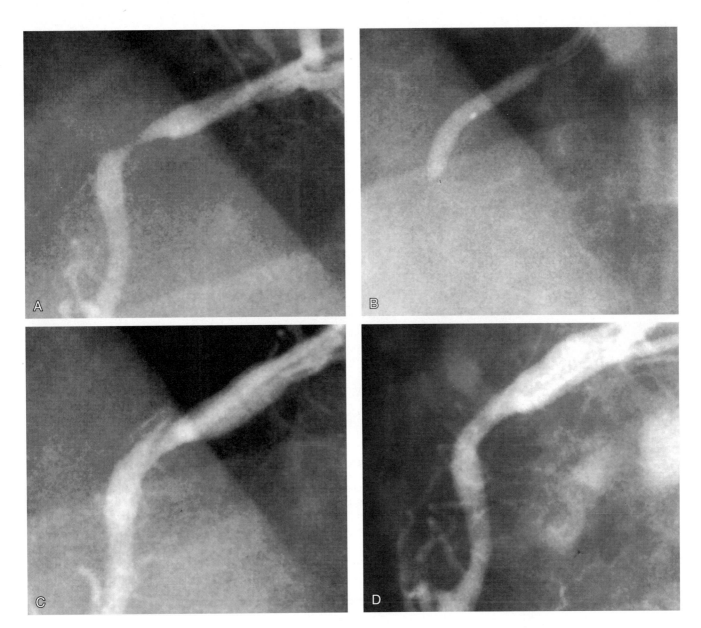

Figure 12–12
This angulated, eccentric lesion in the proximal portion of the right coronary artery *(Panel A)* was treated with a 2.5-mm balloon dilatation catheter *(Panel B)*. A localized dissection (NHLBI type B) developed and persisted despite several prolonged balloon inflations *(Panel C)*. Because the patient was asymptomatic and anterograde perfusion was not compromised, intravenous administration of heparin was continued after the procedure. Repeat angiography 6 months later demonstrated remodeling of the dissection flap and a widely patent lumen at the site of prior coronary angioplasty *(Panel D)*.

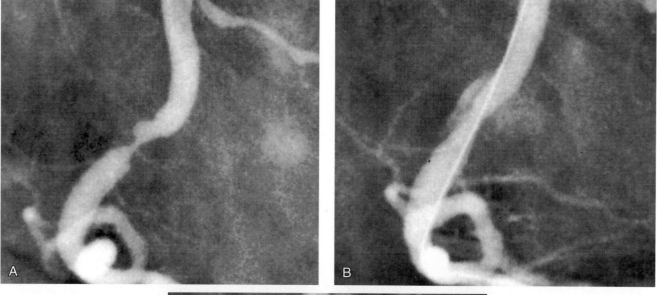

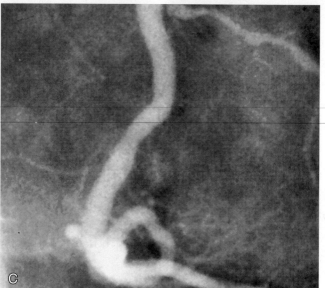

Figure 12–13

An ulcerated lesion in the distal segment of the right coronary artery *(Panel A)* was treated with a 3.0-mm balloon dilatation catheter. After the initial balloon inflation, an 8-mm localized dissection (NHLBI type C) developed *(Panel B)*. Although additional balloon inflations were performed with larger balloons and prolonged inflations, the localized dissection persisted. The patient remained asymptomatic, and heparin was administered after the procedure. Repeat coronary angiography 6 months later demonstrated a widely patent lumen at the angioplasty site *(Panel C)*.

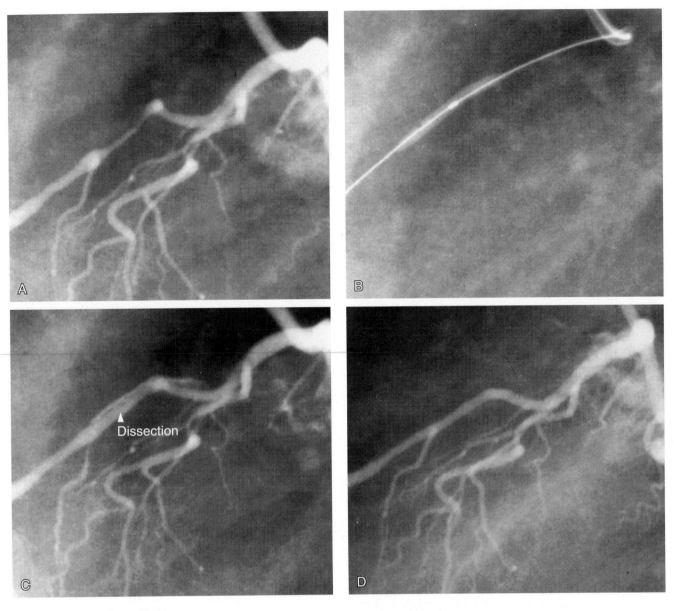

Figure 12–14
A tubular, angulated lesion in the midsegment of the left anterior descending artery *(Panel A)* was treated with a 2.5-mm balloon dilatation catheter *(Panel B)*. After two inflations, a long (20-mm) spiral dissection developed *(Panel C)*. Additional balloon inflations were used but did not bring about significant change in the dissection morphology. Because the patient remained asymptomatic and had no compromise of anterograde coronary perfusion, and since the residual lumen diameter was >2.0 mm, no further therapy (e.g., intracoronary stenting) was pursued. Angiography performed 6 months later demonstrated complete remodeling of the dissection and a widely patent lumen at the site of coronary angioplasty *(Panel D)*.

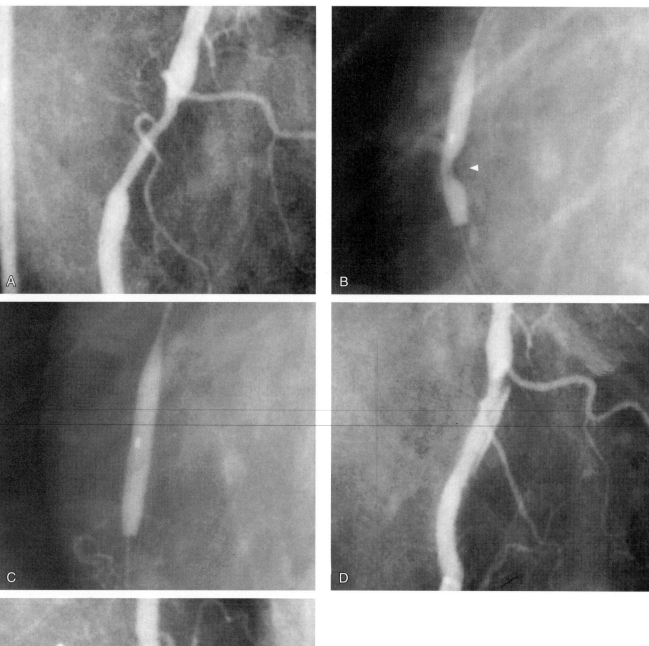

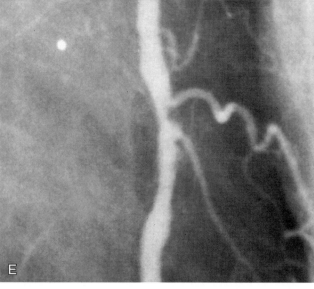

Figure 12–15

A tubular lesion in the midportion of the right coronary artery *(Panel A)* was dilated with a 2.5-mm balloon catheter *(arrow)*. The lesion appeared initially rigid, with a significant residual waist at a nominal balloon inflation pressure (6 atm). Sustained oscillation of the balloon inflation pressures resulted in symmetric balloon expansion at 8 atm *(Panel C)*. A 15-mm dissection refractory to additional balloon dilatation developed *(Panel D)*. Symptoms recurred 8 weeks later, and repeat angiography demonstrated resolution of the localized dissection. However, a focal stenosis was noted just distal to the origin of the acute marginal branch on the angiogram, which showed little progression relative to the immediate postprocedural angiogram.

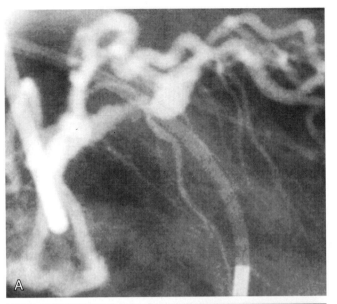

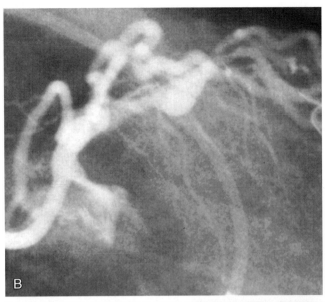

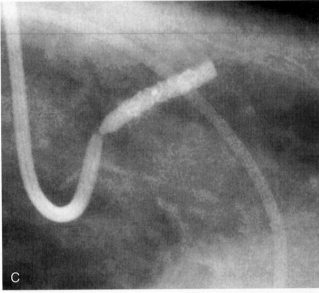

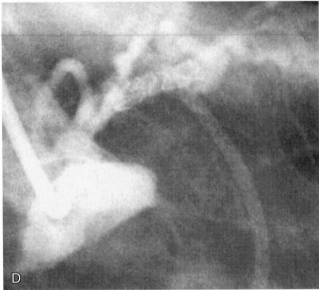

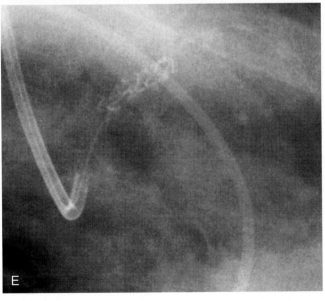

Figure 12–16
A complex lesion was noted in the proximal left anterior descending artery *(Panel A)* and was treated with balloon angioplasty. A linear dissection developed *(Panel B)* that propagated and was associated with reduced anterograde perfusion. A 3.5-mm Wiktor stent was placed *(Panel C)*, resulting in a "tacking up" of the dissection *(Panel D)*. The tantalum stent is clearly visualized on fluoroscopy *(Panel E)*.

Localized or nonlocalized coronary perforations occur infrequently (in <1% of patients) after balloon or new device angioplasty. Coronary perforation with balloon angioplasty generally occurs when the coronary guide wire becomes subintimal and is advanced through the coronary artery into the pericardial space. Localized coronary perfo- rations can be managed with prolonged balloon inflations across the site of perforation and with reversal of anticoag- ulation. Coronary perforations associated with clinical tam- ponade should be treated with pericardiocentesis and emer- gency operative repair if the bleeding cannot be controlled with conservative measures.

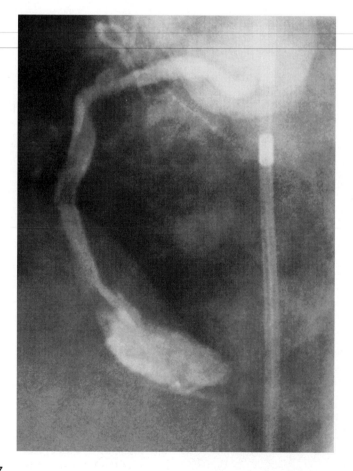

Figure 12–17
Attempted intubation of the right coronary artery using a left Amplatz guiding catheter resulted in a spiral dissection within the right coronary artery. Attempts to recanalize the vessel using a coronary guide wire resulted in passage of the guide wire and balloon catheter into the false channel. Balloon inflation resulted in localized extravasation of contrast medium.

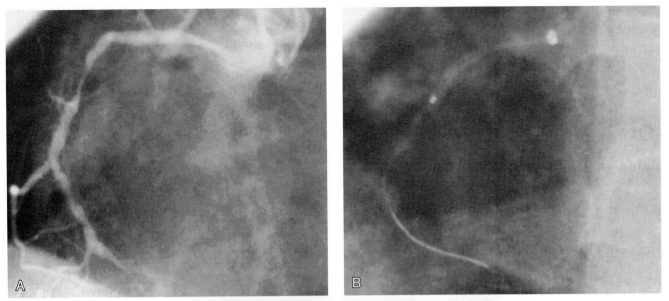

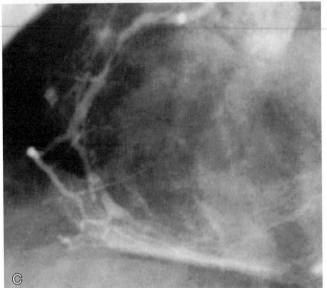

Figure 12–18
Sequential stenosis of 60% in the midsegment of the right coronary artery and total occlusion of the distal segment of the right coronary artery were treated with standard balloon angioplasty *(Panel A)*. A 3.0-mm balloon catheter was inflated across the midsegment lesion *(Panel B)*. With attempts to advance the coronary guide wire across the total occlusion, the guide wire became subintimal, and localized coronary perforation developed *(Panel C)*.

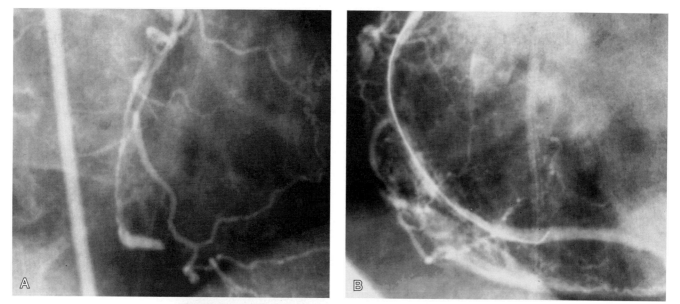

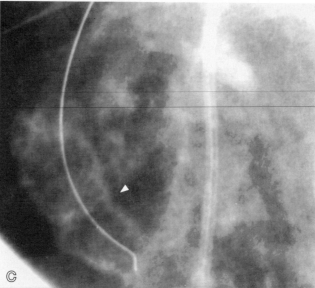

Figure 12–19

After coronary angioplasty of a long lesion in the midportion of the right coronary artery, an extensive dissection developed. The dissection resulted in abrupt closure 3 hours later. Repeat angiography demonstrated a long spiral dissection of the right coronary artery *(Panel A).* Attempts to cross the dissection using a 0.014-inch standard coronary guide wire resulted in subintimal dissection and extravasation of contrast medium into the pericardial space *(Panel B).* Retained contrast medium was noted in the pericardium *(arrow, Panel C).*

Air embolism, an infrequent complication of coronary angioplasty, may occur more often when multiple guiding catheter and balloon catheter exchanges are performed during a procedure. Although death is a rare occurrence, air embolism may result in significant chest pain, electrocardiographic changes consistent with transmural ischemia, and delayed myocardial perfusion. The treatment of choice for air embolism is 100% oxygen therapy, which accelerates the resorption of the nitrogen-rich air from the distal coronary bed. Rapid saline flush or blood perfusion and intracoronary nitroglycerin administration may be considered.

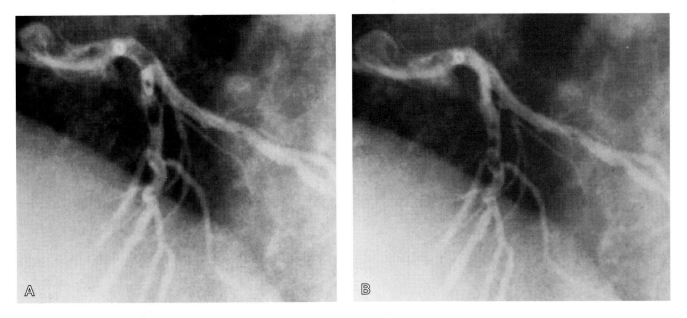

Figure 12–20
After successful coronary angioplasty of the midsegment of the left anterior descending artery, air bubbles were inadvertently injected into the left coronary artery *(Panels A and B)*. The patient developed severe chest pain associated with ST segment elevation in the anterior precordium. These ischemic changes resolved after 10 minutes without associated myocardial necrosis as assessed by serial cardiac isoenzyme analysis.

Coronary vasoconstriction and spasm occur commonly after balloon and new device angioplasty. Owing to this, the routine use of frequently administered intracoronary nitroglycerin boluses has been advocated to reduce the incidence of these complications. On occasion, a focal stenosis that mimicks coronary spasm is seen during coronary angioplasty of markedly tortuous vessels. Straightening of the segment by the coronary guide wire results in an "accordion" effect on the vessel contour. After removal of the coronary guide wire, the focal stenosis may no longer be noted.

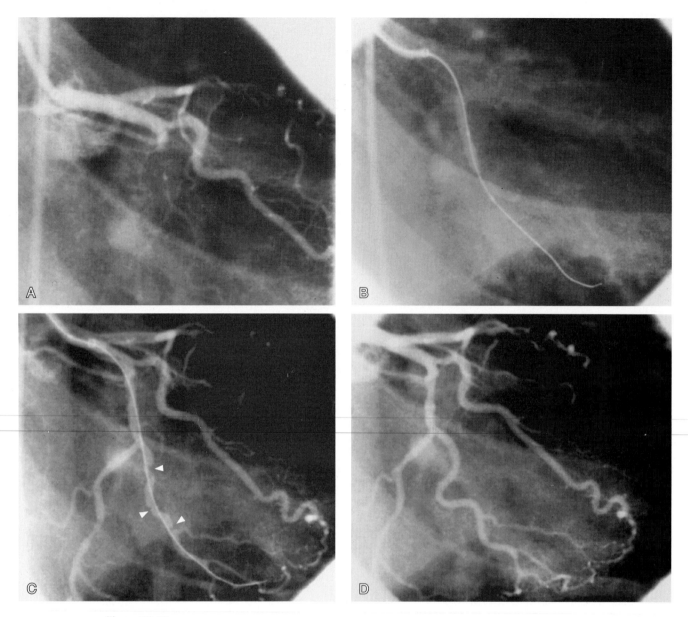

Figure 12–21
A total occlusion of the midsegment of the left circumflex coronary artery *(Panel A)* was crossed with
a 0.014-inch intermediate coronary guide wire. A 3.0-mm balloon catheter was inflated *(Panel B)*, and
the left circumflex was successfully recanalized *(Panel C)*. However, focal regions of coronary
vasoconstriction were noted *(arrows)*; these persisted despite repeat intracoronary administration of
nitroglycerin boluses. After removal of the coronary guide wire, however, the focal regions of stenosis
were no longer noted *(Panel D)*.

Late angiographic complications have been noted after
coronary angioplasty. The development of a pseudoaneurysm late after the procedure suggests disruption of the
intima and media with progressive expansion of the underlying adventitia. Depending on its size, the time course of
its expansion, and associated atherosclerotic involvement,
the pseudoaneurysm may be treated conservatively or with
intracoronary stenting. On occasion, coronary artery bypass
grafting is required.

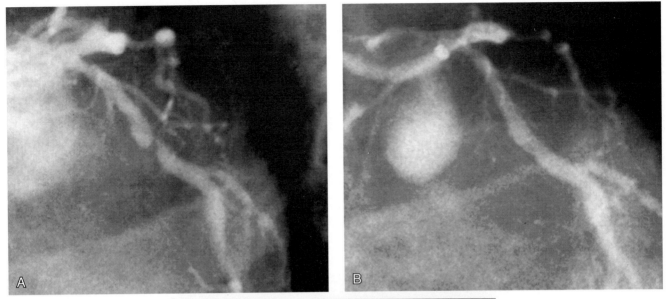

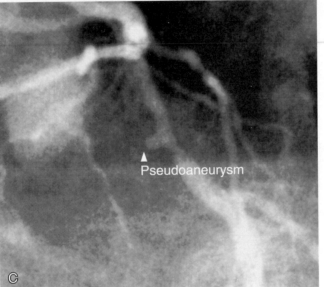

Figure 12–22
An eccentric ulcerated lesion of the midportion of the left circumflex *(Panel A)* was treated with standard balloon angioplasty. An excellent anatomic result was obtained with mild ectasia but no localized dissection *(Panel B)*. At routine angiographic follow-up 6 months later, a focal expansion at the angioplasty site *(arrowhead)* consistent with coronary pseudoaneurysm formation was observed *(Panel C)*.

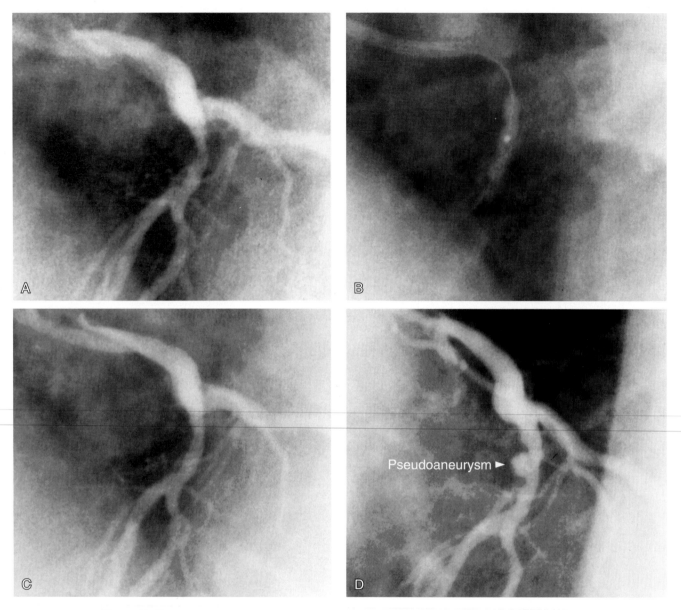

Figure 12–23
A concentric stenosis in the midsegment of the left anterior descending artery *(Panel A)* was treated with standard balloon angioplasty *(Panel B)*. After final balloon inflation *(Panel C)*, a 20% residual stenosis was noted *(Panel C)*. At the 6-month angiographic follow-up, a focal expansion of the lesion site, again consistent with a localized pseudoaneurysm, was observed *(Panel D)*.

SELECTED REFERENCES

Bell M, Garratt K, Bresnahan J, et al. Relation of deep arterial resection and coronary artery aneurysms after directional coronary atherectomy. J Am Coll Cardiol 1992; 20:1474–1481.

Black A, Namay D, Niederman A, et al. Tear or dissection after coronary angioplasty: Morphologic correlates of an ischemic complication. Circulation 1989; 79:1035–1042.

Cowley M, Dorros G, Kelsey S, et al. Acute coronary events associated with percutaneous transluminal coronary angioplasty. Am J Cardiol 1984; 53:12C–16C.

Dorros G, Cowley M, Simpson J, et al. Percutaneous transluminal coronary angioplasty: Report of complications from the National Heart, Lung and Blood Institute PTCA Registry. Circulation 1983; 67:723–730.

Ellis S, Vandormael M, Cowley M, et al. Coronary morphologic and clinical determinants of procedural outcome with angioplasty for multivessel coronary disease: Implications for patient selection. Circulation 1990; 82:1193–1202.

Ellis S, Roubin G, King S III, et al. Angiographic and clinical predictors of acute closure after native vessel coronary angioplasty. Circulation 1988; 77:372–379.

Hermans W, Rensing B, Foley D, et al. Therapeutic dissection after successful coronary balloon angioplasty: No influence on restenosis or on clinical outcome in 693 patients. J Am Coll Cardiol 1992; 20:767–780.

Holmes D, Vlietstra R, Mock M, et al. Angiographic changes produced by percutaneous transluminal coronary angioplasty. Am J Cardiol 1983; 51:676–683.

Krolick M, Bugni W, Walsh J. Coronary artery aneurysm formation following directional coronary atherectomy. Cathet Cardiovasc Diagn 1992; 27:117–121.

Preisack M, Voelker W, Haase K, Karsch M. Case report: Formation of vessel aneurysm after stand alone excimer laser angioplasty. Cathet Cardiovasc Diagn 1992; 27:122–124.

Rab S, King S III, Roubin G, et al. Coronary aneurysms after stent placement: A suggestion of altered vessel wall healing in the presence of anti-inflammatory agents. J Am Coll Cardiol 1991; 18:1524–1528.

Ryan T, Faxon D, Gunnar R, et al. Guidelines for percutaneous transluminal coronary angioplasty. J Am Coll Cardiol 1988; 12:529–545.

Walford G, Midei M, Aversano T, et al. Coronary artery aneurysm formation following percutaneous transluminal coronary angioplasty: Treatment of associated restenosis with repeat percutaneous transluminal coronary angioplasty. Cathet Cardiovasc Diagn 1990; 20:77–83.

Waller B, Orr C, Pinkerton C, et al. Coronary balloon angioplasty dissections: "The good, the bad and the ugly." J Am Coll Cardiol 1992; 20:701–706.

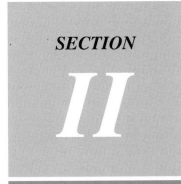

A TECHNIQUE APPROACH TO CORONARY INTERVENTION

Directional Coronary Atherectomy

Directional coronary atherectomy is the most widely applied atherectomy technique, having been performed in more than 100,000 patients worldwide. The unilateral cutting window of the atherectomy catheter allows directed resection of biopsy-sized fragments of atherosclerotic plaque (total: 10–25 mg), potentially without the risk of excessive barotrauma induced after standard balloon angioplasty. Several studies have suggested that larger initial lumen dimensions can be obtained with the use of directional atherectomy rather than standard balloon angioplasty. How this finding impacts on late clinical recurrence and restenosis remains an unsettled issue.

Unique features of the directional atherectomy device include (1) a multilumen catheter with a cylindrical cutter and a unilateral balloon mounted opposite the cutting window (9 mm in length); (2) a flexible distal nose cone that facilitates passage of the rigid housing device across the lesion and that stores the resected atherosclerotic plaque (Figure 13–1); and (3) a motor drive unit that rotates the cutting blade at approximately 2000 rpm.

The principal advantage of directional atherectomy is its capacity to remove bulky atherosclerotic plaque, which is not significantly affected when standard balloon dilatation methods are used. Thus, directional atherectomy may be well suited for the treatment of eccentric lesions in large vessels and of those lesions with an irregular border or localized dissection flap. As with other devices, an operator "learning curve" has been noted with the use of directional coronary atherectomy devices. Owing to this, guidelines for lesion complexity have been provided (Table 13–1).

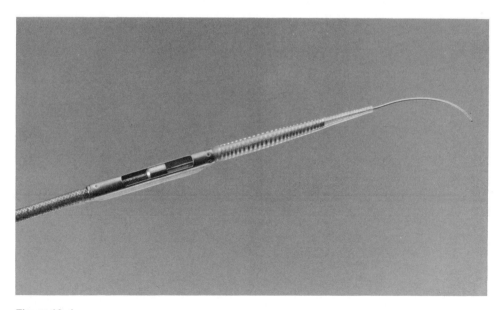

Figure 13–1
The directional atherectomy catheter.

Table 13–1   Complexity Level for Directional Coronary Atherectomy

Level 1: Highly Favorable for Directional Coronary Atherectomy

- Proximal/mid-LAD
- Proximal left circumflex with short left main and shallow takeoff
- Vessel size: 3.0–3.5 mm
- Restenosis lesions
- Eccentric lesions

Level 2: Favorable for Directional Coronary Atherectomy

- Proximal/mid-RCA
- SVG without thrombus or calcification
- Accessible mid–left circumflex
- Tubular length (11–20 mm)
- Vessel size: 2.5–4.0 mm in diameter
- De novo lesion
- Concentric morphology
- Ulcerative plaque

Level 3: Moderate Risk for Directional Coronary Atherectomy

- Distal LAD/RCA $\geq$ 2.5 mm
- Aorto-ostial location
- Protected left main
- Moderate angulation/takeoff
- Moderate proximal tortuosity
- Thrombus present
- Diffuse length (>20 mm)
- Flaps
- Minor dissection
- Adjacent distal lesion
- Moderate calcification

Level 4: Not Recommended for Directional Coronary Atherectomy

- Unprotected left main
- Highly angulated segment
- Vessel <2.5 mm in diameter
- Degenerated SVG with friable lesions
- Long/spiral dissections
- Heavy calcification
- Disease in ileofemoral arteries
- Moderate disease in left main

Abbreviations: LAD = left anterior descending artery; RCA = right coronary artery; SVG = saphenous vein graft.

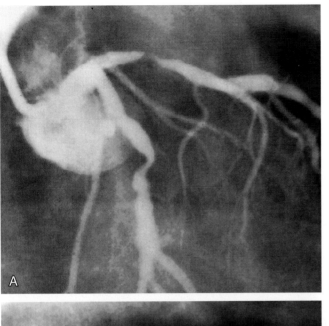

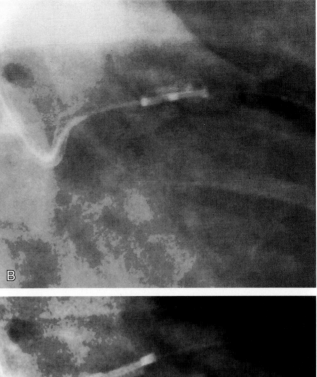

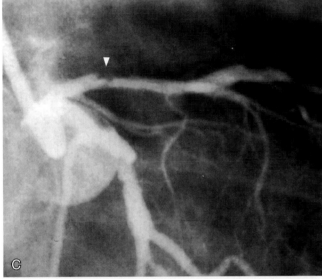

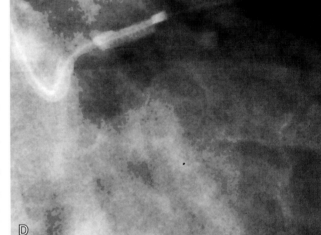

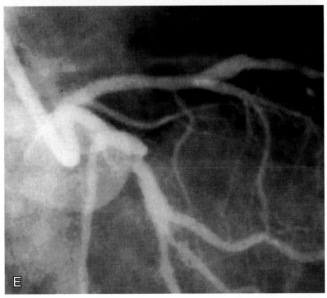

Figure 13–2
A discrete stenosis of the proximal left anterior descending artery
was treated with directional atherectomy *(Panel A)*. A 6-French DVI
SCA atherectomy device was advanced across the lesion, and the
unilateral positioning balloon was inflated to 20 psi with the cutting
window facing downward *(Panel B)*. After six inferior and lateral
cuts were made, residual atheroma was demonstrated in the
superior aspect of the lesion *(arrow, Panel C)*. The 6-French
atherectomy device was then repositioned with the cutting window
facing upward, and directed cuts of tissue were taken from the
superior aspect *(Panel D)*. After retrieval of an abundant amount of
tissue (30 mg), no residual stenosis was seen at the site of
atherectomy *(Panel E)*.

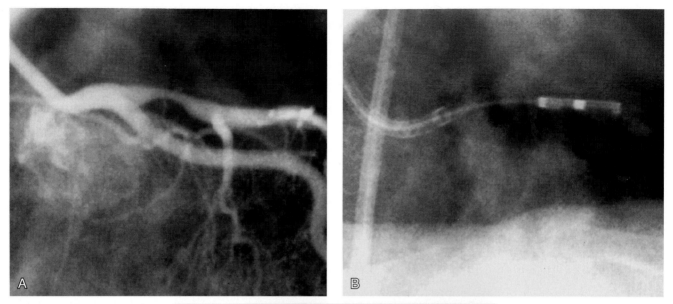

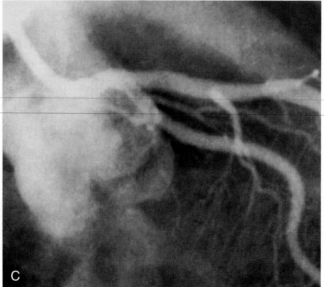

Figure 13–3
An eccentric lesion of the proximal segment of the left anterior descending artery *(Panel A)* was treated with a 7-French DVI EX directional atherectomy device with inflation pressures as high as 30 psi *(Panel B)*. Directed cuts along the inferior border resulted in a moderate amount of tissue retrieval. After directional atherectomy, a smooth lumen contour and a minimal residual stenosis were demonstrated *(Panel C)*.

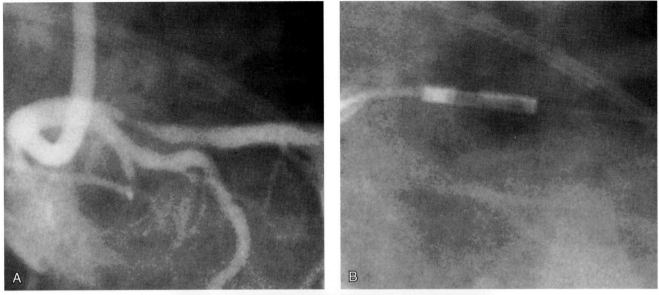

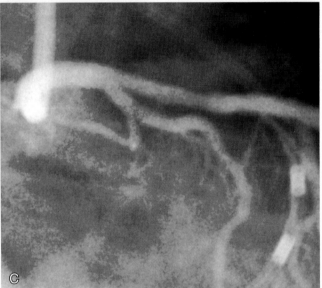

Figure 13–4
Directional atherectomy was selected to treat this patient with a relatively concentric lesion that involved the ostium of the left anterior descending artery *(Panel A).* A 7-French DVI EX atherectomy device was used *(Panel B).* After circumferential cuts were performed, an excellent angiographic result and a smooth lumen contour were obtained *(Panel C).*

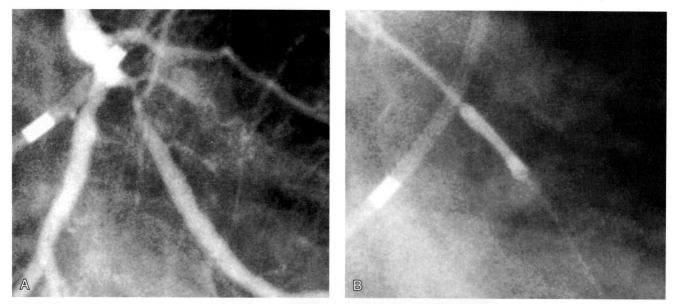

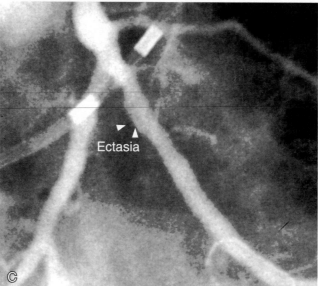

Figure 13–5
An eccentric bifurcation stenosis of the origin of the first obtuse marginal branch was noted *(Panel A)*. A 6-French DVI EX atherectomy device was advanced across the stenosis, and circumferential cuts were made at a maximum pressure of 30 psi *(Panel B)*, resulting in abundant retrieval of tissue. After atherectomy, a moderate degree of ectasia *(arrowheads)* was demonstrated at the atherectomy site *(Panel C)*.

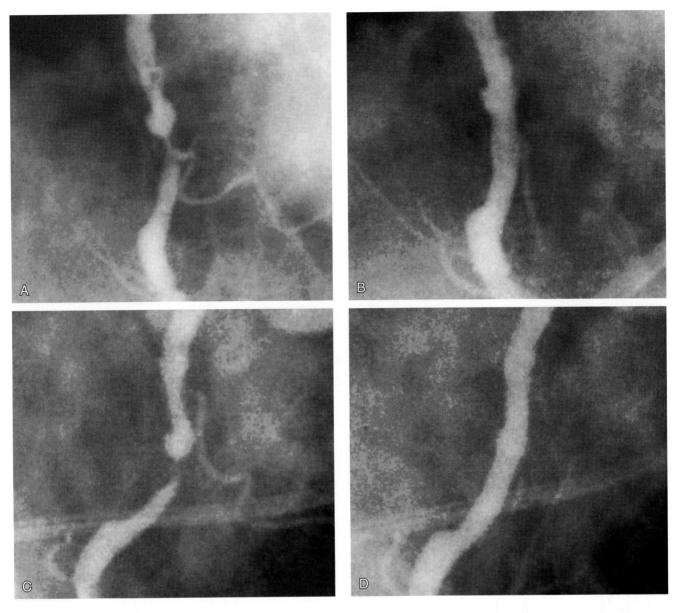

Figure 13–6
An irregular, concentric stenosis with proximal aneurysmal dilatation in the midportion of the right coronary artery was demonstrated in the left *(Panel A)* and right *(Panel C)* anterior oblique projections. After circumferential atherectomy with a 7-French DVI EX device, an acceptable angiographic result and a smooth lumen contour were obtained in both the left *(Panel B)* and right *(Panel D)* anterior oblique projections.

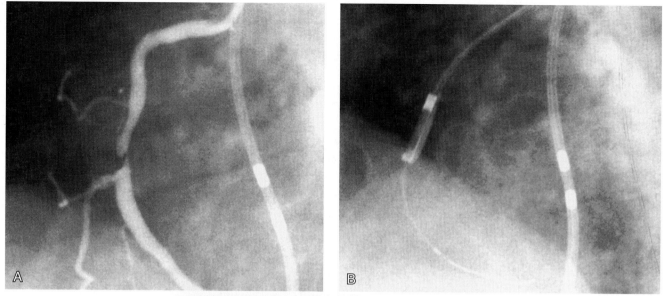

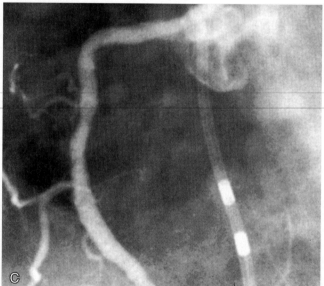

Figure 13–7

An eccentric, ulcerated stenosis in the midportion of the right coronary artery was located just proximal to a large right ventricular branch *(Panel A)*. A 7-French DVI EX atherectomy device was advanced across the lesion, and directed lateral cuts were performed *(Panel B)*. After 10 cuts, the device was withdrawn, and angiography demonstrated a 20% residual stenosis *(Panel C)*.

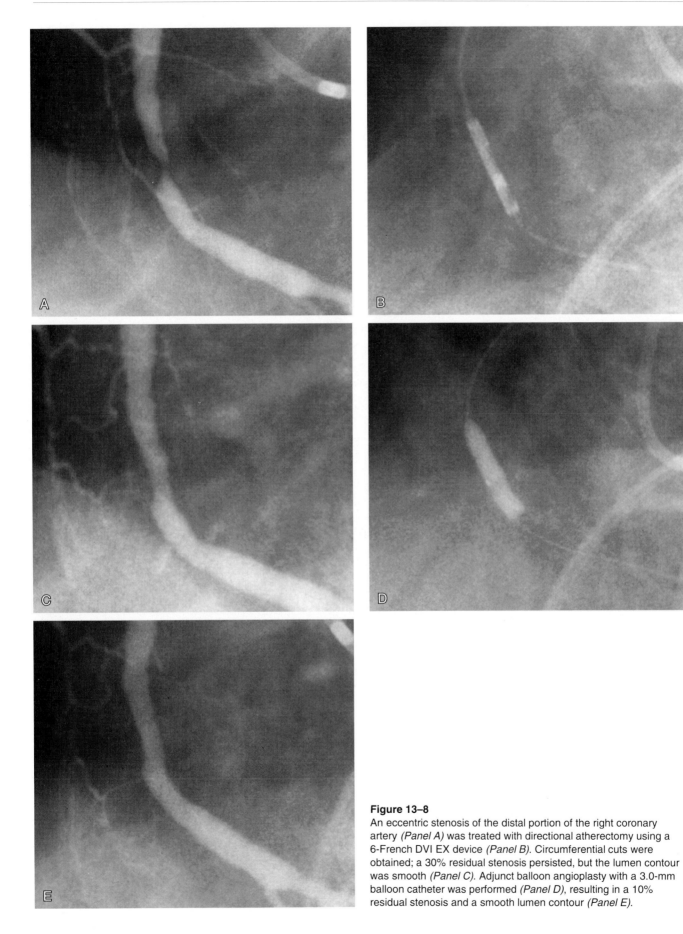

Figure 13–8
An eccentric stenosis of the distal portion of the right coronary artery *(Panel A)* was treated with directional atherectomy using a 6-French DVI EX device *(Panel B)*. Circumferential cuts were obtained; a 30% residual stenosis persisted, but the lumen contour was smooth *(Panel C)*. Adjunct balloon angioplasty with a 3.0-mm balloon catheter was performed *(Panel D)*, resulting in a 10% residual stenosis and a smooth lumen contour *(Panel E)*.

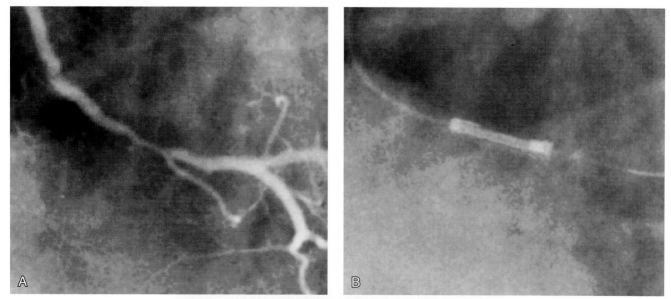

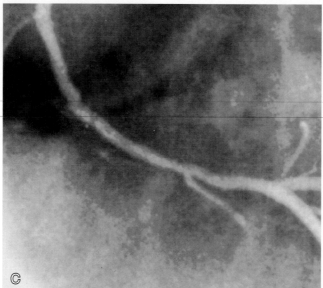

Figure 13–9
Arteriography performed in this patient 2 months after balloon angioplasty of the distal right coronary artery demonstrated restenosis at the site of prior dilatation *(Panel A)*. A 6-French DVI EX atherectomy device was advanced across the stenosis, and six circumferential excisions were performed at a maximum of 30 psi *(Panel B)*. Following atherectomy, a <10% residual stenosis was obtained, without evidence of dissection or side branch occlusion *(Panel C)*.

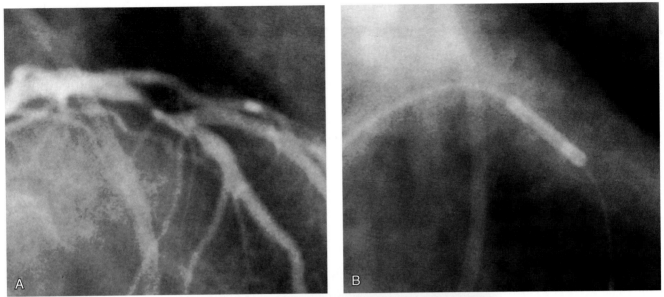

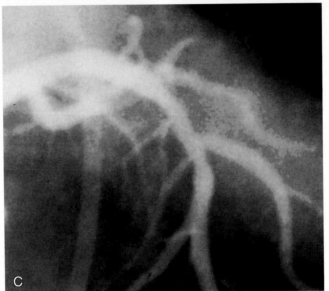

Figure 13–10
Coronary arteriography demonstrated a concentric stenosis involving the proximal portion of the left anterior descending artery just proximal to a large second diagonal branch *(Panel A)*. A 7-French DVI EX atherectomy device was advanced across the stenosis *(Panel B)*, and circumferential cuts were performed. After stand-alone atherectomy, an excellent anatomic result was obtained without significant residual stenosis *(Panel C)*.

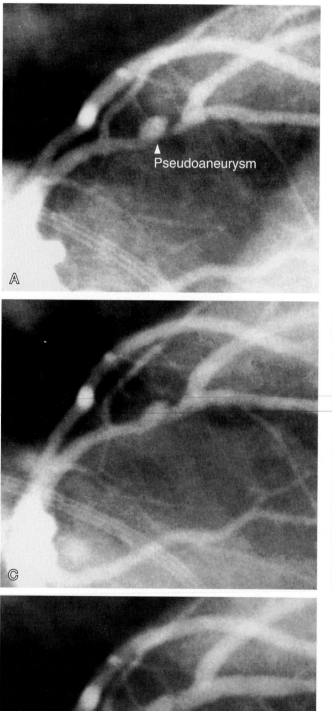

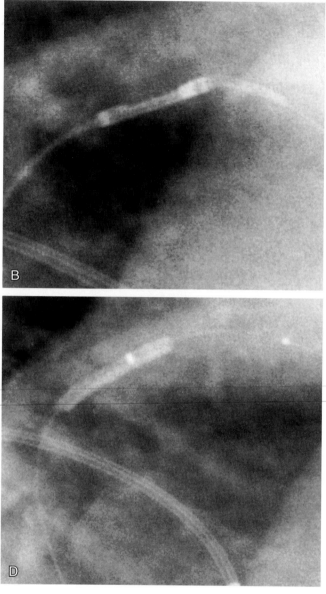

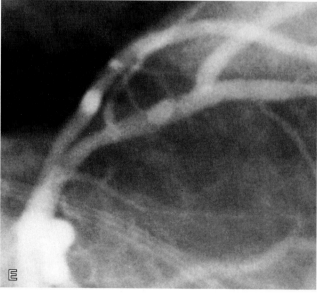

Figure 13–11

Coronary angiography demonstrated a severe stenosis in the proximal segment of the left anterior descending artery at a site of prior coronary angioplasty. Notably, a pseudoaneurysm was present *(Panel A)*. A 6-French DVI SCA atherectomy device *(Panel B)* was used to perform directed cuts toward the asymmetric plaque; a 30% residual stenosis was obtained *(Panel C)*. Oversizing of the atherectomy device in the region of aneurysm formation was avoided. A 3.0-mm balloon catheter was used to dilate the residual stenosis *(Panel D)*. Following balloon deflation, a <10% residual stenosis was obtained. Note the change in the appearance of the pseudoaneurysm *(Panel E)*.

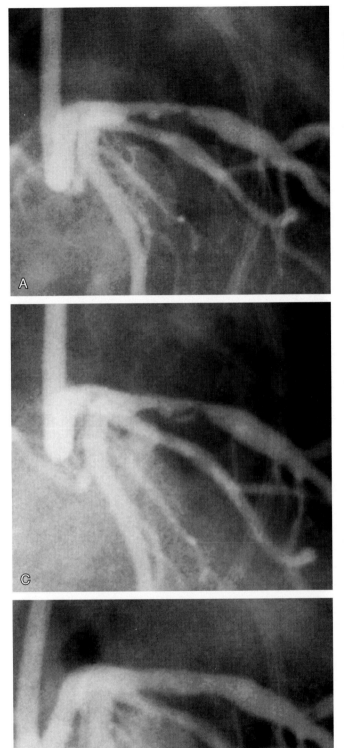

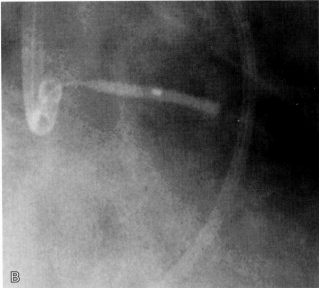

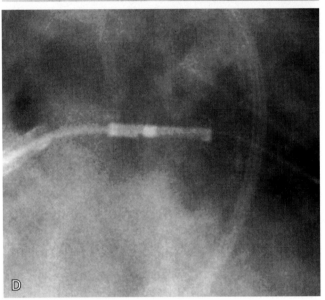

Directional coronary atherectomy has also been used to resect localized dissection flaps that occur after standard balloon angioplasty. It is important that directional atherectomy only be used in this setting if the dissection is focal (<10 mm) and does not extend beyond the initial lesion boundaries. A more conservative approach with the use of undersized devices initially is recommended. Coronary perforation has occurred with salvage directional atherectomy of more extensive dissections.

Figure 13–12
This tubular, ulcerated stenosis of the proximal left anterior descending artery *(Panel A)* was initially treated using an undersized 2.5-mm balloon dilatation catheter *(Panel B)*. After inflation to 10 atm, a localized dissection flap developed at the site of balloon dilatation *(Panel C)*; this flap was refractory to prolonged balloon inflations. A 7-French DVI atherectomy device was advanced across the localized dissection *(Panel D)*, and directed cuts to 30 psi were performed *(Panel D)*. Following excision of a moderate amount of white glistening tissue (15 mg), an excellent anatomic result was obtained *(Panel E)*.

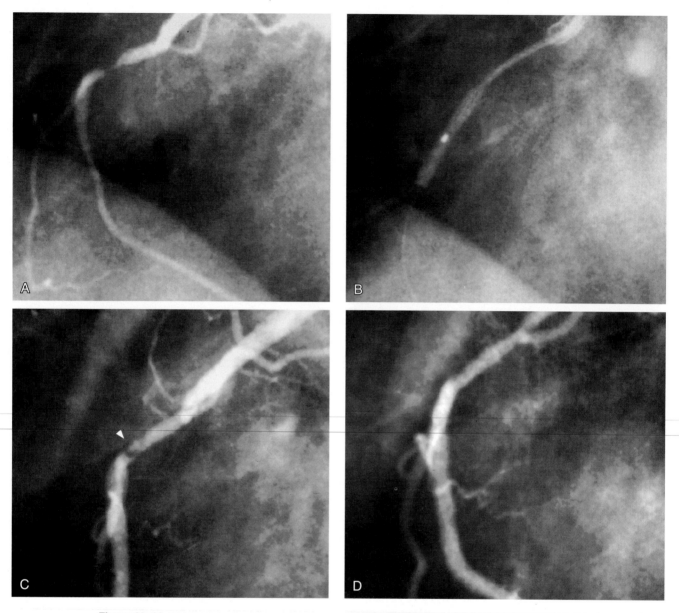

Figure 13–13

An eccentric stenosis involving the proximal right coronary artery *(Panel A)* was treated with standard balloon angioplasty using a 2.5-mm balloon catheter *(Panel B)*. Following balloon dilatation, a residual intimal flap developed *(arrow, Panel C)*; the flap was refractory to further conventional angioplasty methods. A 6-French DVI EX atherectomy device was positioned across the intimal flap, and five directed cuts were performed (not shown). After atherectomy, an excellent anatomic result was obtained, and only mild residual intraluminal haziness was observed *(Panel D)*.

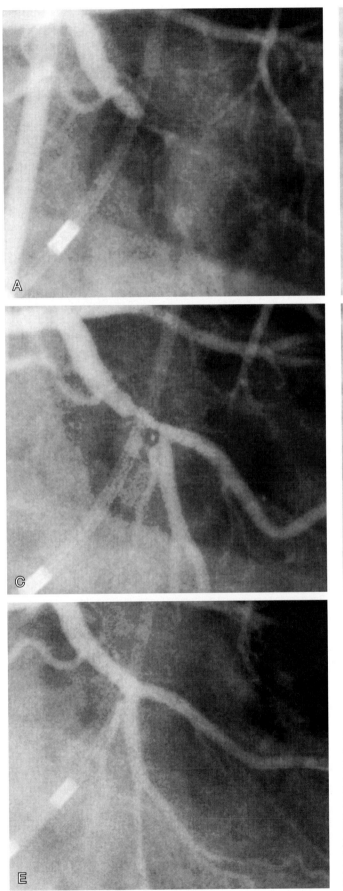

Figure 13–14

A total coronary occlusion of the proximal left circumflex artery *(Panel A)* was crossed with a 0.014-inch intermediate guide wire. Predilatation with a 2.0-mm balloon dilatation catheter *(Panel B)* recanalized the large left circumflex artery and first obtuse marginal branch *(Panel C)*. A significant amount of bulky plaque remained after initial balloon dilatation *(Panel C)*. For this reason, a 7-French DVI EX atherectomy device was advanced across the bifurcation lesion and positioned in the inferior branch of the obtuse marginal branch *(Panel D)*. Circumferential cuts were performed in both the inferior and, subsequently, superior branches *(Panel D)*. After eight cuts at 30 psi, an excellent anatomic result was achieved *(Panel E)*.

Restenosis after directional coronary atherectomy occurs in 32% to 50% of patients who undergo the procedure. The risk for restenosis appears to be related to both clinical factors (e.g., presence of diabetes mellitus and unstable angina) and procedural factors (final per cent diameter ste- nosis). It appears that a lower risk for restenosis may exist if a low residual stenosis (<10%) is obtained. However, the effect of this aggressive approach on periprocedural complications requires further prospective study.

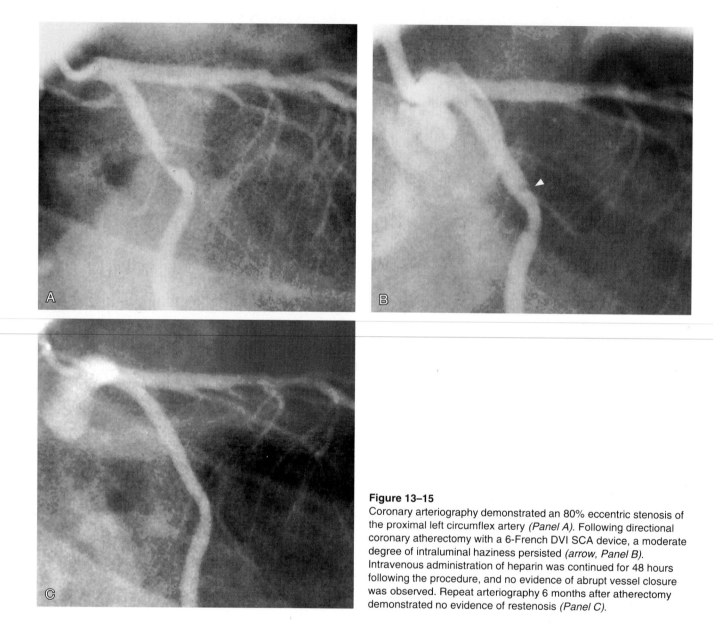

Figure 13–15
Coronary arteriography demonstrated an 80% eccentric stenosis of the proximal left circumflex artery *(Panel A)*. Following directional coronary atherectomy with a 6-French DVI SCA device, a moderate degree of intraluminal haziness persisted *(arrow, Panel B)*. Intravenous administration of heparin was continued for 48 hours following the procedure, and no evidence of abrupt vessel closure was observed. Repeat arteriography 6 months after atherectomy demonstrated no evidence of restenosis *(Panel C)*.

Figure 13–16
An eccentric stenosis of the midsegment of the left anterior descending artery was demonstrated in the right anterior *(Panel A)* and left anterior *(Panel B)* oblique projections. A 7-French DVI EX atherectomy device was advanced across the stenosis *(Panel C)*, and directed cuts were performed. An excellent anatomic result was noted in the right anterior oblique projection *(Panel D)*; however, a moderate degree of ectasia and localized dissection were observed in the left anterior oblique projection *(Panel E)*. Symptoms recurred 3 months later, and repeat angiography demonstrated restenosis at the atherectomy site *(Panel F)*.

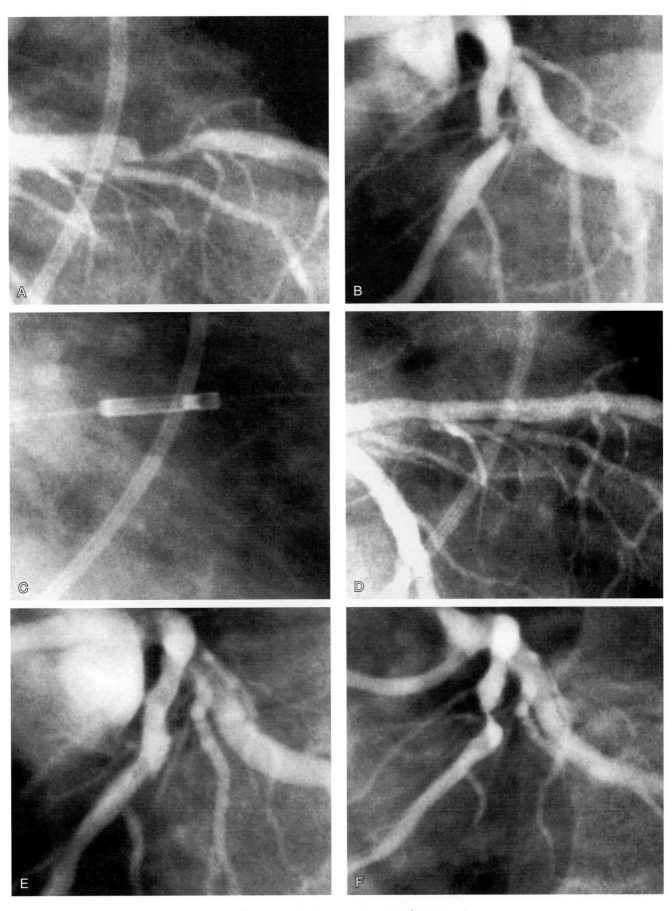

Figure 13–16. *See legend on opposite page*

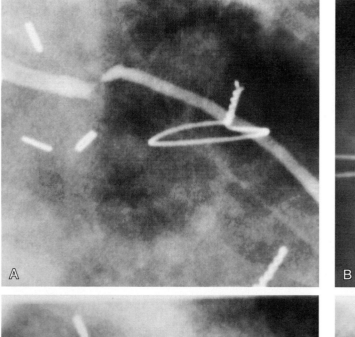

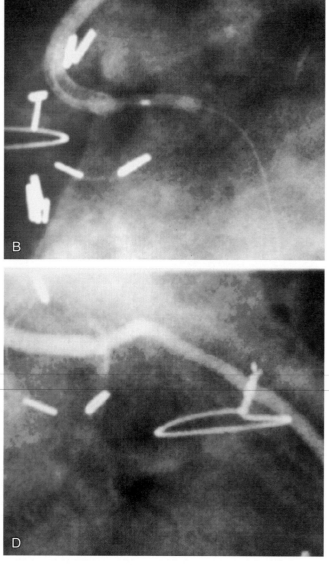

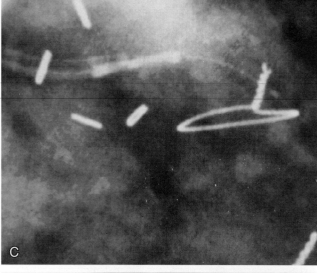

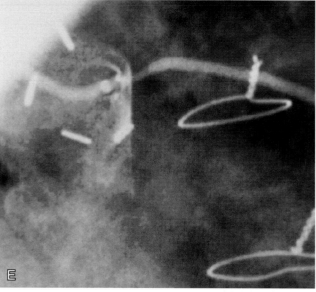

Figure 13–17

A restenotic, ostial lesion of a saphenous vein graft to the left anterior descending artery *(Panel A)* was predilated with a 2.5-mm balloon catheter *(Panel B)*. A 7-French DVI SCA atherectomy device was positioned across the ostial lesion, and circumferential cuts were performed *(Panel C)*. Although an excellent initial stand-alone result was obtained *(Panel D)*, the patient's symptoms recurred 3 months later. Repeat angiography demonstrated partial restenosis (50% residual stenosis) at the atherectomy site *(Panel E)*.

Major angiographic complications after directional atherectomy include coronary dissection (due to guiding catheter positioning, nose cone trauma, or deep resection), abrupt closure, distal embolization, and coronary perforation. The incidence of these complications is relatively low and does appear to differ significantly from complication rates for balloon angioplasty. Improved case selection and continued evolution of guiding catheter designs and device configuration may promote even lower rates of complications.

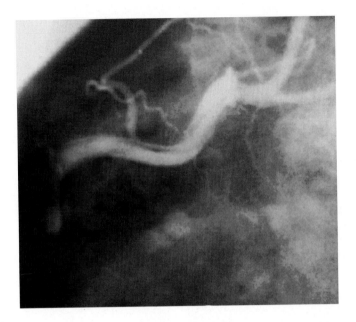

Figure 13–18
Coronary arteriography demonstrated a 90% eccentric stenosis in the midportion of the right coronary artery in this patient with unstable angina. Following intubation of the right coronary artery using an 11-French guiding catheter, an extensive guiding catheter dissection was noted. Resultant abrupt vessel closure culminated in referral for emergency coronary artery bypass surgery.

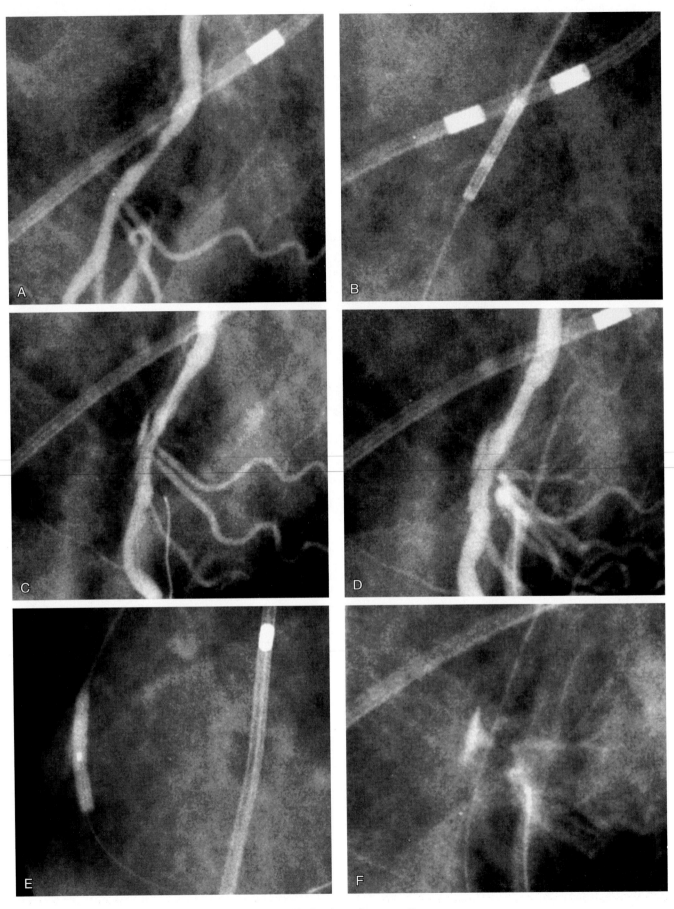

Figure 13–19. *See legend on opposite page*

Figure 13–19
An eccentric lesion of the midsegment of the right coronary artery *(Panel A)* was treated with directional atherectomy using a 6-French DVI SCA device *(Panel B)*. After initial circumferential atherectomy, a localized dissection was demonstrated *(Panel C)*. Prolonged balloon inflation using a 2.5-mm balloon catheter *(Panel D)* failed to improve the extent of the dissection *(Panel E)*. Contrast medium staining was noted *(Panel F)*. The patient underwent aggressive anticoagulation therapy with heparin for 48 hours and did not experience clinical sequelae.

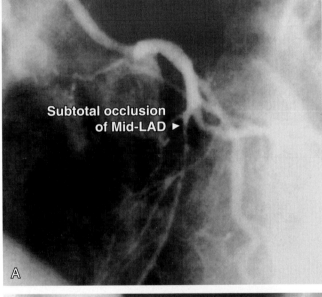

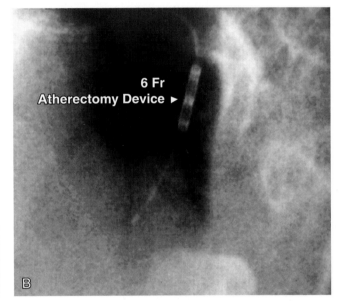

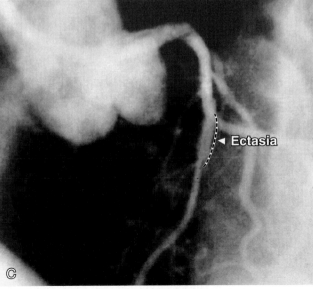

Figure 13–20
Coronary arteriography demonstrated a subtotal occlusion of the midportion of the left anterior descending artery *(Panel A)*. A 6-French directional atherectomy device was positioned across the stenosis, and four passes were performed at 20 psi *(Panel B)*. Following sequential circumferential cuts, a moderate degree of ectasia was noted *(Panel C)*. (Reprinted from DeCesare N, Popma J, Holmes D, et al. Clinical angiographic and histologic correlates of ectasia after directional coronary atherectomy. Am J Cardiol 1992; 69:314–319, with permission.)

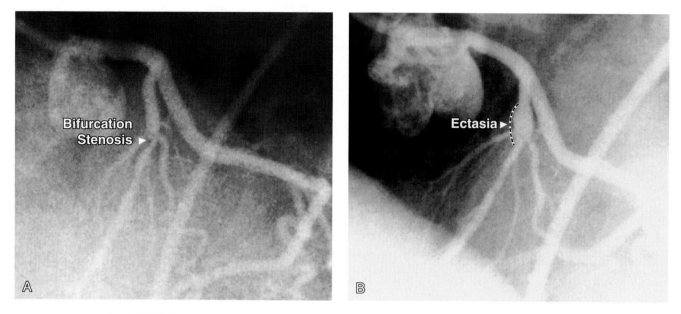

Figure 13–21
A complex bifurcation lesion involving the midportion of the left anterior descending artery *(Panel A)* was treated with a 7-French directional atherectomy device. After directional atherectomy, severe ectasia was noted in the proximal portion of the left anterior descending artery *(Panel B)*. This aneurysmal dilatation was observed to progressively increase during the period of follow-up, and coronary artery bypass grafting was eventually performed. (Reprinted from DeCesare N, Popma J, Holmes D, et al. Clinical angiographic and histologic correlates of ectasia after directional coronary atherectomy. Am J Cardiol 1992; 69:314–319, with permission.)

Coronary vasoconstriction and vasospasm have been demonstrated after balloon angioplasty, presumably due to platelet activation and the subsequent release of vasoactive amines. This vasoconstriction is generally responsive to intracoronary nitroglycerin, which should be administered liberally during coronary interventional procedures. A similar vasoconstrictor phenomenon may be noted after directional atherectomy.

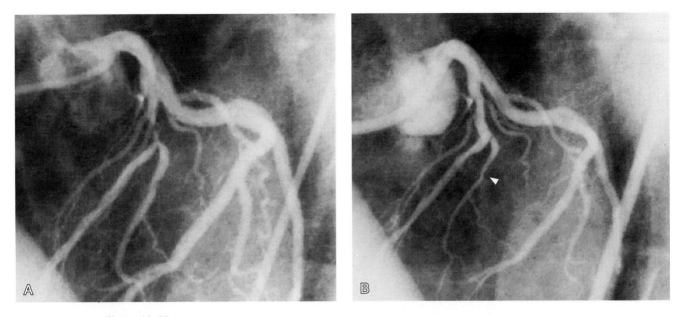

Figure 13–22
A concentric stenosis was noted in the midportion of the left anterior descending artery prior to the origin of a large first diagonal branch *(Panel A)*. Following directional atherectomy, coronary vasoconstriction occurred within the diagonal branch *(arrows, Panel B)*. Vasoconstriction was subsequently relieved with intracoronary administration of nitroglycerin, 200 μg.

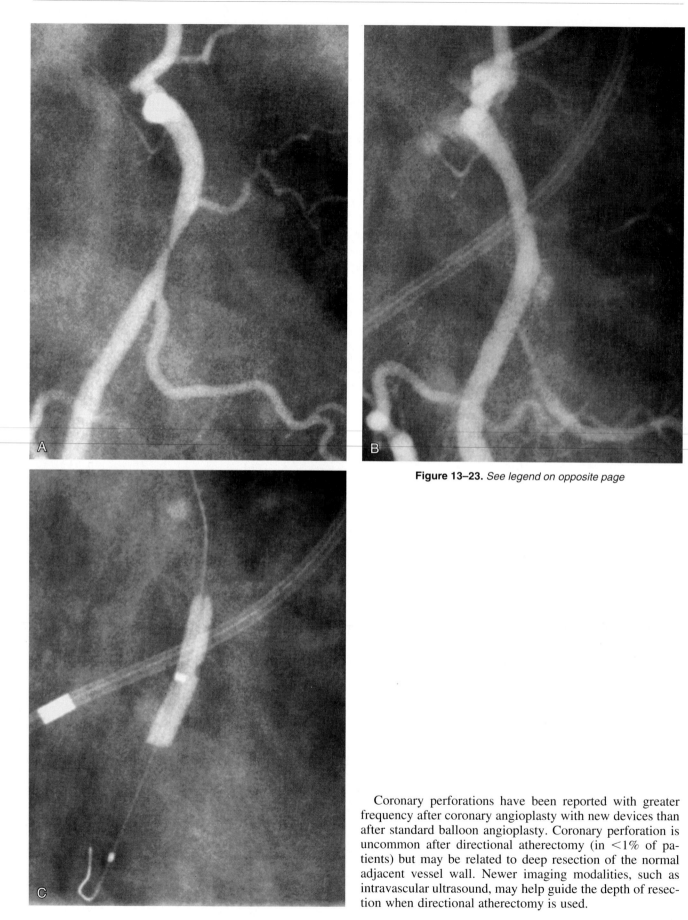

Figure 13–23. *See legend on opposite page*

Coronary perforations have been reported with greater frequency after coronary angioplasty with new devices than after standard balloon angioplasty. Coronary perforation is uncommon after directional atherectomy (in <1% of patients) but may be related to deep resection of the normal adjacent vessel wall. Newer imaging modalities, such as intravascular ultrasound, may help guide the depth of resection when directional atherectomy is used.

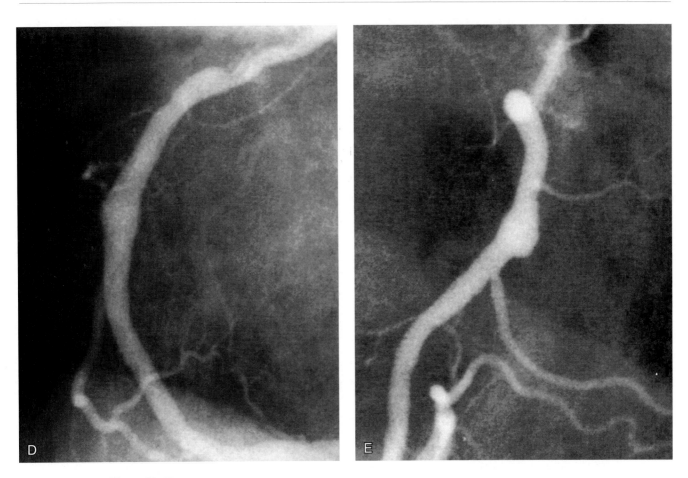

Figure 13–23
A tubular, concentric stenosis in the midportion of the right coronary artery *(Panel A)* was treated with directional atherectomy using a 7-French DVI EX device (not shown). After the initial passes, contrast extravasation was noted just proximal to the origin of the right ventricular branch *(Panel B)*. Prolonged balloon inflation using a 3.0-mm balloon catheter was performed to seal the perforation and prevent tamponade *(Panel C)*. After a 15-minute balloon inflation, a moderate degree of ectasia was noted at the atherectomy site; however, no further extravasation of contrast medium was observed *(Panel D)*. Repeat angiography 24 hours later demonstrated expansion of the pseudoaneurysm *(Panel E)*; as a result, the patient was referred for coronary bypass surgery.

SELECTED REFERENCES

Adelman A, Cohen E, Kimball B, et al. A comparison of directional atherectomy with balloon angioplasty for lesions of the left anterior descending coronary artery. N Engl J Med 1993; 329:228–233.

Altmann D, Popma J, Pichard A, et al. Impact of directional atherectomy on adjacent branch vessels. Am J Cardiol 1993; 72:351–353.

Bell M, Garratt K, Bresnahan J, et al. Relation of deep arterial resection and coronary artery aneurysms after directional coronary atherectomy. J Am Coll Cardiol 1992; 20:1474–1481.

DeCesare N, Popma J, Holmes D, et al. Clinical angiographic and histologic correlates of ectasia after directional coronary atherectomy. Am J Cardiol 1992; 69:314–319.

Dick R, Haudenschild C, Popma J, et al. Directional atherectomy for total coronary occlusions. Coron Artery Dis 1991; 2:189–199.

Ellis S, DeCesare N, Pinkerton C, et al. Relation of stenosis morphology and clinical presentation to the procedural results of directional coronary atherectomy. Circulation 1991; 84:644–653.

Fishman R, Kuntz R, Carrozza J, et al. Long-term results of directional coronary atherectomy: Predictors of restenosis. J Am Coll Cardiol 1992; 20:1101–1110.

Garratt K, Edwards W, Kaufmann U, et al. Differential histopathology of primary atherosclerotic and restenotic lesions in coronary arteries and saphenous vein bypass grafts: Analysis of tissue obtained from 73

patients by directional atherectomy. J Am Coll Cardiol 1991; 17:442–448.

Garratt K, Edwards W, Vlietstra R, et al. Coronary morphology after percutaneous directional coronary atherectomy in humans: Autopsy analysis of three patients. J Am Coll Cardiol 1990; 16:1432–1436.

Garratt K, Holmes D, Bell M, et al. Restenosis after directional coronary atherectomy: Differences between primary atheromatous and restenosis lesions and influence of subintimal resection. J Am Coll Cardiol 1990; 16:1665–1671.

Garratt K, Holmes D, Bell M, et al. Results of directional atherectomy of primary atheromatous and restenotic lesions in coronary arteries and saphenous vein grafts. Am J Cardiol 1992; 1992:449–454.

Hinohara T, Robertson G, Selmon M, et al. Restenosis after directional coronary atherectomy. J Am Coll Cardiol 1992; 20:623–632.

Hinohara T, Rowe M, Robertson G, et al. Effect of lesion characteristics on outcome of directional coronary atherectomy. J Am Coll Cardiol 1991; 17:1112–1120.

Hinohara T, Rowe M, Robertson G, et al. Directional coronary atherectomy for the treatment of coronary lesions with abnormal contour. J Invasive Cardiol 1990; 2:57–63.

Hofling B, Gonschior P, Simpson L, et al. Efficacy of directional coronary atherectomy in cases unsuitable for percutaneous transluminal coronary angioplasty (PTCA) and after unsuccessful PTCA. Am Heart J 1992; 124:341–348.

Jackman J, Hermiller J, Sketch M, et al. Combined rotational and directional atherectomy guided by intravascular ultrasound in an occluded vein graft. Am Heart J 1992; 124:214–216.

Kuntz R, Hinohara T, Robertson G, et al. Influence of vessel selection on the observed restenosis rate after endoluminal stenting or directional atherectomy. Am J Cardiol 1992; 70:1101–1108.

Kuntz R, Hinohara T, Safian R, et al. Restenosis after directional coronary atherectomy: Effects of luminal diameter and deep wall excision. Circulation 1992; 86:1394–1399.

Mansour M, Fishman R, Kuntz R, et al. Feasibility of directional atherectomy for the treatment of bifurcation lesions. Coron Artery Dis 1992; 3:761–765.

Pomerantz R, Kuntz R, Carrozza J, et al. Acute and long-term outcome of narrowed saphenous venous grafts treated by endoluminal stenting and directional atherectomy. Am J Cardiol 1992; 70:161–167.

Popma J, DeCesare N, Ellis S, et al. Clinical, angiographic and procedural correlates of quantitative coronary dimensions after directional coronary atherectomy. J Am Coll Cardiol 1991; 18:1183–1189.

Popma J, DeCesare N, Pinkerton C, et al. A quantitative analysis of factors influencing late lumen loss and restenosis after directional coronary atherectomy. Am J Cardiol 1993; 71:552–557.

Popma J, Topol E, Hinohara T, et al. Abrupt vessel closure after directional coronary atherectomy. J Am Coll Cardiol 1992; 19:1372–1379.

Rowe M, Hinohara T, White N, et al. Comparison of dissection rates and angiographic results following directional coronary atherectomy and coronary angioplasty. Am J Cardiol 1990; 66:49–53.

Serruys P, Umans V, Strauss B, et al. Quantitative angiography after directional coronary atherectomy. Br Heart J 1991; 66:122–129.

Topol E, Leya F, Pinkerton C, et al. A comparison of directional atherectomy with coronary angioplasty in patients with coronary artery disease. N Engl J Med 1993; 329:221–227.

Umans V, Beatt K, Rensing B, et al. Comparative quantitative angiographic analysis of directional coronary atherectomy and balloon coronary angioplasty. Am J Cardiol 1991; 68:1556–1563.

Rotational Coronary Atherectomy

Rotational coronary atherectomy involves the ablation of fibrocalcific plaque into microparticles that pass downstream into the distal microcirculation. Unique technical features of the rotational atherectomy device include (1) a 310-cm 0.009-inch stainless steel wire with a radiopaque platinum spring tip that is 0.014 inches in diameter; (2) rotational atherectomy burrs that range in size from 1.25 to 2.5 mm, contain miniature diamond chips, and rotate at 150,000 to 200,000 rpm (Figure 14–1); and (3) a high-speed compressed gas turbine connected to the saline infusion apparatus that lubricates and cools the system.

Differential forward cutting with the rotational atherectomy burr results in ablation of the diseased plaque, leaving the normal, uninvolved arterial wall intact. The principle of the technique is based on the observation that elastic tissue (normal vessel wall) moves away from the diamond chip burrs, whereas inelastic tissue (calcified or fibrous) is frac-

tured into microparticles. In addition, the high rotational speeds of the burrs displace frictional components in an orthogonal vector; this markedly enhances burr and catheter axial movement over the guide wire and results in excellent tracking over tortuous vessel segments.

Multicenter registry results have demonstrated that high procedural success rates (>90%) and low rates of major complications (<3%) can be attained in complex lesion subsets with rotational coronary atherectomy. Since approval of rotational coronary atherectomy devices for marketing by the Food and Drug Administration Device Panel in May 1993, their use has been incorporated at a number of clinical centers. To enable operators to safely surmount a "learning curve" associated with the use of new devices, guidelines for lesion complexity have been recommended (Table 14–1).

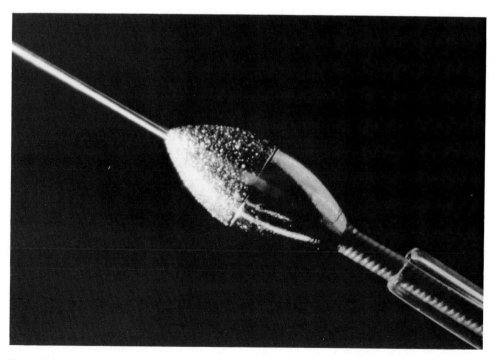

Figure 14–1
A rotational atherectomy device burr.

Table 14–1   Lesion Complexity and the Level of Experience for Rotational Coronary Atherectomy

	Level 1	Level 2	Level 3
Number of cases	0–10	10–20	20+
Location within vessel	Medial and distal	Proximal, medial, and distal	All lesions, except SVG lesions
Lesion length	Discrete (<10 mm)	Tubular (<20 mm)	Diffuse (<25 mm)
Lesion angulation	<45°	<90°	Any
Lesion morphology	Concentric	Mildly eccentric	Eccentric or concentric
Restenotic lesion	Yes	Yes or no	Yes or no
Lesion calcification	None	Mild-moderate	Moderate-heavy
Total occlusion	No	No	Crossable with wire
Side branch narrowed	No	Yes, proceed with caution	Yes
Left ventricular function	LVEF ≥50%	LVEF ≥40%	LVEF ≥30%
Diabetic patient, small vessel	No	Yes; proceed with caution	Yes; proceed with caution
Ostial lesions	No	No	Yes; proceed with caution

Abbreviations: SVG = saphenous vein graft; LVEF = left ventricular ejection fraction.

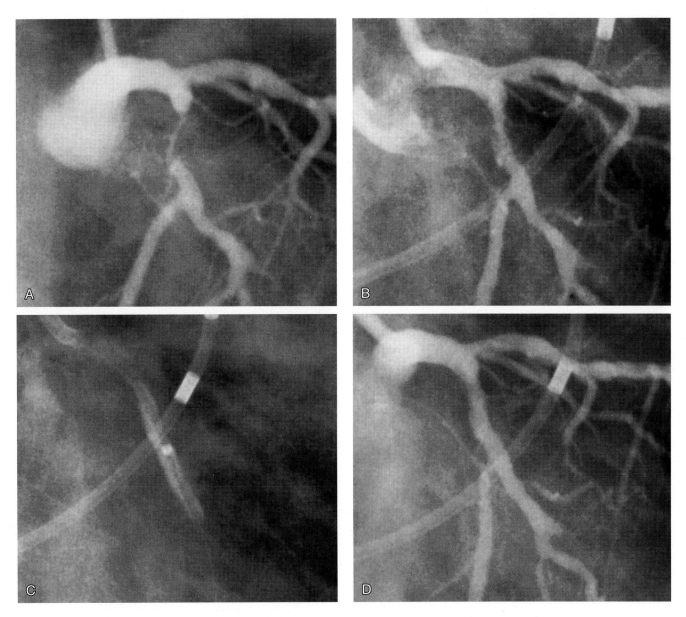

Figure 14–2
A long lesion in the proximal portion of the left circumflex artery *(Panel A)* was treated with rotational coronary atherectomy and adjunct balloon angioplasty. Using a "stepped approach" to burr selection, sequential rotational atherectomy was performed with 1.5- and 2.0-mm burrs (not shown), yielding a 40% residual stenosis with mild lumen irregularities *(Panel B)*. Adjunct balloon dilatation was performed with a 2.5-mm balloon catheter *(Panel C)*, resulting in a 20% residual stenosis and a smooth lumen contour *(Panel D)*.

Rotational atherectomy is particularly useful for the treatment of calcified lesions, lesions on bends, and lesions in small vessels as well as in selected patients with prior restenosis.

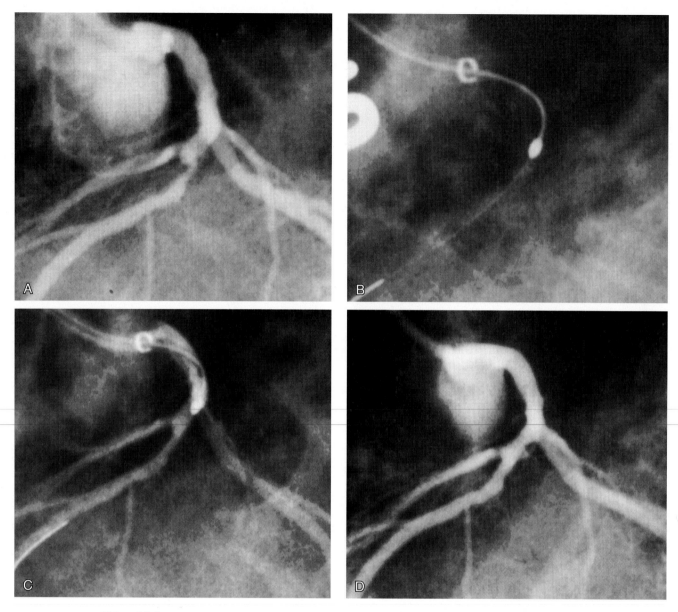

Figure 14–3
A calcified, eccentric stenosis in the midsegment of the left anterior descending artery *(Panel A)* was treated with a 1.5-mm burr *(Panels B and C)*. Multiple passes with a 1.75-mm burr (not shown) resulted in an excellent stand-alone result without dissection or reduced distal flow *(Panel D)*.

Figure 14–4
An eccentric, angulated stenosis that involved the midsegment of the left anterior descending artery *(Panel A)* was notable for intralesion calcium *(arrowheads, Panel B)*. Sequential rotational atherectomy was performed with 1.5-, 2.0-, and 2.5-mm burrs *(Panel C)*. After rotational atherectomy, a <20% residual stenosis was obtained; however, a mild degree of intraluminal haziness was observed *(Panel D)*. A 3.0-mm balloon was inflated to 6 atm *(Panel E)* to smooth the lumen contour and maximize the final lumen diameter. After final balloon deflation, a <10% residual stenosis and a smoother lumen contour were obtained *(Panel F)*.

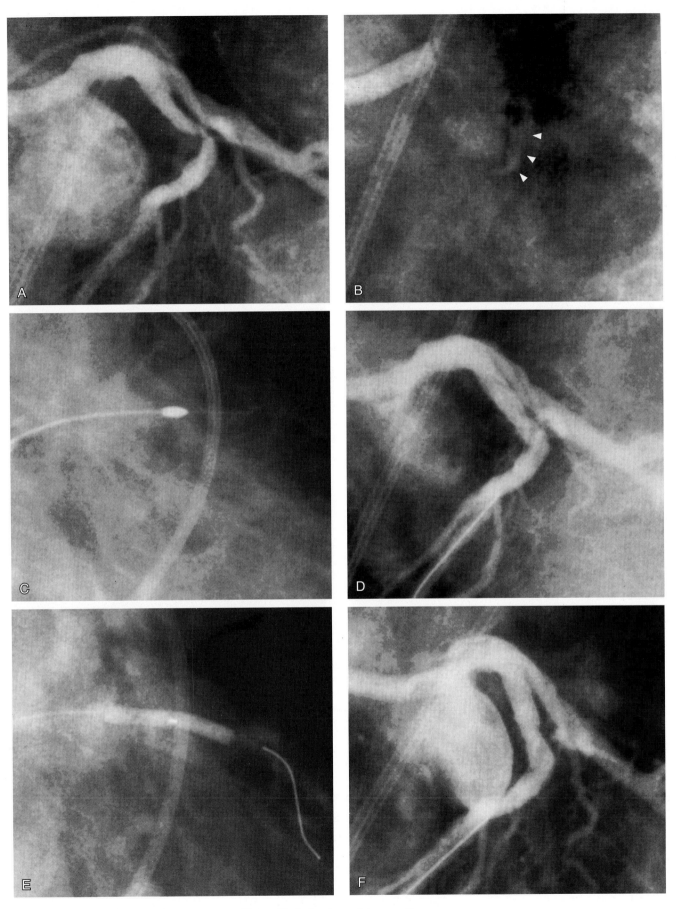

Figure 14–4. *See legend on opposite page*

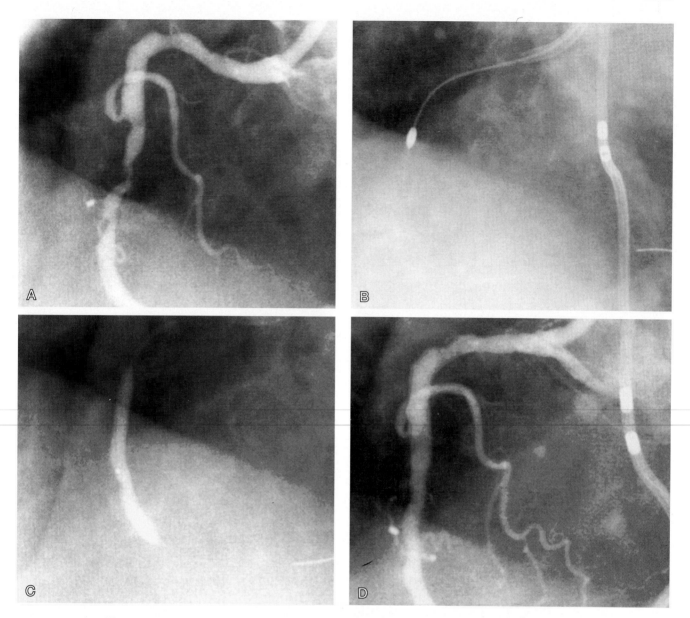

Figure 14–5
A tubular, calcified, eccentric stenosis of the midportion of the right coronary artery *(Panel A)* was treated with rotational atherectomy using 1.5- and 2.0-mm burrs *(Panel B)*. The patient developed transient bradycardia and required temporary pacemaker support. A 40% residual stenosis was treated with 2.5- and 3.0-mm balloon catheters *(Panel C)*. After final balloon inflation, an improved lumen contour was achieved, and a <30% residual stenosis was demonstrated *(Panel D)*.

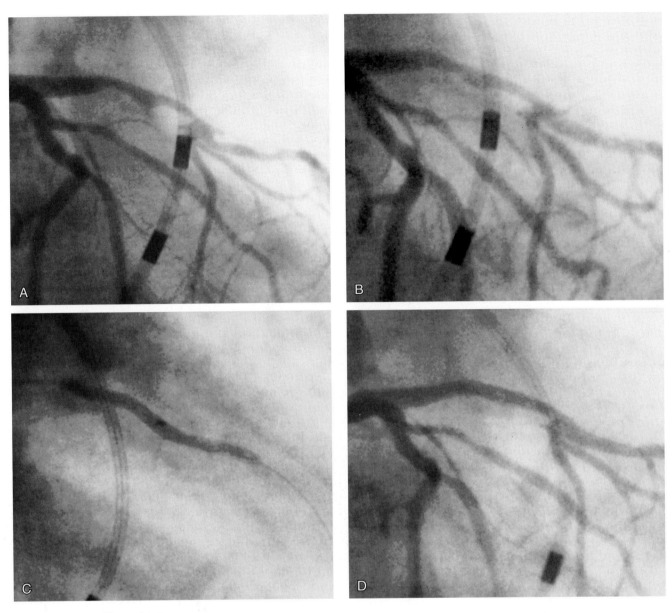

Figure 14–6
An eccentric stenosis in the midportion of the left anterior descending artery *(Panel A)* was treated with 1.5- and 2.0-mm burrs. After sequential atherectomy, a smooth lumen contour was noted, but a 40% to 50% residual stenosis remained *(Panel B)*. Adjunct balloon dilatation was performed with a 2.5-mm long (30-mm) balloon *(Panel C)*, and a 30% residual stenosis was obtained *(Panel D)*.

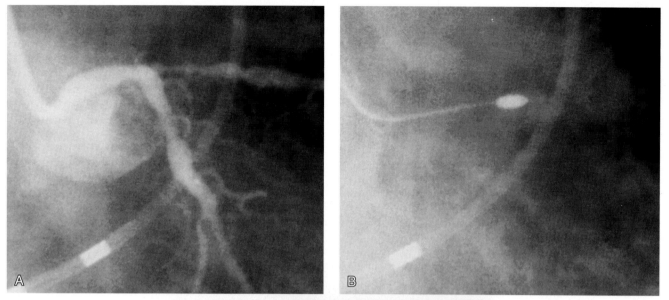

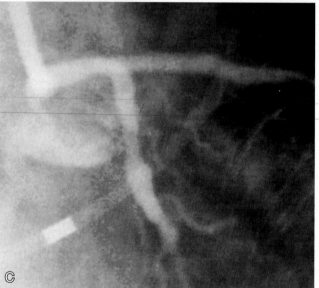

Figure 14–7

A calcified ostial lesion of the left anterior descending artery *(Panel A)* was treated with 1.75- and 2.15-mm burrs *(Panel B)*. Adjunct balloon dilatation with a 3.0-mm balloon was used to manage a 40% residual stenosis. An excellent angiographic result was obtained *(Panel C)*.

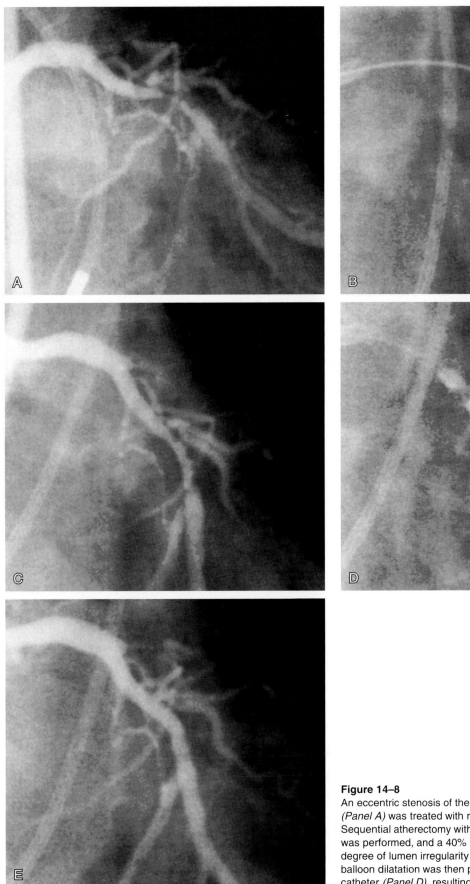

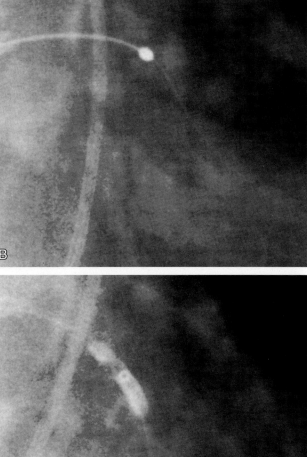

Figure 14–8
An eccentric stenosis of the midsegment of the left circumflex *(Panel A)* was treated with rotational coronary atherectomy. Sequential atherectomy with 1.75- and 2.25-mm burrs *(Panel B)* was performed, and a 40% residual stenosis with a moderate degree of lumen irregularity was obtained *(Panel C)*. Adjunct balloon dilatation was then performed with a 3.0-mm balloon catheter *(Panel D)*, resulting in a <10% residual stenosis *(Panel E)*.

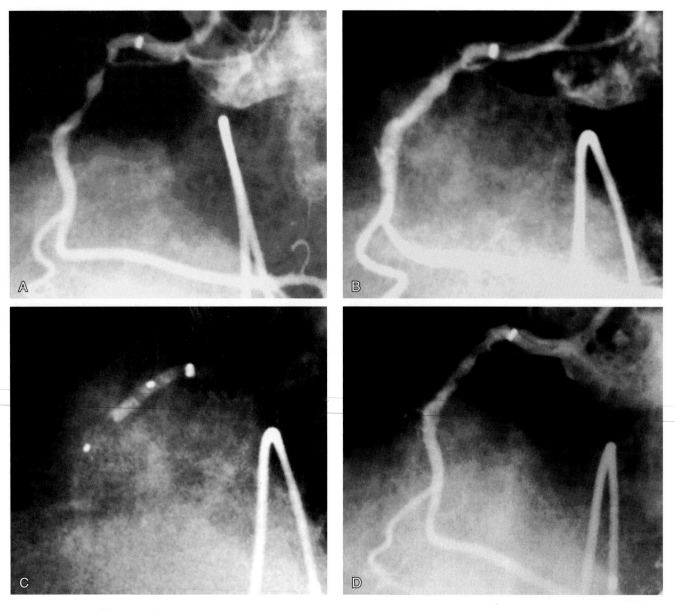

Figure 14–9
Tandem lesions in the proximal and midsegments of the right coronary artery were treated with rotational atherectomy using 1.5- and 2.0-mm burrs (not shown). A 40% residual stenosis in the proximal lesion *(Panel B)* was treated with a prolonged balloon inflation using a 2.5-mm balloon catheter *(Panel C)*. After final balloon inflation, a 20% residual stenosis was obtained with a mild degree of residual intraluminal haziness *(Panel D)*.

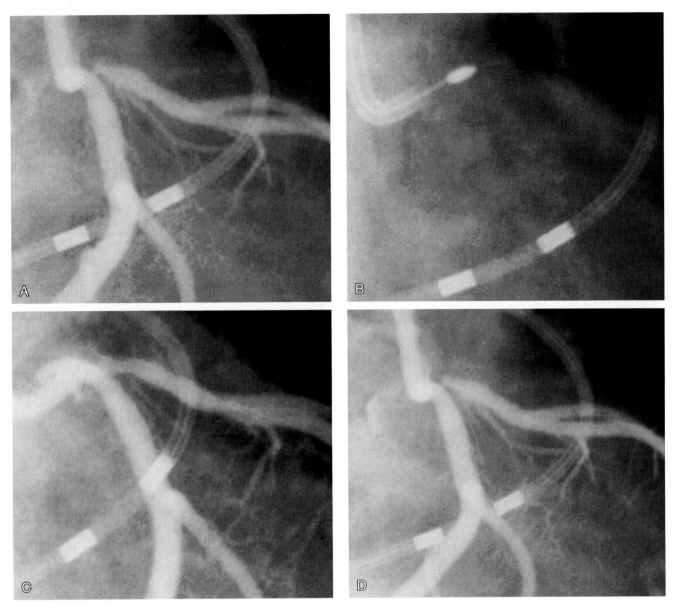

Figure 14–10
A calcified, ostial lesion of the left anterior descending artery *(Panel A)* was treated with stand-alone rotational coronary atherectomy using 1.75- and 2.15-mm burrs *(Panel B)*. A 40% residual stenosis was obtained *(Panel C)*. The patient's symptoms recurred 6 weeks later, and repeat angiography demonstrated a recurrence of the ostial stenosis *(Panel D)*.

Major angiographic complications (dissection ≥10mm, perforations) are uncommon (≤5%) after rotational atherectomy. A transient reduction in anterograde coronary perfusion may develop in 10% to 20% of patients who undergo rotational atherectomy, attributable to the development of distal microembolization or severe vasoconstriction, or both. Factors that affect the amount of embolic plaque burden are lesion length, the size of the rotational atherectomy burr, severity of the stenosis, perfusion pressure, and distal coronary run-off. In most circumstances, the "delayed" filling of the distal coronary bed is transient and responsive to intracoronary nitroglycerin or verapamil administration.

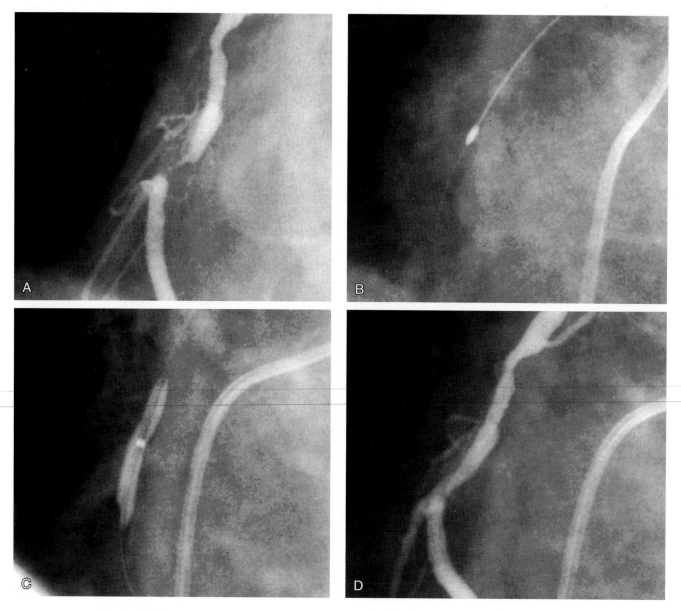

Figure 14–11

A discrete lesion in the midportion of the right coronary artery *(Panel A)* was treated with rotational atherectomy using 1.25- and 1.75-mm burrs *(Panel B)*. Vasospasm developed just distal to the treatment site; the vasospasm was refractory to intracoronary nitroglycerin administration and was treated with a 2.5-mm balloon catheter *(Panel C)*. Anterograde flow was promptly re-established, and a 30% residual stenosis was noted *(Panel D)*. A mild degree of intraluminal haziness was observed, but no subsequent clinical sequelae occurred.

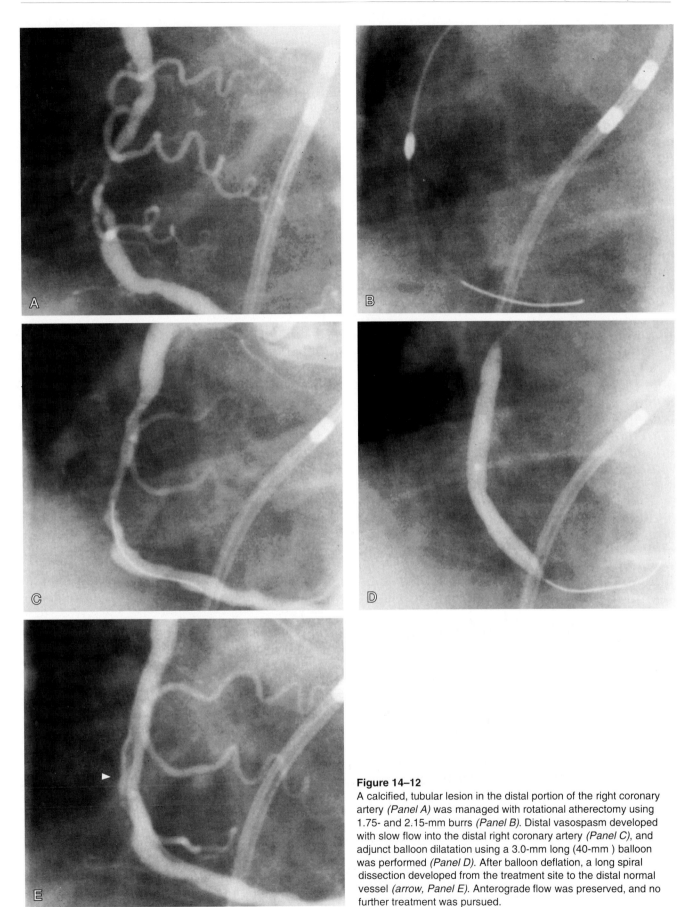

Figure 14–12
A calcified, tubular lesion in the distal portion of the right coronary artery *(Panel A)* was managed with rotational atherectomy using 1.75- and 2.15-mm burrs *(Panel B)*. Distal vasospasm developed with slow flow into the distal right coronary artery *(Panel C)*, and adjunct balloon dilatation using a 3.0-mm long (40-mm) balloon was performed *(Panel D)*. After balloon deflation, a long spiral dissection developed from the treatment site to the distal normal vessel *(arrow, Panel E)*. Anterograde flow was preserved, and no further treatment was pursued.

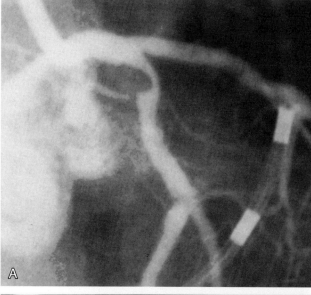

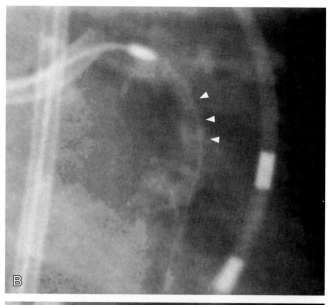

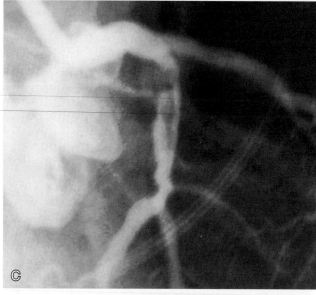

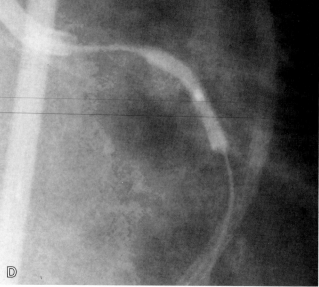

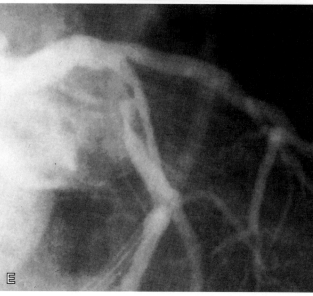

Figure 14–13

A heavily calcified eccentric stenosis involving the ostium of the left circumflex coronary artery *(Panel A)* was treated with rotational atherectomy. The heavy cast of calcium was notable *(arrows)*, and stepped rotational atherectomy was performed using 1.50- and 2.0-mm burrs *(Panel B)*. After rotational atherectomy, a long, spiral dissection of the proximal left circumflex artery developed *(Panel C)*; this was managed with the use of a 2.5-mm balloon catheter *(Panel D)*. Although a significant residual stenosis persisted *(Panel E)*, it remained stable at repeat angiography 24 hours later.

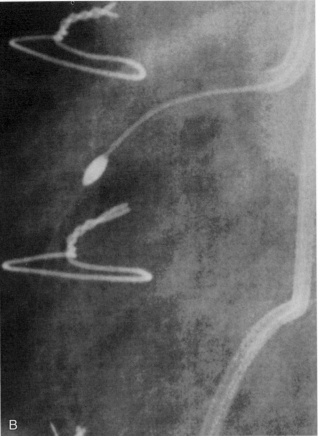

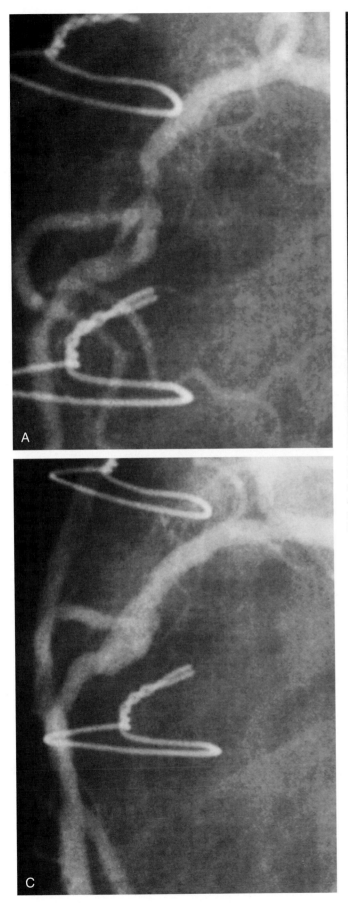

Figure 14–14
Rotational atherectomy was performed in the calcified lesion of the midsegment of the right coronary artery *(Panel A)*. Sequential atherectomy with 1.75- and 2.15-mm burrs *(Panel B)* resulted in marked ectasia at the treatment site *(Panel C)*. Repeat angiography 24 hours later demonstrated no progression of the ectasia.

The currently available 0.009-inch rotablator wire is difficult to torque and maneuver; it has fractured on rare occasions, related to failure to control rotation of the wire during burr exchanges. For adjunct balloon angioplasty, consideration of switching to a conventional wire at the time of exchange may be prudent.

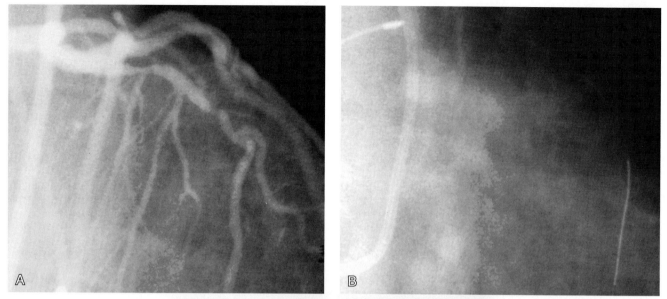

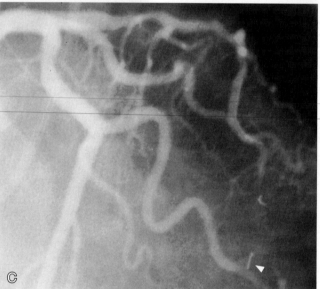

Figure 14–15
Sequential lesions of the midportion of the left anterior descending artery *(Panel A)* were treated with rotational coronary atherectomy. Atherectomy using 1.25- and 1.75-mm burrs was performed *(Panel B)*. During the final burr exchange, the distal tip of the guide wire drifted distally into a septal branch, and inadvertent guide wire fracture occurred *(arrow, Panel C)*. Vasospasm in the distal left anterior descending artery was not responsive to intracoronary nitroglycerin administration *(Panel C)*. Attempts to remove the coronary guide wire using percutaneous methods were unsuccessful.

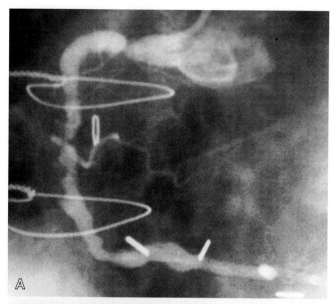

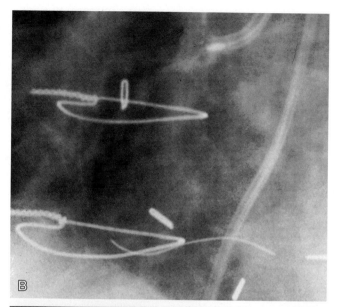

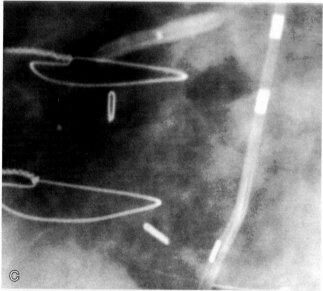

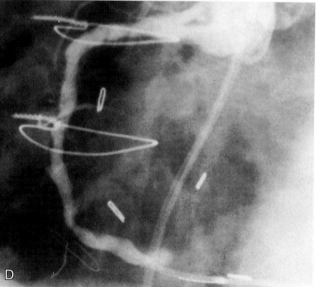

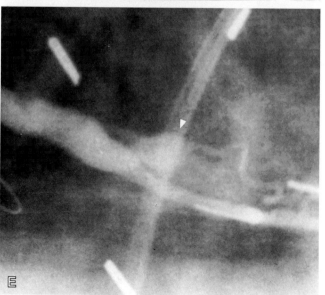

Figure 14–16
A calcified, concentric stenosis of the proximal segment of the right coronary artery *(Panel A)* was treated with rotational atherectomy *(Panel B)* and adjunct balloon dilatation *(Panel C)*. Although an excellent anatomic result was obtained *(Panel D)*, a localized guide wire perforation was noted in the distal right coronary artery *(arrow, Panel E)*.

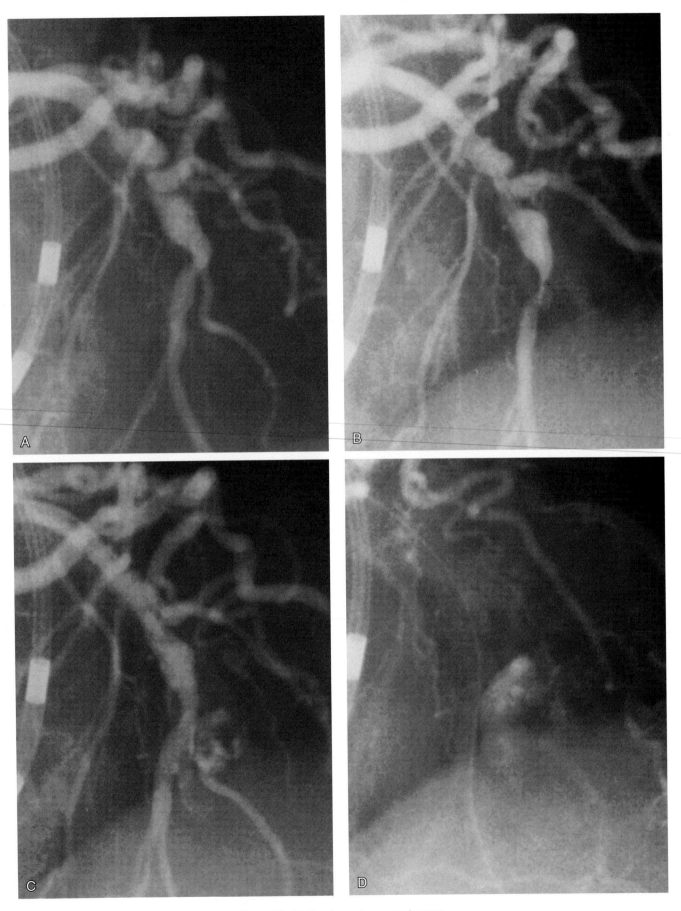

Figure 14–17. *See legend on opposite page*

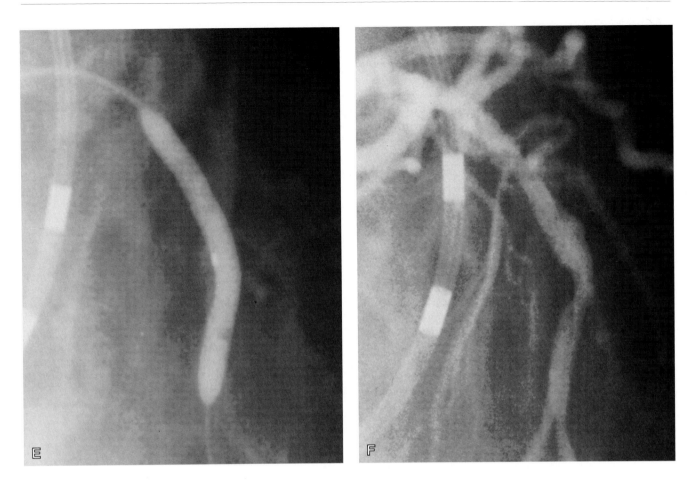

Figure 14-17
A complex, bifurcation stenosis of the distal portion of the left anterior descending artery *(Panel A)* was treated with rotational atherectomy using a 1.5-mm burr (not shown). After the initial pass, a significant residual stenosis was noted *(Panel B)*. Although no evidence of coronary dissection was observed, the small diagonal branch became transiently occluded. Repeat angiography demonstrated a localized perforation at the bifurcation site *(Panel C)* associated with contrast medium staining *(Panel D)*. A 3.5-mm long (40-mm) balloon was used to seal the perforation *(Panel E)*; however, the diagonal branch was again occluded *(Panel F)*. An echocardiogram did not demonstrate significant pericardial fluid accumulation.

SELECTED REFERENCES

Brogan W, Popma J, Pichard A, et al. Rotational coronary atherectomy after unsuccessful coronary balloon angioplasty. Am J Cardiol 1993; 71:794–798.

Brown R, Penn I. Coronary rotational ablation for unsuccessful angioplasty due to failure to cross the stenosis with a dilatation catheter. Cathet Cardiovasc Diagn 1992; 26:110–112.

Dorros G, Iyer S, Zaitoun R, et al. Acute angiographic and clinical outcome of high speed percutaneous rotational atherectomy (Rotablator®). Cathet Cardiovasc Diagn 1991; 22:157–166.

Gibb M, Buchbinder M. High speed coronary rotational ablation. Coron Artery Dis 1992; 3:908–913.

Iyer S, Hall P, King J, Dorros G. Successful rotational coronary ablation following failed balloon angioplasty. Cathet Cardiovasc Diagn 1991; 24:65–68.

Jackman J, Hermiller J, Sketch M, et al. Combined rotational and directional atherectomy guided by intravascular ultrasound in an occluded vein graft. Am Heart J 1992; 124:214–216.

Mintz G, Pichard A, Popma J, et al. Preliminary experience with adjunct directional coronary atherectomy following high-speed rotational atherectomy in the treatment of calcific coronary artery disease. Am J Cardiol 1993; 71:799–804.

Mintz G, Potkin B, Keren G, et al. Intravascular ultrasound evaluation of the effect of rotational atherectomy in obstructive atherosclerotic coronary artery disease. Circulation 1992; 86:1383–1393.

Popma J, Brogan W, Pichard A, et al. Rotational coronary atherectomy of ostial stenoses. Am J Cardiol 1993; 71:436–438.

Rosenblum J, Stertzer S, Shaw R, et al. Rotational ablation of balloon angioplasty failures. J Invasive Cardiol 1992; 4:312–318.

Teirstein P, Warth D, Haq N, et al. High speed rotational coronary atherectomy for patients with diffuse coronary artery disease. J Am Coll Cardiol 1991; 18:1694–1701.

Umans V, Strauss B, Rensing B, et al. Comparative angiographic quantitative analysis of the immediate efficacy of coronary atherectomy with balloon angioplasty, stenting, and rotational ablation. Am Heart J 1991; 122:836–843.

Zacca N, Kleiman N, Rodriguez A, et al. Rotational ablation of coronary artery lesions using single, large burrs. Cathet Cardiovasc Diagn 1992; 26:92–97.

Transluminal Extraction Atherectomy

Transluminal extraction atherectomy is another alternative atherectomy method that has been approved for marketing by the Food and Drug Administration Device Panel. Because transluminal extraction atherectomy cuts the atheromatous material into macroparticulate debris and removes the slurry with vacuum suction, the technique may be useful in the management of patients with lesions in saphenous vein grafts (SVGs), particularly those with degeneration or those that contain thrombus. It may also be used in the treatment of ostial lesions, proximal lesions, and those lesions of excessive length in both native coronaries and SVGs. The transluminal extraction catheter (TEC) device is available in 5.5 French, 6 French, 6.5 French, 7 French, and 7.5 French sizes and comprises an open, cone-shaped cutter attached to a motor-driven torque tube that rotates at 750 rpm (Figure 15–1). When the cutter is rotated, a vacuum is applied within the torque tube. A slurry of diluted blood and small fragments of particulate debris is extracted and stored in a glass reservoir attached to the rear of the control piece. Adjunct coronary angioplasty is recommended when a >50% stenosis remains following extraction atherectomy with the largest device size appropriate for the vessel; this may be required in >80% of patients.

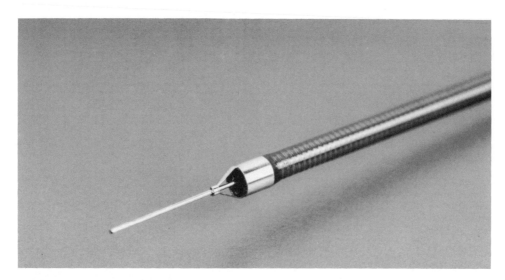

Figure 15–1
A transluminal extraction atherectomy catheter.

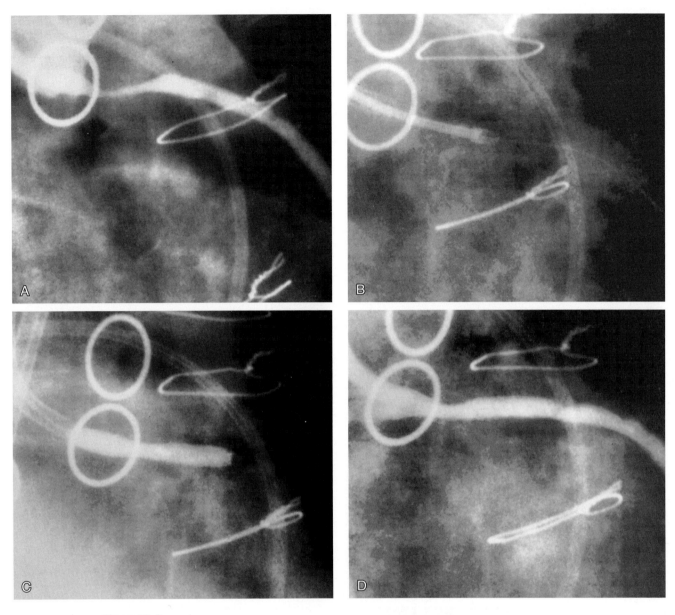

Figure 15–2
An eccentric stenosis in the ostium of a SVG to the left anterior descending artery *(Panel A)* was
treated with extraction atherectomy. Progressive atherectomy using 6.5-French and 7-French devices
was performed *(Panel B)*, and a 50% residual stenosis was obtained. Adjunct balloon dilatation was
performed with a 3.5-mm balloon catheter and was notable for incomplete balloon expansion at the
site of the stenosis *(Panel C)*. A 30% residual stenosis remained at the site of lesion rigidity or dense
plaque accumulation *(Panel D)*.

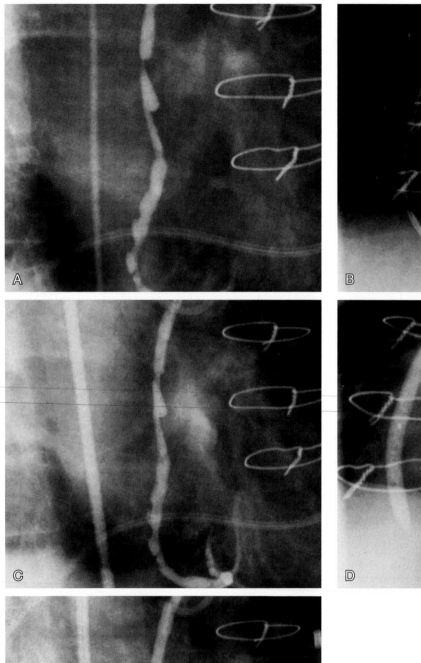

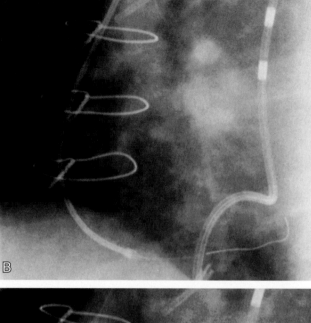

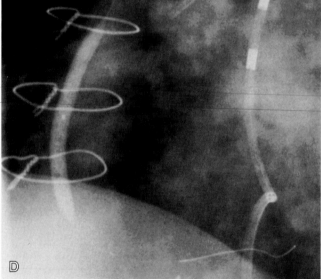

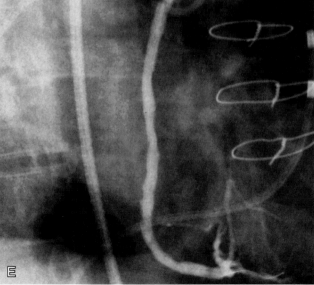

Figure 15–3
Extraction atherectomy was used to treat a diffusely diseased SVG to the distal portion of the right coronary artery *(Panel A)*. Sequential passes with a 2.5-mm TEC device were performed throughout the entire extent of the diseased SVG. A larger channel was obtained within the midsegment of the SVG, particularly in the more proximal aspect *(Panel C)*, and adjunct balloon dilatation was performed using a 4.0-mm long (40-mm) balloon *(Panel D)*. After adjunct dilatation, a smooth SVG contour was obtained without evidence of distal embolization or reduction in anterograde perfusion *(Panel E)*. (Reprinted from Popma J, Leon M, Mintz G, et al. Results of coronary angioplasty using the transluminal extraction catheter. Am J Cardiol 1992; 70:1526–1532, with permission.)

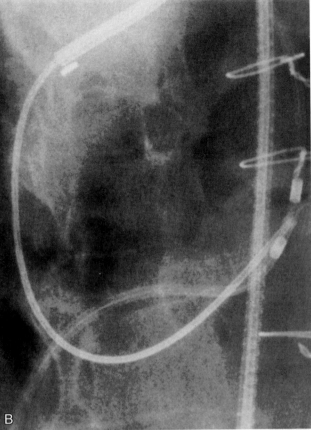

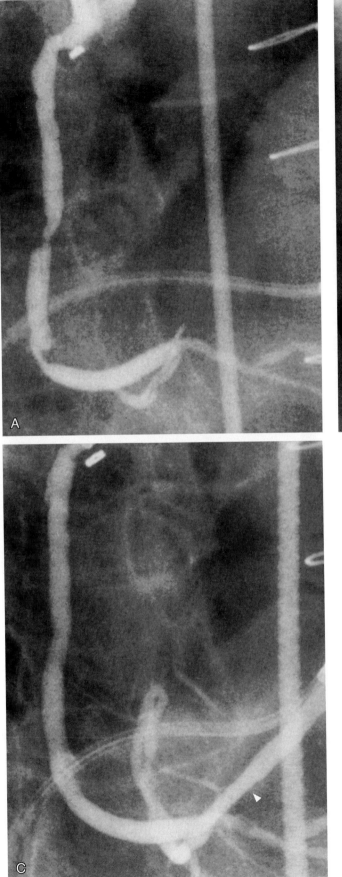

Figure 15–4
Sequential stenoses of the midsegment and distal segment of the SVG to the posterior descending artery and posterolateral branches *(Panel A)* were treated with sequential passes using progressively larger 6.5-French and 7-French TEC devices *(Panel B)*. After adjunct balloon angioplasty using a 4.0-mm long (40-mm) balloon (not shown), an excellent angiographic result was obtained, and no evidence of distal embolization was observed *(Panel C)*. Note that the totally occluded sequential limb to the posterolateral branch was widely patent after extraction atherectomy *(arrow, Panel C)*.

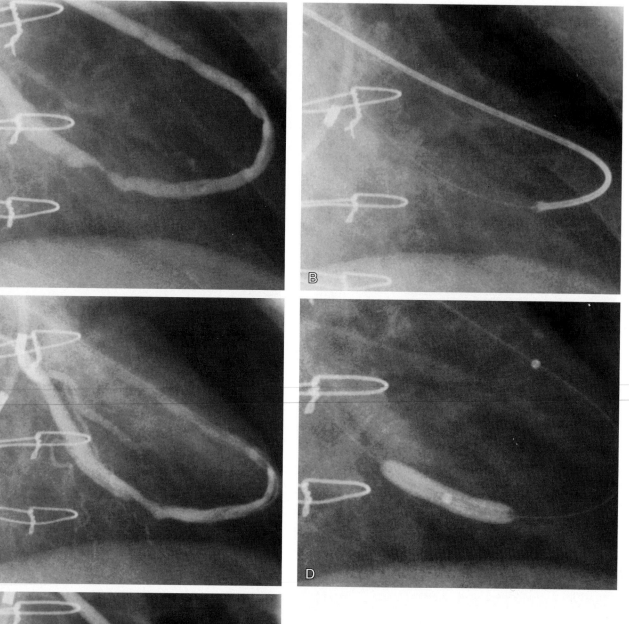

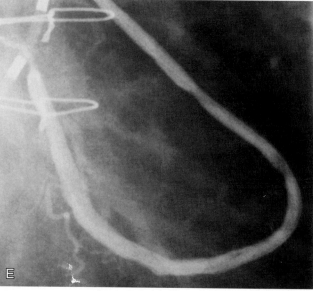

Figure 15–5

An eccentric stenosis of a degenerated "beltway" SVG *(Panel A)* was treated with extraction atherectomy using a 7-French TEC device *(Panel B)*. After extraction atherectomy, a modest improvement in stenosis severity occurred *(Panel C)*. Adjunct balloon dilatation was performed with a 3.5-mm balloon *(Panel D)*, resulting in a minimal residual stenosis at the treatment site and no evidence of distal embolization *(Panel E)*.

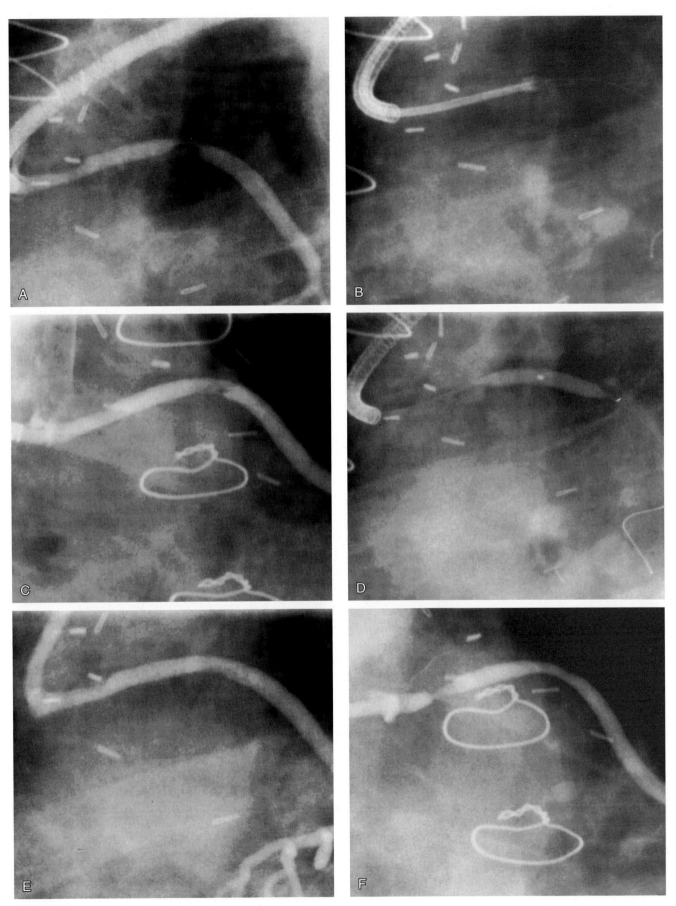

Figure 15–6
An eccentric lesion in a moderately diseased SVG to the left anterior descending artery *(Panel A)* was treated with a 7-French TEC device *(Panel B)*. A mild degree of lumen irregularity was observed after extraction atherectomy *(Panel C)*; this was treated using a 3.0-mm balloon catheter *(Panel D)*. After balloon dilatation, an excellent angiographic result was obtained *(Panel E)*. Symptoms recurred 3 months later, and repeat angiography demonstrated progression of SVG disease proximal to the original treatment site *(Panel F)*.

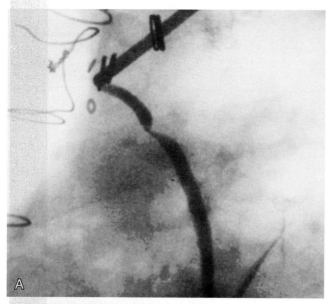

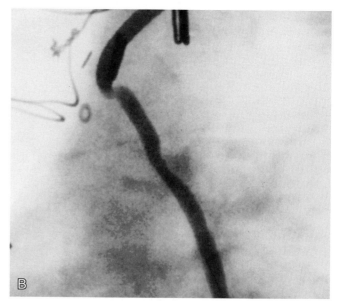

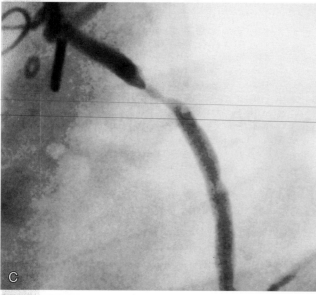

Figure 15–7

An eccentric stenosis of the midsegment of the SVG to the left anterior descending artery *(Panel A)* was treated with stand-alone extraction atherectomy using a 2.5-mm device (not shown). After atherectomy, a 30% residual stenosis was obtained *(Panel B)*. The patient's symptoms recurred 2 months later, and repeat angiography demonstrated recurrence at the site of prior atherectomy *(Panel C)*.

Although transluminal extraction atherectomy has been targeted for the treatment of degenerated SVGs, it has also been used successfully in native coronary arteries, particularly those that contain thrombus.

Figure 15–8

A recent total occlusion of the proximal segment of the right coronary artery *(Panel A)* was crossed with a 0.014-inch guide wire. Residual thrombus was demonstrated at the site of occlusion. After positioning the guide wire in the distal vessel, a 6-French TEC device was advanced across the total occlusion *(Panel B)*, and recanalization of the right coronary artery was achieved *(Panel C)*. A 3.0-mm balloon was inflated across the 50% residual stenosis *(Panel D)*, and a 30% to 40% residual stenosis was obtained *(Panel E)*. Notably, symptoms recurred 3 months later, and repeat angiography demonstrated total occlusion at the site of extraction atherectomy *(Panel F)*.

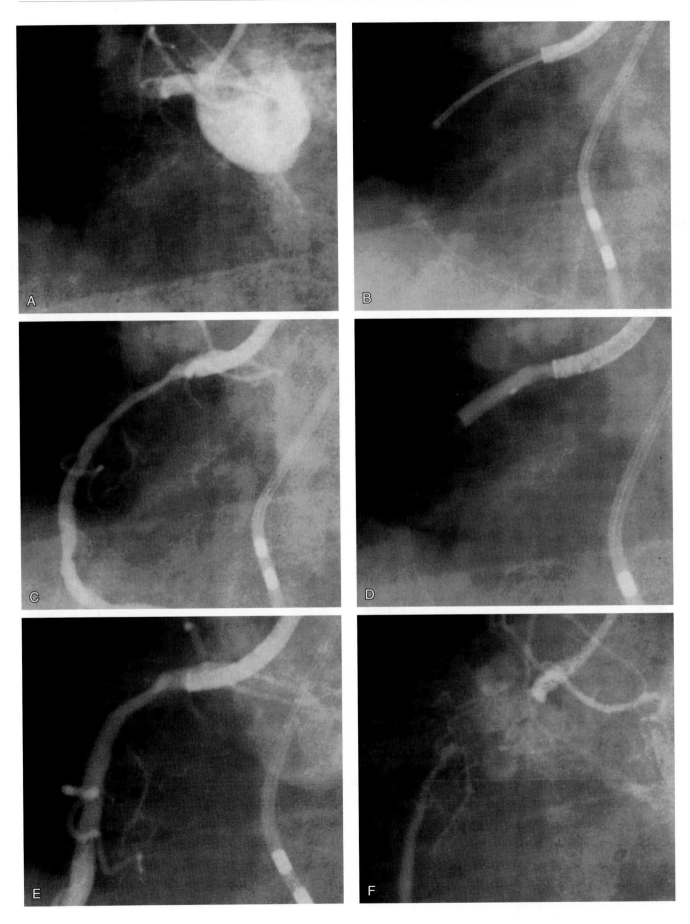

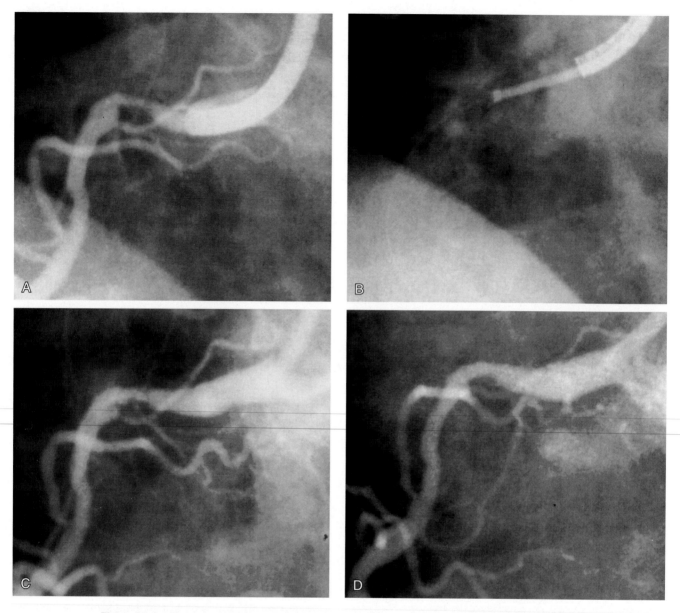

Figure 15–9

An angulated, eccentric stenosis in the proximal segment of the right coronary artery *(Panel A)* was treated with sequential passes of 6.0-French and 6.5-French TEC devices *(Panel B)*. After adjunct balloon angioplasty was used to treat a 60% residual stenosis (not shown), a 40% residual stenosis with a localized linear dissection was demonstrated *(Panel C)*. Despite the 40% residual stenosis, no loss in lumen diameter occurred during the 4 month follow-up period *(Panel D)*.

Although extraction atherectomy removes macroparticles through the use of continuous vacuum suction, distal embolization may still occur. Distal embolization during extraction atherectomy may develop in one of three settings: (1) after passage of the guide wire across the friable stenosis; (2) after passage of the TEC device; or, most often, (3) after adjunct balloon dilatation to maximize the final lumen diameter or treat complications. As a result, adjunct balloon angioplasty should be performed cautiously after extraction atherectomy, particularly in patients with degenerated SVGs; in high-risk patients, adjunct angioplasty should potentially be deferred for several days or weeks after the initial TEC device procedure.

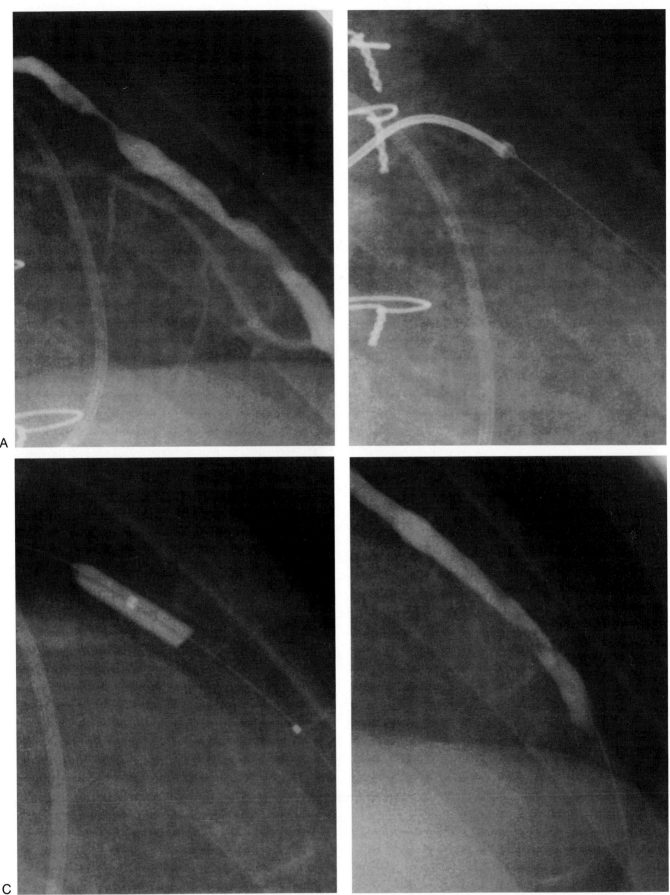

A

B

C

D

Figure 15–10
A tubular stenosis in the midsegment of a degenerated SVG to the left anterior descending artery *(Panel A)* was treated with sequential passes of a 2.5-mm TEC device *(Panel B)*. After extraction atherectomy, a 40% residual stenosis persisted; however, no evidence of distal embolization was seen (not shown). A 3.5-mm perfusion balloon was inflated across the residual lesion *(Panel C)*. Immediately after balloon deflation, the patient developed severe chest pain associated with anterior ST segment elevation. Repeat angiography demonstrated reduced flow into the distal vessel as well as intraluminal filling defects consistent with distal embolization *(Panel D)*.

SELECTED REFERENCES

Lasorda D, Incorvati D, Randall R. Extraction atherectomy during myocardial infarction in a patient with prior coronary artery bypass surgery. Cathet Cardiovasc Diagn 1992; 26:117–121.

Mehta S, Kramer B, Margolis J, Trautwein R. Transluminal extraction. Coron Artery Dis 1992; 3:887–896.

Popma J, Leon M, Mintz G, et al. Results of coronary angioplasty using the transluminal extraction catheter. Am J Cardiol 1992; 70:1526–1532.

Sketch M, Phillips H, Lee M, Stack R. Coronary transluminal extraction-endarterectomy. J Invasive Cardiol 1991; 3:13–18.

CHAPTER

16

Palmaz-Schatz Stents

A number of intracoronary stents have been introduced to scaffold the arterial lumen and reduce elastic recoil, which accounts for an initial 30% loss of the maximal lumen dimensions achieved with balloon angioplasty. The Palmaz-Schatz stent (PS stent) was first used in human coronary arteries in 1988 and has now been deployed in over 10,000 patients worldwide. The PS stent is a balloon-expandable stent constructed from cylindrical 0.08-mm stainless steel tubing. The slots of the tubing are offset, giving a diamond shaped appearance to the stent struts in the stent's fully expanded position. The PS stent was designed to render the arterial lumen resistant to radial collapse. The PS stent is 15 mm in length and has a single 1-mm articulation strut at its center; this provides maximum flexibility within the arterial lumen. Although investigators originally deployed the PS stent by crimping it onto a balloon dilatation catheter and subsequently delivering it through a 5-French Schneider delivery sheath, current PS stent designs now incorporate a dedicated stent, balloon catheter, and delivery sheath.

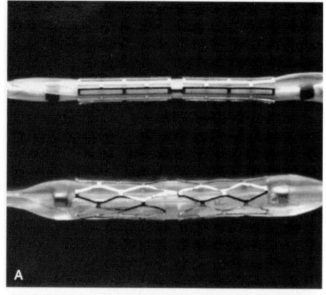

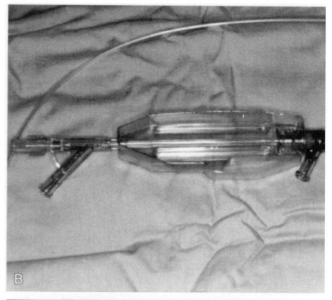

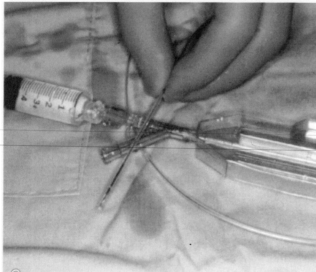

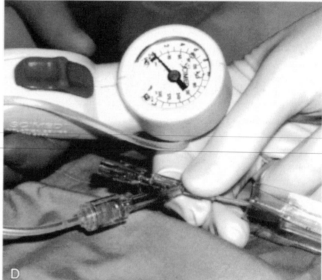

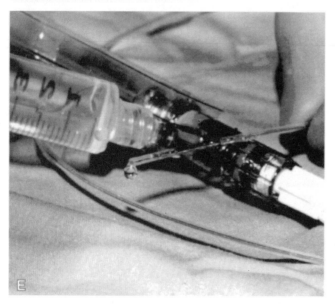

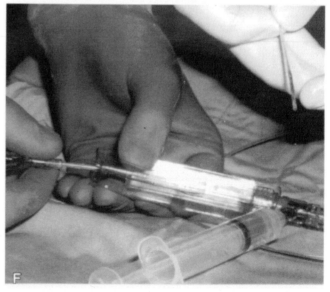

Figure 16–1

The PS stent is a 15-mm tubular slotted stent with a single 1-mm articulation strut. After balloon inflation, the tubular slotted stent struts take on a diamond-shaped appearance *(Panel A)*. The delivery system consists of a proximally placed sheath with a retaining sleeve that prevents retraction of the sheath proximally and inadvertent stent deployment *(Panel B)*. The central wire lumen is flushed with normal saline *(Panel C)*. A drop of a 50% mixture of iodinated contrast medium and normal saline is used to prepare the balloon catheter for the stent delivery system, but negative suction is not performed. Using a running "connection," the indeflator is connected to the balloon inflation port *(Panel D)*. The delivery sheath is then flushed in the proximal port *(Panel E)*. On positioning of the stent across the lesion, the retaining membrane is withdrawn *(Panel F)*.

Focal lesions in vessels greater than 3 mm in size are generally considered suitable for intracoronary stenting. It is essential that adequate coronary guiding catheter backup be obtained to provide maximum support for delivery of the PS stent. In addition, predilatation with an undersized balloon catheter is generally recommended. The size of the stent should be selected to approximate a 1:1 ratio to the normal reference segment adjacent to the coronary stenosis. Occasionally, offsetting the articulation strut from the cor-

onary stenosis may be necessary to allow full stent expansion and to avoid evagination of the stenosis into the 1-mm articulation strut. In general, adjunct balloon angioplasty after stent deployment should be performed with an appropriately sized noncompliant balloon dilatation catheter. Maximum stent deployment (residual stenosis <10%) is generally recommended in order to optimize long-term angiographic outcome.

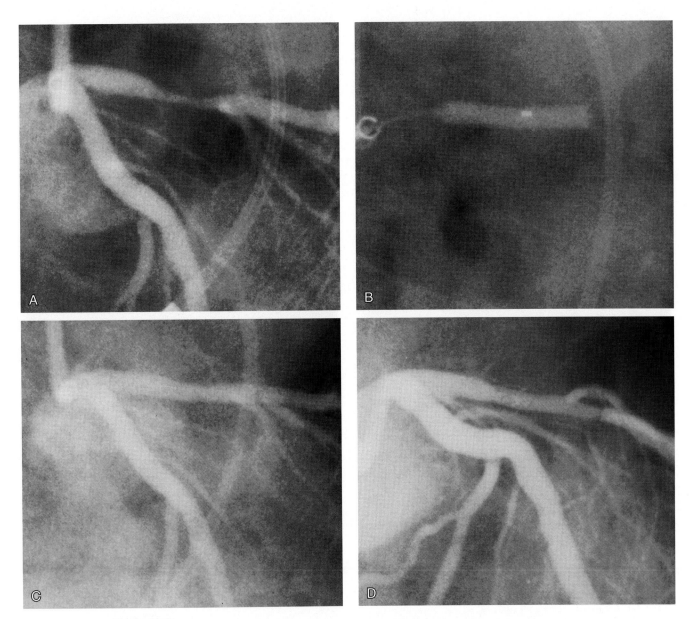

Figure 16–2
An eccentric lesion of the proximal left anterior descending artery *(Panel A)* was predilated with a 2.5-mm balloon. A 3.0-mm PS stent was deployed across the stenosis *(Panel B)* and resulted in a <10% residual stenosis *(Panel C)*. Adjunct balloon dilatation was performed with a noncompliant balloon. Although little change was noted in the residual diameter stenosis, intravascular ultrasound studies have demonstrated that adjunct balloon dilatation with the use of a noncompliance balloon results in more symmetric stent deployment and in firmer embedding of the stent struts into the vessel wall *(Panel D)*.

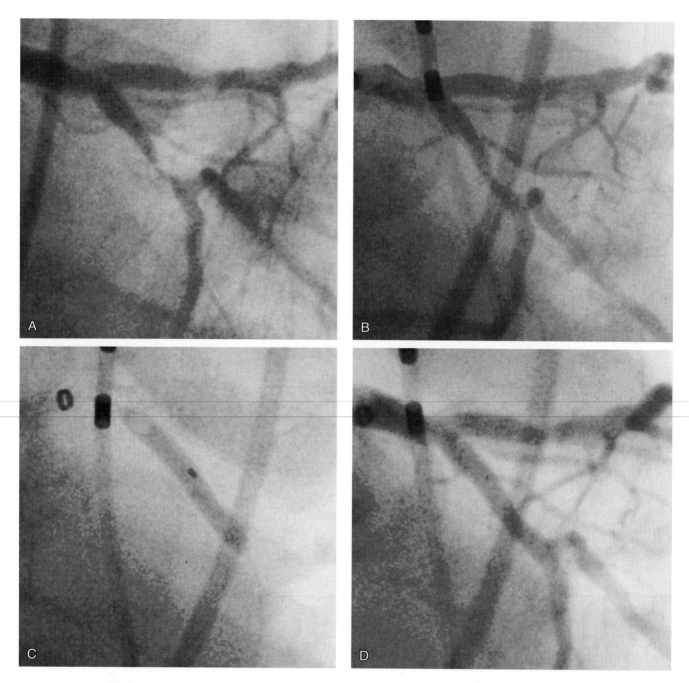

Figure 16–3
An eccentric stenosis of the proximal segment of the left circumflex *(Panel A)* was predilated with a
2.5-mm balloon *(Panel B)*. A 3.0-mm PS stent was deployed across the stenosis *(Panel C)* and
resulted in a <10% residual stenosis *(Panel D)*.

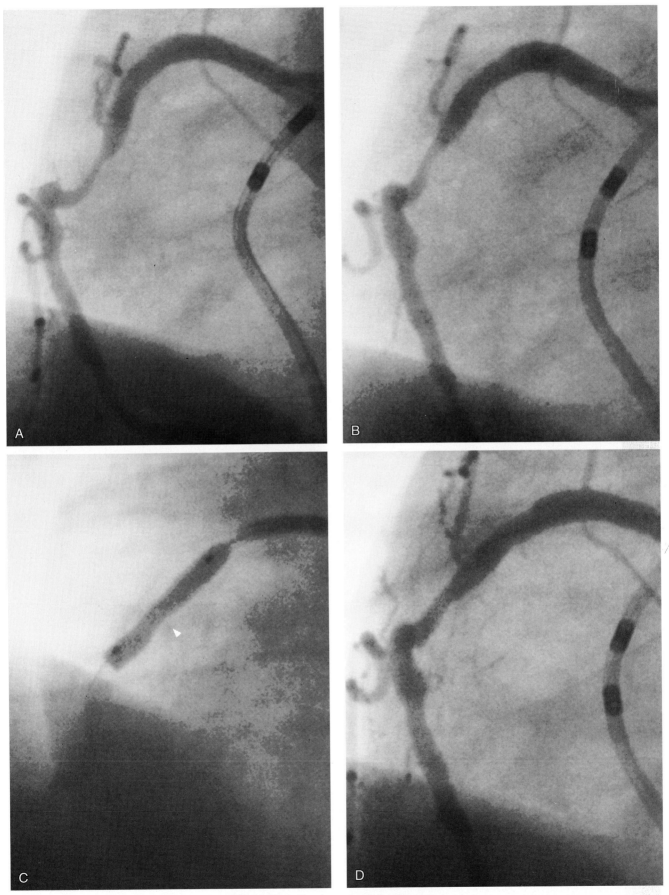

Figure 16–4. *See legend on following page*

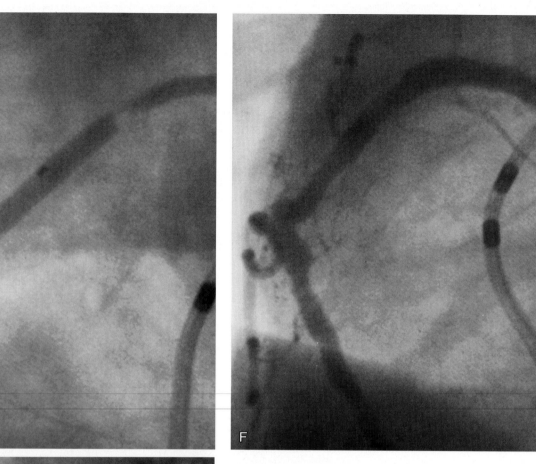

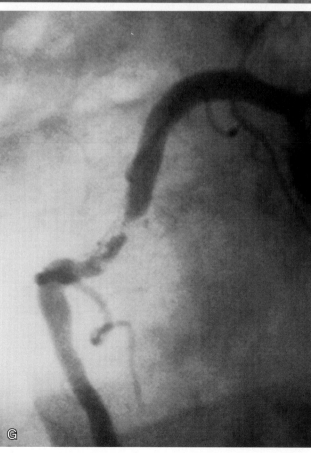

Figure 16–4

A tubular stenosis in the midportion of the right coronary artery *(Panel A)* was predilated with a 2.5-mm balloon catheter. After predilatation, a 50% residual stenosis was noted *(Panel B)*. A 3.0-mm PS stent was deployed; however, a significant waist was noted at the dilatation site *(arrow, Panel C)*. After stent deployment, a 30% residual stenosis remained *(Panel D)*. Adjunct balloon dilatation was performed to obtain a better initial result, but the lesion did not respond to high balloon pressures *(Panel E)*, and a 30% residual stenosis persisted *(Panel F)*. Two months later, the patient's symptoms recurred, and repeat angiography demonstrated restenosis within the stent *(Panel G)*.

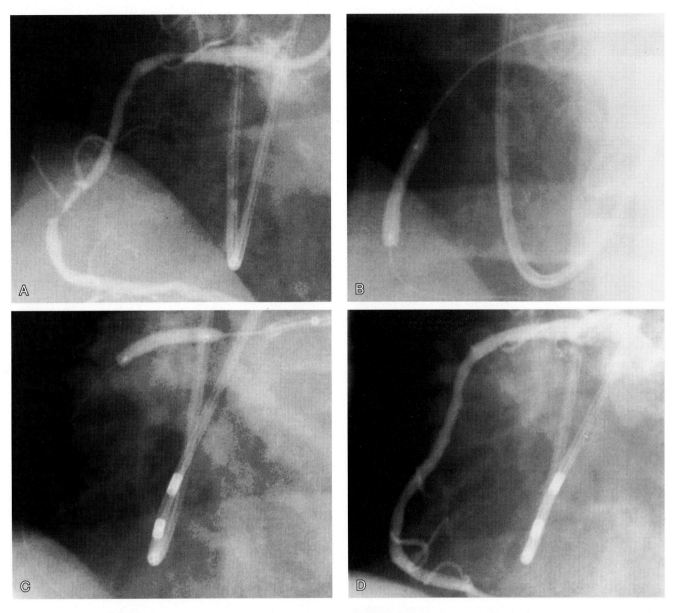

Figure 16–5
Two stenoses in the proximal and distal portions of the right coronary artery *(Panel A)* were predilated with a 2.5-mm balloon catheter. A 3.5-mm PS stent was deployed across the distal lesion *(Panel B)*, and 3.0-mm PS stent was deployed across the proximal stenosis *(Panel C)*. Following the stent deployments, an excellent angiographic result was obtained *(Panel D)*.

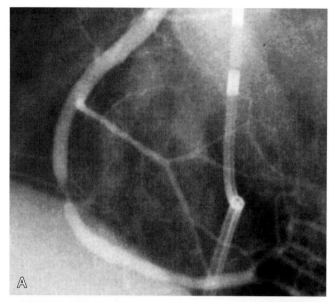

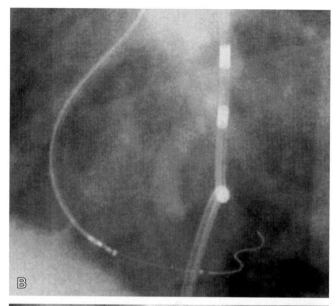

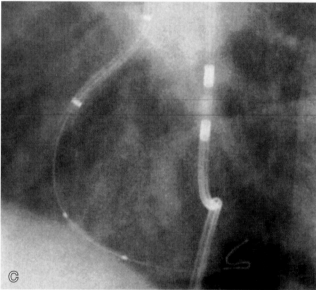

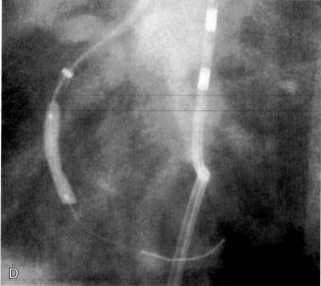

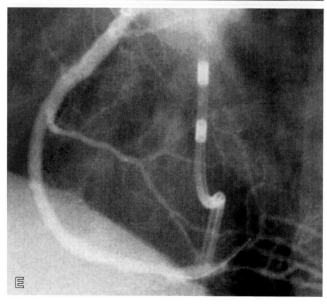

Figure 16–6

A 35-year-old heart transplant recipient developed accelerated atherosclerosis of the right coronary artery. Restenosis developed after two prior angioplasty attempts. Coronary arteriography demonstrated recurrent stenosis in the midportion of the right coronary artery *(Panel A)*. Intracoronary ultrasound was performed *(Panel B)* and demonstrated mild atherosclerotic involvement of the proximal and distal segments adjacent to the coronary stenosis. Following predilatation with a 2.5-mm balloon catheter, a 3.5-mm PS stent was advanced across the stenosis *(Panel C)* and inflated to 6 atm *(Panel D)*. An excellent anatomic result was obtained *(Panel E)*.

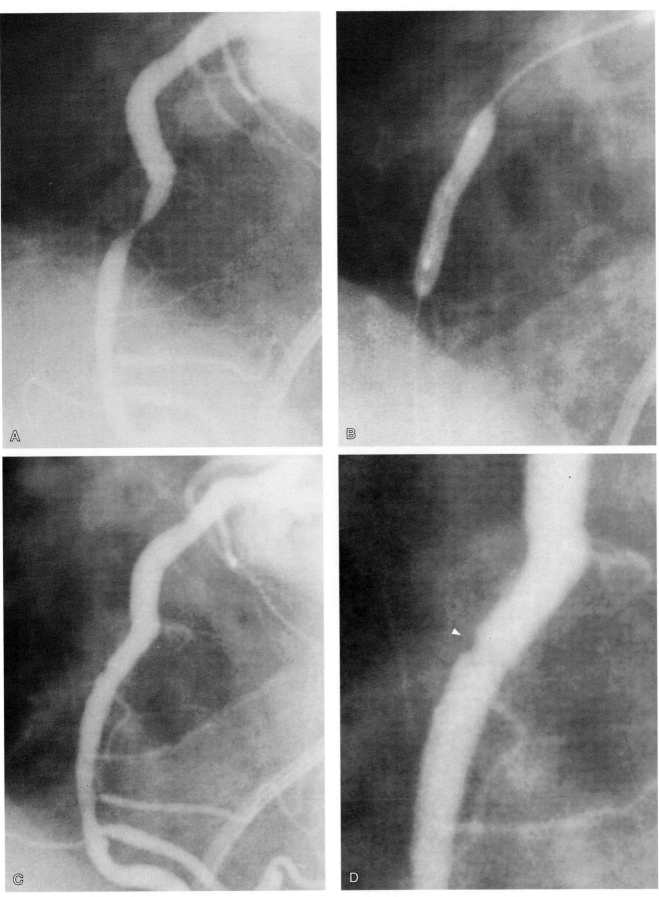

Figure 16–7
A concentric stenosis in the midportion of the right coronary artery *(Panel A)* was predilated with a
2.5-mm balloon catheter. A 3.0-mm PS stent was advanced across the stenosis and inflated to 6 atm
(Panel B). Although a <10% visual stenosis was obtained *(Panel C)*, a residual stenosis was noted at
the articulation strut on a magnified view *(arrow, Panel D)*.

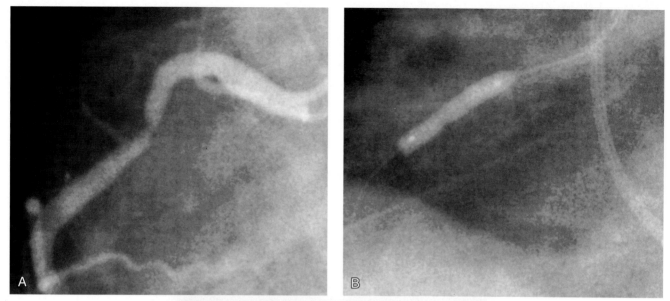

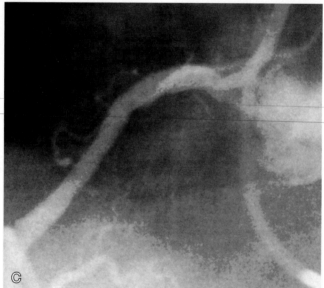

Figure 16–8
An eccentric stenosis in the midportion of the right coronary artery *(Panel A)* was predilated with a 2.5-mm balloon catheter. A 3.0-mm PS stent was deployed across the stenosis *(Panel B)*, resulting in a 20% residual stenosis *(Panel C)*. Note the straightening of the vessel after stent implantation.

Figure 16–9
Sequential stenoses in the midbody of a SVG to the left anterior descending artery *(Panel A)* were predilated with a 2.5-mm balloon catheter. Two 3.0-mm PS stents were placed in the distal and proximal stenoses *(Panel B)*, resulting in a 20% residual stenosis at the articulation strut in the more proximal lesion *(Panel C)*. Four months later, the patient's symptoms recurred, and repeat angiography demonstrated restenosis in the proximal stent *(Panel D)*. Repeat dilatation was performed with a 3.5-mm balloon catheter *(Panel E)*, resulting in a 20% residual stenosis *(Panel F)*.

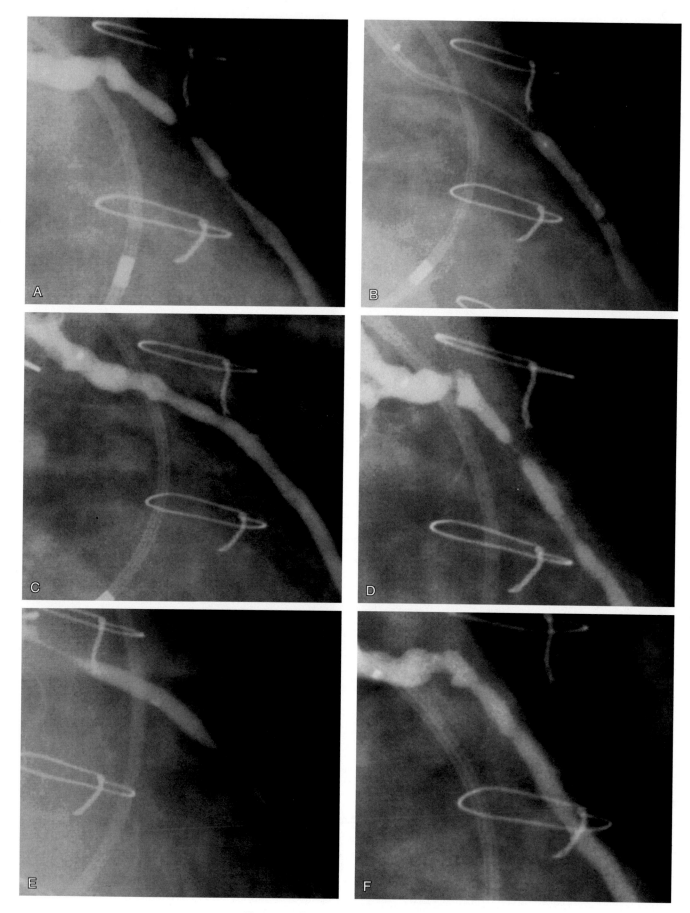

Figure 16–9. *See legend on opposite page*

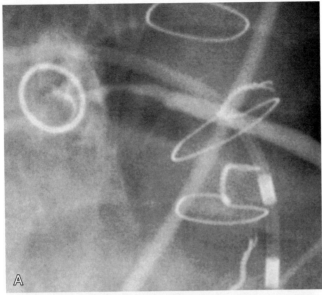

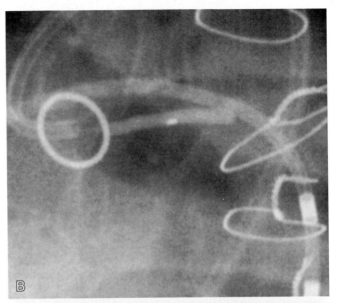

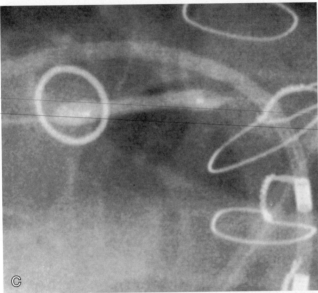

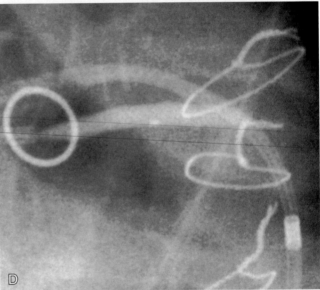

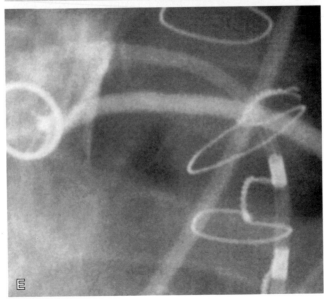

Figure 16–10
An ostial stenosis of the SVG to the obtuse marginal branch *(Panel A)* was treated with a 2.5-mm balloon catheter *(Panel B)*. A 3.0-mm PS stent was inflated across the ostial stenosis; however, incomplete stent expansion due to lesion rigidity or extensive plaque was noted *(Panel C)*. A 3.5-mm noncompliant balloon was inflated across the ostial stenosis and inflated to 14 atm *(Panel D)*. After final balloon deflation, a 10% residual stenosis was obtained *(Panel E)*.

Subacute thrombosis occurs in 2% to 5% of patients who undergo stent placement, developing more often in those patients receiving the procedure emergently. Subacute thrombosis is related to the size of the vessel, the presence of residual dissection following stent deployment, outflow obstruction, and the presence of thrombus. It can be managed with repeat dilatation and intracoronary thrombolytic agents; however, myocardial infarction may occur.

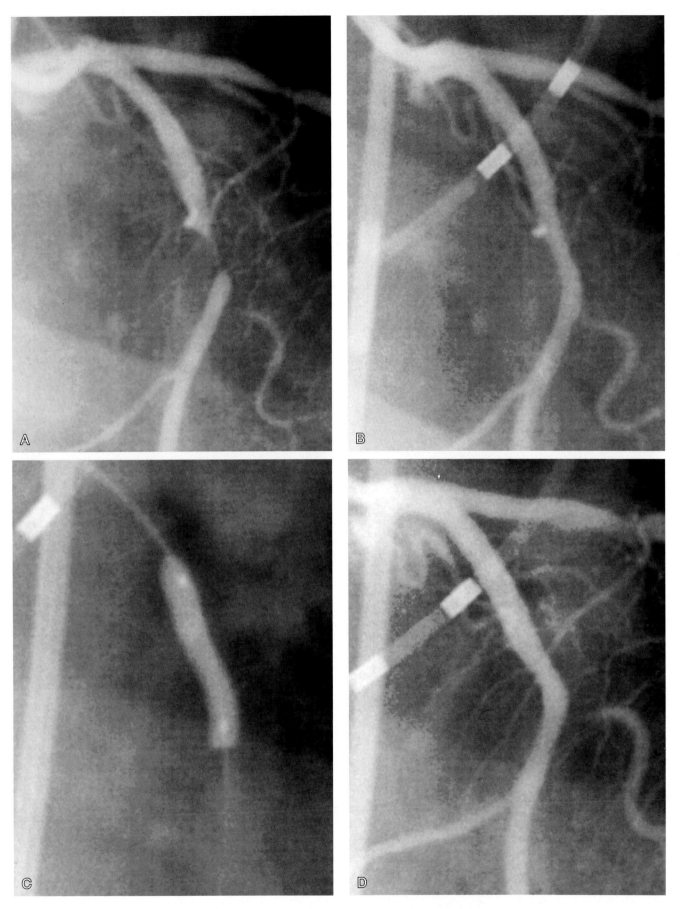

Figure 16–11. *See legend on following page*

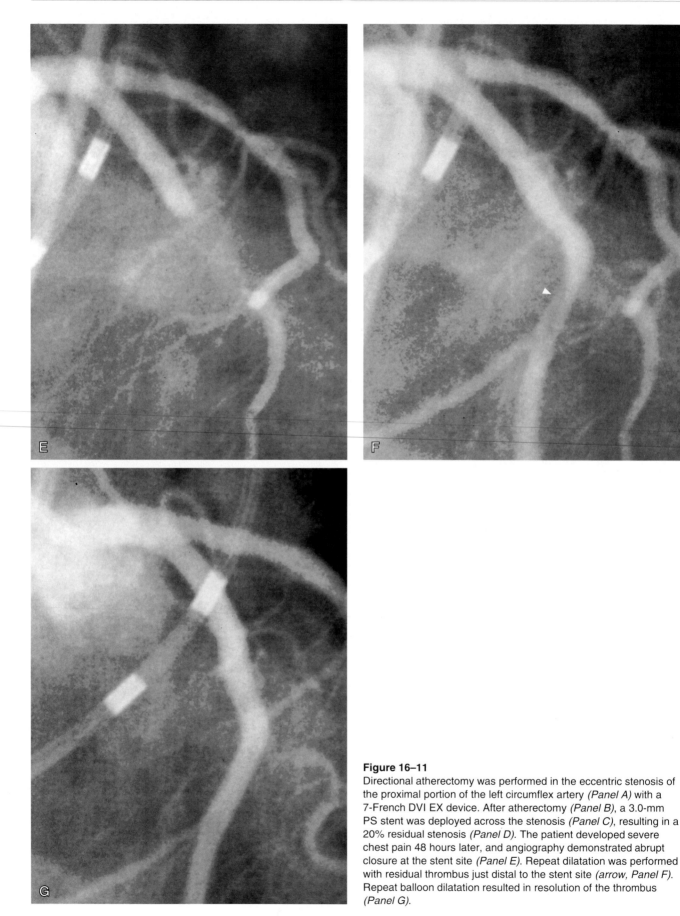

Figure 16–11
Directional atherectomy was performed in the eccentric stenosis of
the proximal portion of the left circumflex artery *(Panel A)* with a
7-French DVI EX device. After atherectomy *(Panel B)*, a 3.0-mm
PS stent was deployed across the stenosis *(Panel C)*, resulting in a
20% residual stenosis *(Panel D)*. The patient developed severe
chest pain 48 hours later, and angiography demonstrated abrupt
closure at the stent site *(Panel E)*. Repeat dilatation was performed
with residual thrombus just distal to the stent site *(arrow, Panel F)*.
Repeat balloon dilatation resulted in resolution of the thrombus
(Panel G).

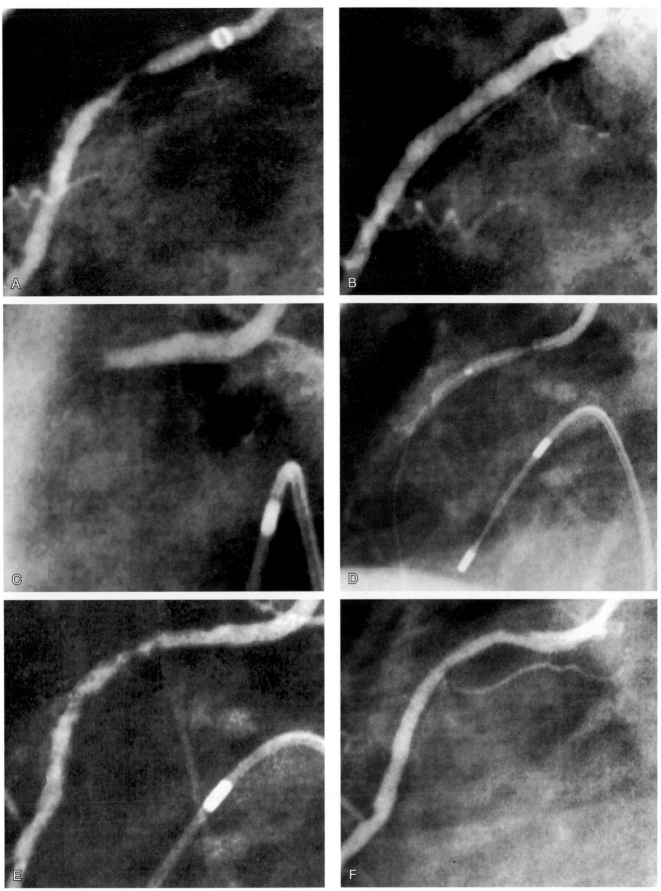

Figure 16–12

A restenotic lesion in the proximal portion of the right coronary artery *(Panel A)* of this patient was treated with a 3.0-mm PS stent with an excellent anatomic result *(Panel B)*. Inadvertent discontinuation of heparin administration 12 hours after stent deployment resulted in abrupt vessel closure *(Panel C)*. Repeat angiography demonstrated occlusion in the proximal right coronary artery, and balloon angioplasty was immediately performed *(Panel D)*. Following successful recanalization, intraluminal thrombus remained (multiple small filling defects) *(Panel E)*. Intracoronary urokinase, 250,000 U, was administered, and 24 hours later a patent coronary artery was noted *(Panel F)*; however, the result was not as favorable as the initial outcome *(Panel B)*.

The PS stent has also been used to treat acute and chronic dissections occurring after conventional balloon angioplasty. The tubular slotted stent design scaffolds the dissection flaps onto the vessel wall, improving anterograde flow.

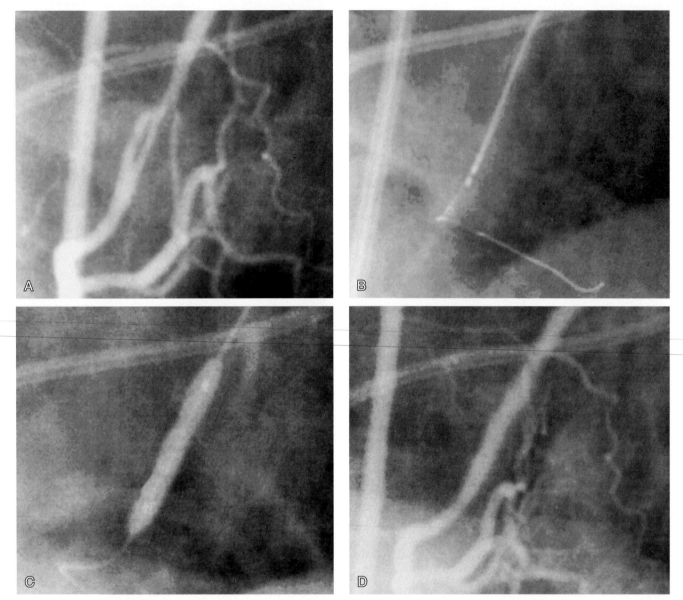

Figure 16–13

Six months after this patient underwent balloon angioplasty of the distal portion of the right coronary artery, "true" and "false" arterial lumens resulted from a chronic dissection *(Panel A)*. Intracoronary ultrasound was used to identify the true lumen *(Panel B)*, and a 3.5-mm stent was deployed across the stenosis *(Panel C)*. After balloon deflation, an excellent residual stenosis was obtained, and the false lumen was obliterated *(Panel D)*. (Reprinted from Schryver T, Popma J, Kent K, et al. Use of intracoronary ultrasound to identify the "true" coronary lumen in chronic coronary dissection treated with intracoronary stenting. Am J Cardiol 1992; 69:1107, with permission.)

Figure 16–14

Coronary arteriography demonstrated a noncalcified stenosis in the ostium of the left anterior descending artery *(Panel A)*. A 7-French DVI EX atherectomy device was advanced across the lesion, and circumferential cuts at 20 psi were performed *(Panel B)*. Although the ostial lesion was successfully treated with directional atherectomy, a distal nose cone dissection was noted *(Panel C)*. Prolonged balloon inflation was performed *(Panel D)*; however, the dissection persisted. A 3.5-mm PS stent was used to "tack up" the nose cone–induced coronary dissection *(Panel E)*. Following stent deployment, an excellent anatomic result was obtained *(Panel F)*.

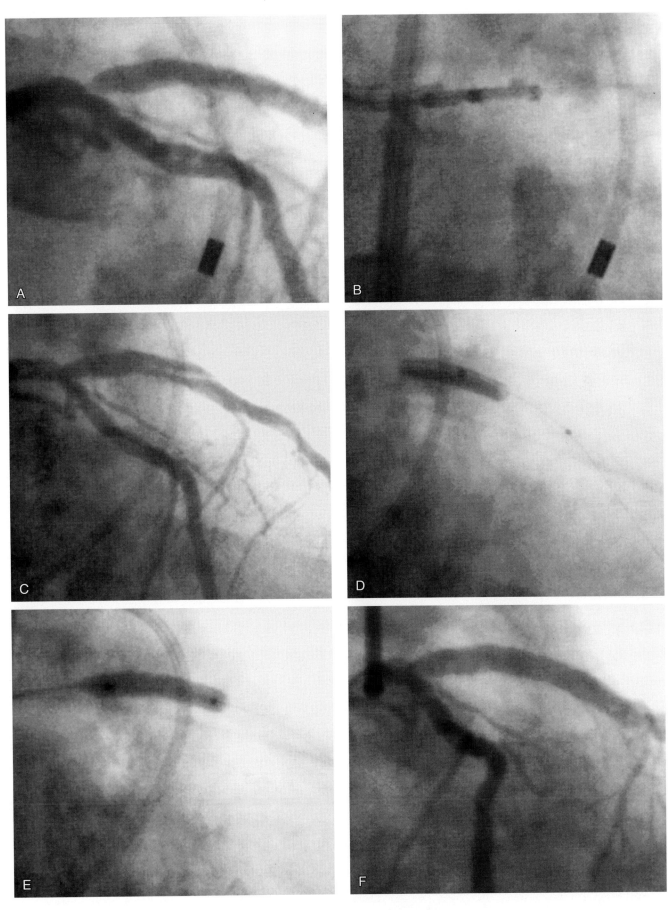

Figure 16–14. *See legend on opposite page*

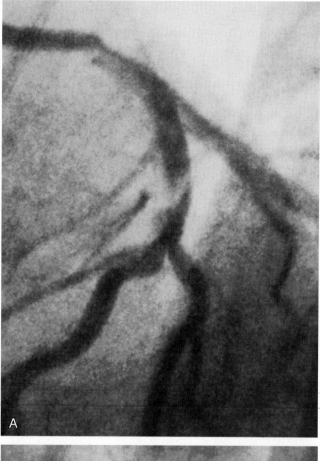

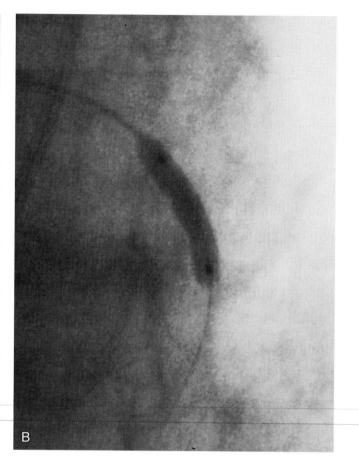

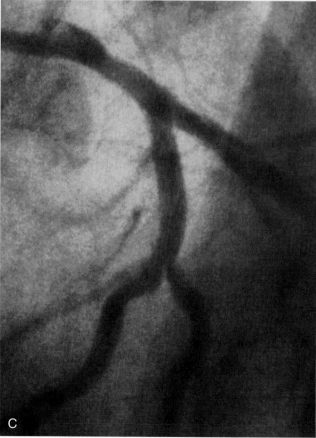

Figure 16–15
Following coronary angioplasty of an eccentric stenosis in the midportion of the left anterior descending artery, a severe coronary dissection developed, limiting anterograde coronary perfusion *(Panel A)*. A 3.5-mm PS stent was deployed across the lesion *(Panel B)*, ''tacking up'' the dissection flap *(Panel C)* and yielding an excellent angiographic result.

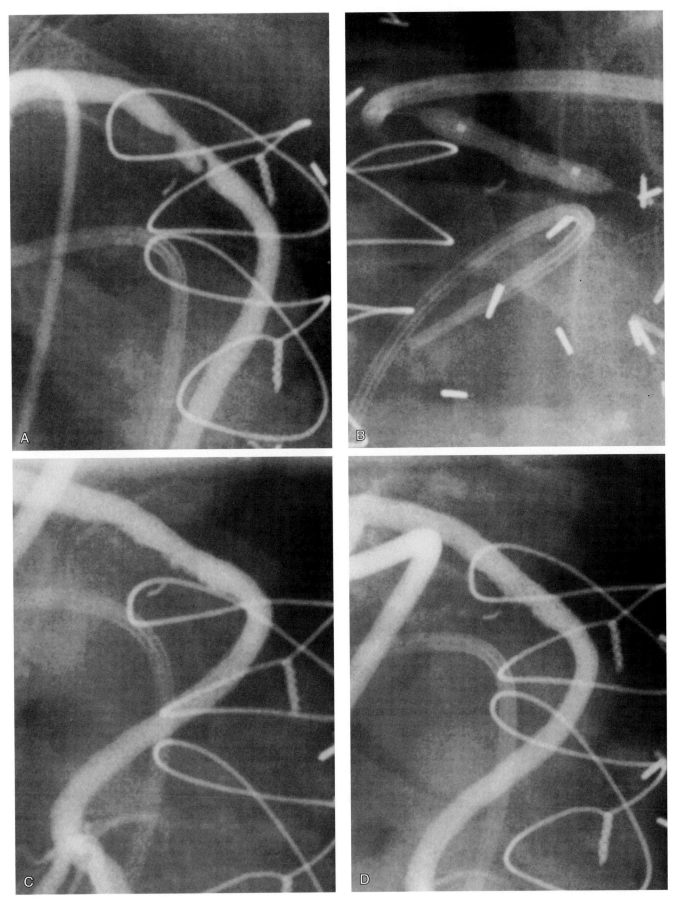

Figure 16–16
An ulcerated stenosis in the midportion of the SVG to the obtuse marginal branch *(Panel A)* was predilated with a 2.5-mm balloon catheter. A 4.0-mm PS 204 stent was positioned across the ulcerated lesion and inflated to 6 atm *(Panel B)*. After stent deployment, a 20% residual stenosis was obtained *(Panel C)*, and adjunct balloon dilatation with a noncompliant balloon was performed to minimize the residual stenosis and to fully deploy the stent struts against the wall of the SVG *(Panel D)*.

Although use of the coronary PS stent has not yet been approved by the Food and Drug Administration, use of the larger ''biliary'' tubular slotted stent in native vessels and in SVGs has been reported at several centers. The biliary stents are generally thicker than the native coronary stents and have a higher radial compressive strength (Table 16–1). Biliary stents are deployed using peripheral balloon catheters that are ≥4.0 mm in diameter. As a result, biliary stents have been used in larger SVGs and native coronary vessels to treat angiographic complications after standard balloon angioplasty and to prevent restenosis by providing a larger initial lumen.

Table 16–1   Coronary and Biliary Stent Configuration

	Coronary PS 153	Biliary PS 204	Biliary PS 104	Biliary PS 154
Expansion range (mm)	3–6	4–7	4–9	4–9
Pre-expansion length (mm)	15.3	20	10	15
Postexpansion length (mm)	11.2–15.0	16.9–19.0	7.8–9.9	11.6–14.7
Stent thickness				
In inches	0.0025	0.0040	0.0055	0.0055
In millimeters	0.635	1.016	1.397	1.397
Average radial force at 4 mm diameter, psi (mm Hg)	6.6 (341)	11.5 (595)	25.2 (1303)	24 (1241)

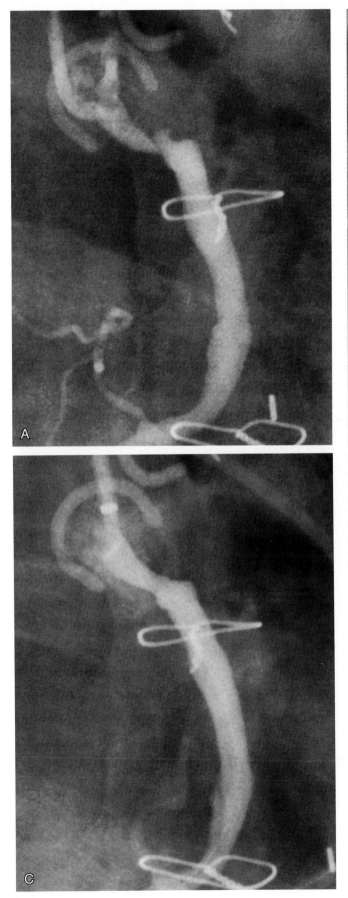

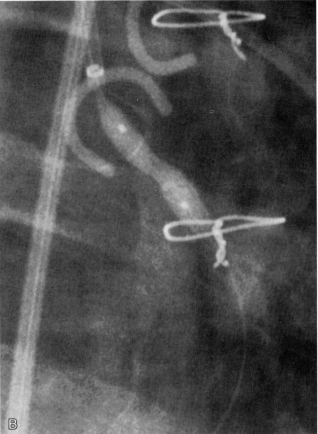

Figure 16–17
An eccentric, ulcerated stenosis involving the ostium of the SVG to the right coronary artery *(Panel A)* was predilated with a 2.5-mm balloon catheter. A PS 204 stent was deployed across the ostium with the guiding catheter withdrawn *(Panel B).* Adjunct balloon dilatation was performed with a 4.0-mm noncompliant balloon catheter; however, a significant waist persisted at the ostium (not shown). After final balloon deflation, a 40% residual stenosis remained *(Panel C).*

In order to alter lesion rigidity or to ''debulk'' extensive plaque typically noted in ostial SVG lesions, partial plaque ''debulking'' using directional atherectomy, extraction atherectomy, or excimer laser angioplasty may be useful prior to stent deployment.

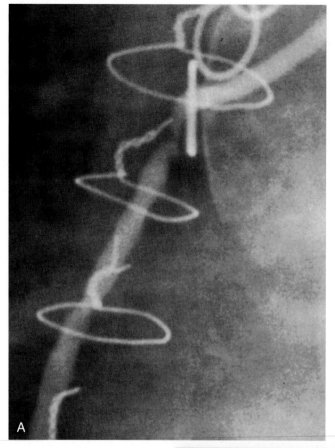
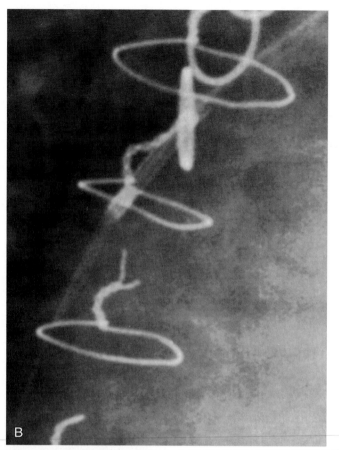
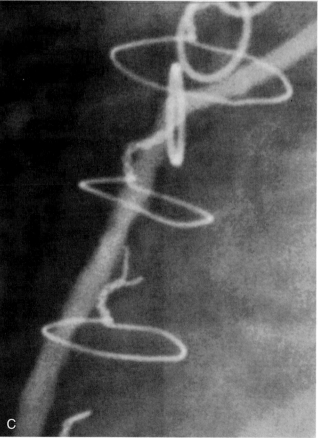

Figure 16–18. *See legend on opposite page*

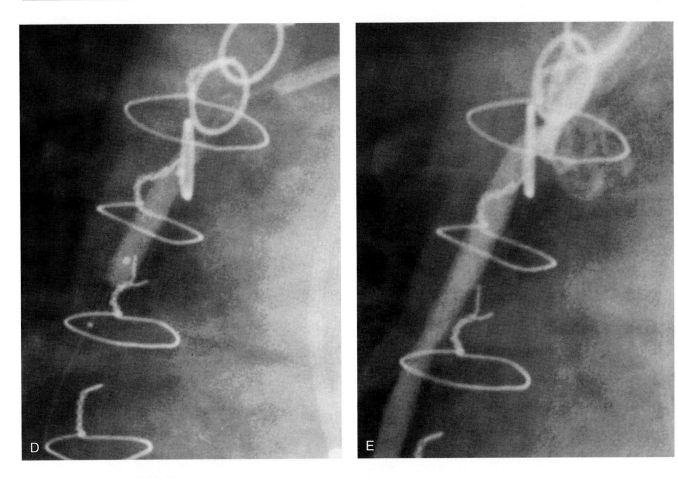

Figure 16–18

An ostial lesion involving the SVG to the posterior descending branch *(Panel A)* was pretreated with directional atherectomy using a 7-French DVI EX device *(Panel B)*. After circumferential cuts were made, a moderate amount of tissue was removed, and a 30% residual stenosis resulted *(Panel C)*. A PS 204 stent was deployed on a 4.5-mm compliant balloon *(Panel D)*, yielding an excellent angiographic result with slight ectasia at the treatment site *(Panel E)*.

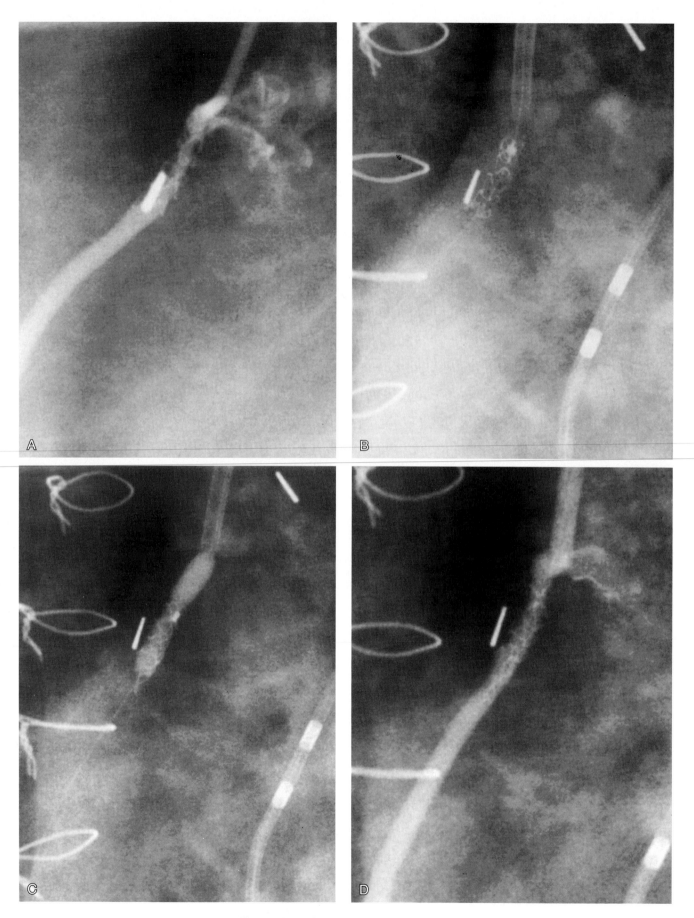

Figure 16–19. *See legend on opposite page*

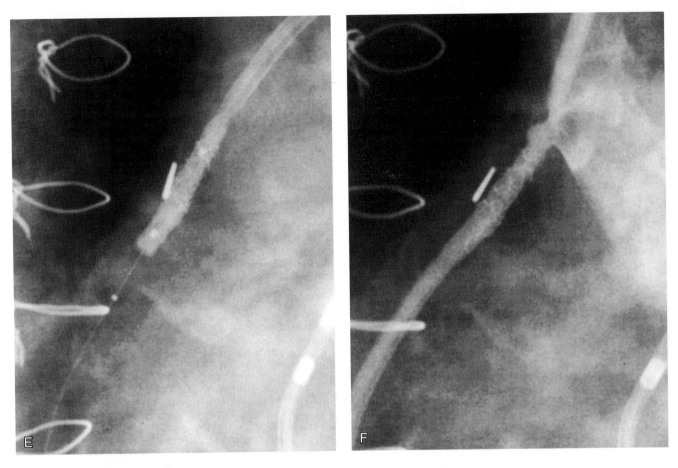

Figure 16–19
Restenosis developed in this patient 3 months after Wiktor stent deployment in the ostium of the SVG to the right coronary artery *(Panel A)*. The radiopaque stent filaments were easily visualized *(Panel B)*. Predilatation with a 2.5-mm balloon catheter *(Panel C)* resulted in a 40% residual stenosis *(Panel D)*. A PS 204 stent was deployed within the lesion with a 4.0-mm compliant balloon *(Panel E)*, resulting in an excellent angiographic outcome *(Panel F)*.

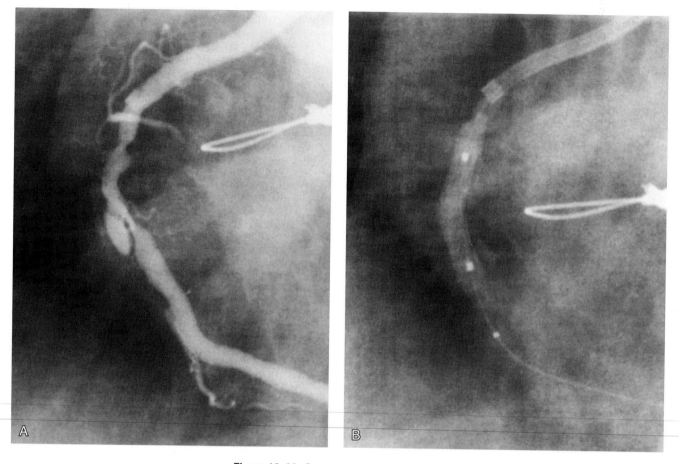

Figure 16–20. *See legend on opposite page*

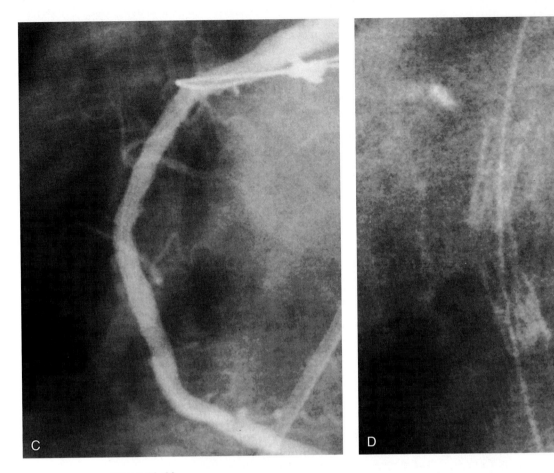

Figure 16–20
A localized pseudoaneurysm developed in this patient 2 months after coronary angioplasty *(Panel A)*.
Predilatation was performed with a 2.5-mm balloon catheter, and a 4.0-mm PS 204 stent was
deployed with the use of a 4.0-mm compliant balloon *(Panel B)*. After balloon deflation, the cavity of
the pseudoaneurysm was obliterated, and excellent flow into the distal vessel was demonstrated
(Panel C). The radiolucent stainless steel stent was visualized angiographically on account of its
thickness (magnified view) *(Panel D)*.

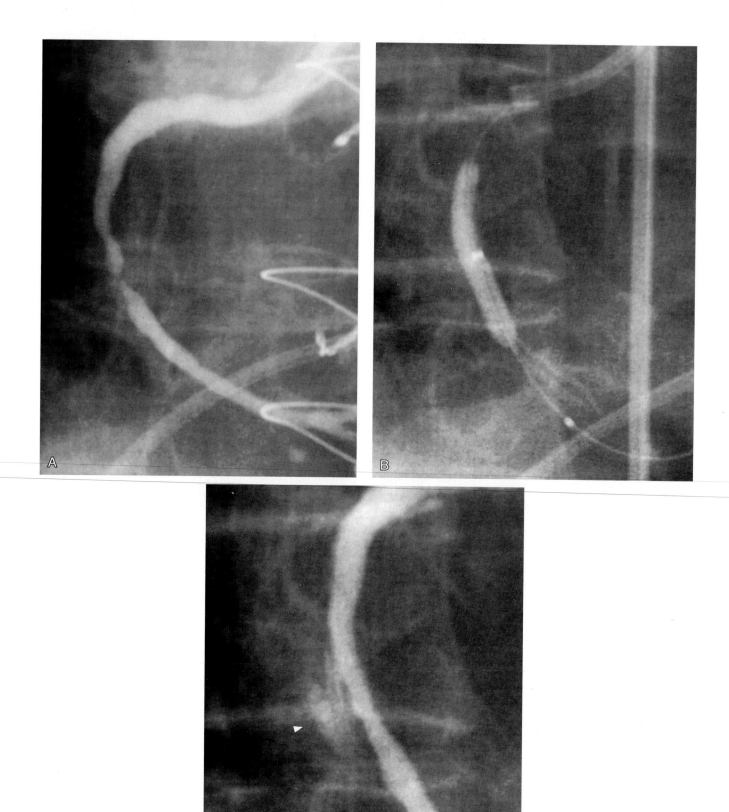

Figure 16–21. *See legend on opposite page*

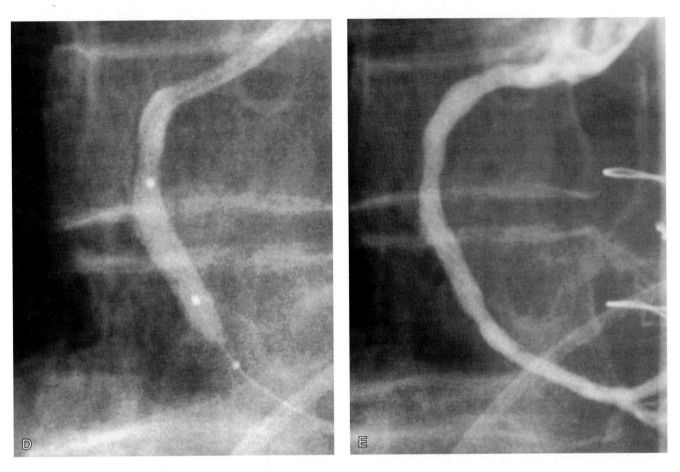

Figure 16–21
A subtotal stenosis in the midportion of the SVG to the posterior descending artery *(Panel A)* was treated with a 3.5-mm balloon dilatation catheter *(Panel B)*. After balloon deflation, mild extravasation of contrast medium was observed at the site of dilatation *(arrow, Panel C)*. Nevertheless, a 4.0-mm PS 204 stent was deployed across the site *(Panel D)*, resulting in an excellent angiographic outcome and in the sealing of the localized perforation *(Panel E)*.

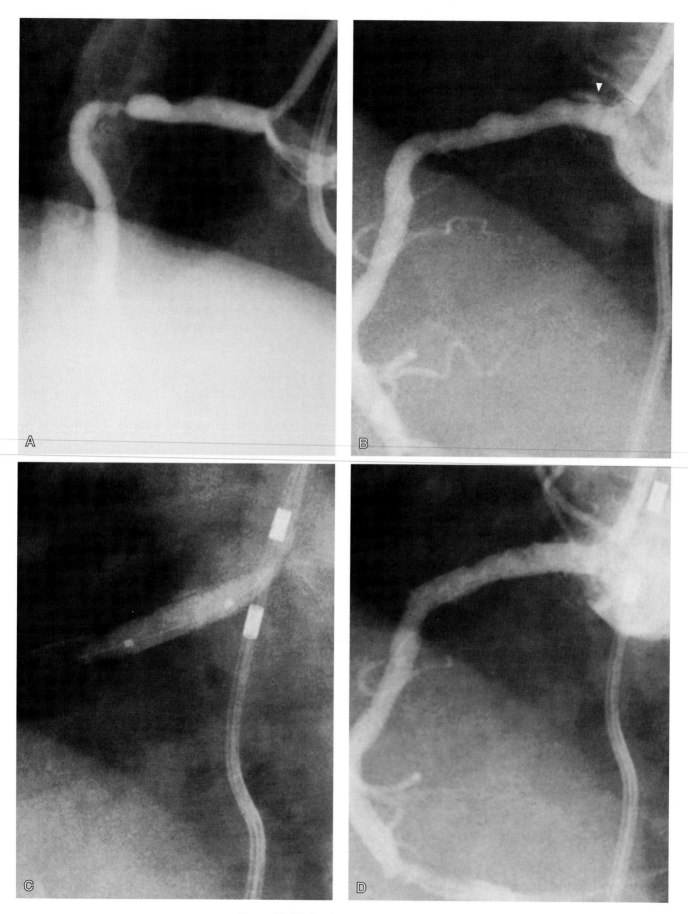

Figure 16–22. *See legend on opposite page*

Figure 16–22

A concentric stenosis in the proximal portion of the right coronary artery was treated with standard balloon angioplasty *(Panel A)*. A guiding catheter dissection developed at the ostium of the right coronary artery *(arrow, Panel B)*. The artery deteriorated, causing a reduction in anterograde perfusion *(Panel C)*. A PS 154 stent was deployed on a 4.0-mm noncompliant balloon within the ostium of the right coronary artery *(Panel D)*, yielding an excellent angiographic result and the restoration of coronary perfusion.

SELECTED REFERENCES

Carrozza J, Kuntz R, Fishman R, et al. Multivessel coronary intervention with a balloon-expandable intracoronary stent. Coron Artery Dis 1992; 3:403–406.

Carrozza J, Kuntz R, Levine M, et al. Angiographic and clinical outcome of intracoronary stenting: Immediate and long-term results from a large single-center experience. J Am Coll Cardiol 1992; 20:328–337.

Colombo A, Hall P, Thomas J, et al. Initial experience with the disarticulated (one-half) Palmaz-Schatz stent: A technical report. Cathet Cardiovasc Diagn 1992; 25:304–308.

Colombo A, Maiello L, Almagor Y, et al. Coronary stenting: Single institution experience with the initial 100 cases using the Palmaz-Schatz stent. Cathet Cardiovasc Diagn 1992; 26:171–176.

Ellis S, Savage M, Fischman D, et al. Restenosis after placement of Palmaz-Schatz stents in native coronary arteries: Initial results of a multicenter experience. Circulation 1992; 86:1836–1844.

Fischman D, Savage M, Leon M, et al. Effect of intracoronary stenting on intimal dissection after balloon angioplasty: Results of quantitative and qualitative coronary analysis. J Am Coll Cardiol 1992; 18:1445–1451.

Jenny D, Robert G, Fajadet J, et al. Intracoronary stent implantation: New approach using a monorail system and new large-lumen 7F catheters from the brachial route. Cathet Cardiovasc Diagn 1992; 25:297–299.

Kuntz R, Hinohara T, Robertson G, et al. Influence of vessel selection on the observed restenosis rate after endoluminal stenting or directional atherectomy. Am J Cardiol 1992; 70:1101–1108.

Kuntz R, Safian R, Carrozza J, et al. The importance of acute luminal diameter in determining restenosis after coronary atherectomy or stenting. Circulation 1992; 86:1827–1835.

Mansour M, Carrozza J, Kuntz R, et al. Frequency and outcome of chest pain after two new coronary interventions (atherectomy and stenting). Am J Cardiol 1992; 69:1379–1382.

Schatz R, Baim D, Leon M, et al. Clinical experience with the Palmaz-Schatz coronary stent: Initial results of a multicenter study. Circulation 1991; 83:148–161.

Schryver T, Popma J, Kent K, et al. Use of intracoronary ultrasound to identify the "true" coronary lumen in chronic coronary dissection treated with intracoronary stenting. Am J Cardiol 1992; 69:1107–1108.

VerLee P, Muller D, Popma J, et al. A comparison of clinical and quantitative angiographic outcomes of coronary stenting in elective and emergency settings: A single center experience. Coron Artery Dis 1991; 2:945–951.

CHAPTER

17

Gianturco-Roubin Stents

Abrupt closure occurs after coronary angioplasty in 2% to 8% of patients and remains a major limitation of the procedure. Intracoronary stents aid in the management of patients with acute and threatened abrupt closure due to coronary dissection, often obviating the need for emergency bypass surgery. Although the Gianturco-Roubin (GR) stent was initially used as a bridge to surgery in patients with abrupt vessel closure after balloon angioplasty, it is currently used as a definitive treatment for acute or threatened abrupt closure after coronary angioplasty and obviates the need for subsequent urgent bypass surgery. Important contraindications to stenting include a bleeding diathesis that precludes systemic anticoagulation, a vessel size that is

<2.5 mm, significant proximal vessel tortuosity, and the presence of a large amount of thrombus. In addition, vessels with poor distal run-off are generally not suitable for intracoronary stenting.

The GR stent is comprised of a 0.006-inch stainless steel filament shaped into an interdigitating coil and wrapped tightly onto a deflated polyethylene balloon angioplasty catheter. It is 20 mm in length, is available in stent diameters of from 2.0 to 4.0 mm, and is delivered with a 0.016- or 0.018-inch coronary guide wire. Notably, the GR stent is mounted on a compliant balloon that is 0.5 mm larger than the nominal stent size.

Figure 17–1
Preparation of the GR stent *(Panel A)* begins with inspection of the stent to make certain that no frayed stent struts are present *(Panel B)*. The central lumen is flushed with saline *(Panel C)*, and a 10- to 20-mL syringe containing 5 mL of contrast medium is used to apply negative pressure to the balloon lumen *(Panels D and E)*. A stopcock may be used for connection to the inflation device *(Panel F)*.

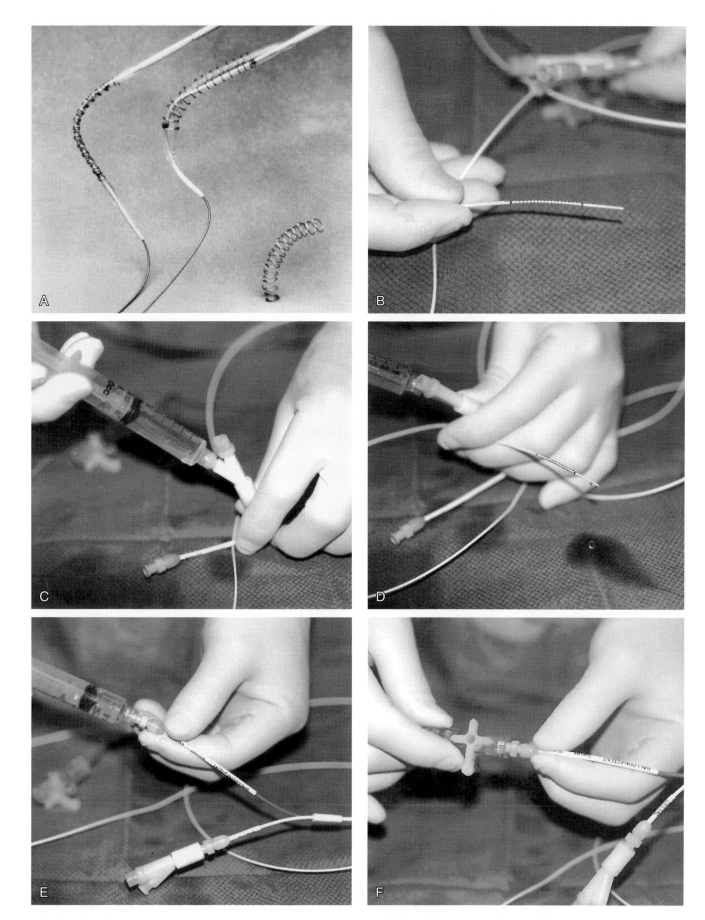

Figure 17–1. *See legend on opposite page*

Currently, the primary indication for the use of the GR stent is the treatment of abrupt or threatened vessel closure due to coronary dissection. Identification of the most distal aspect of the dissection prior to stent deployment is of critical importance, as the most distal stent should always be deployed first. Failure to stent the most distal aspect of the dissection may result in outflow obstruction and stent thrombosis.

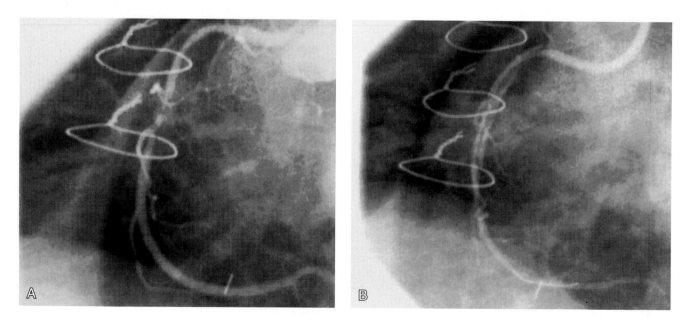

Figure 17–2. *See legend on opposite page*

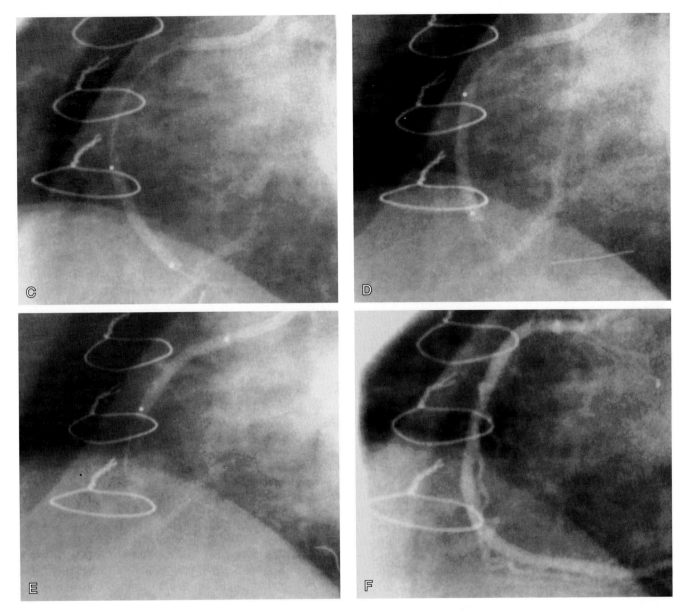

Figure 17–2
A concentric stenosis in the midsegment of the right coronary artery was treated with standard balloon angioplasty *(Panel A)*. This resulted in a spiral dissection that involved the entire right coronary artery *(Panel B)*. Three 2.5-mm GR stents were sequentially deployed in the distal *(Panel C)*, medial *(Panel D)*, and proximal *(Panel E)* segments of the right coronary artery, yielding an excellent anatomic result *(Panel F)*. Repeat arteriography 6 months later demonstrated a widely patent vessel.

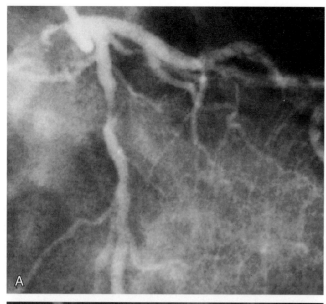

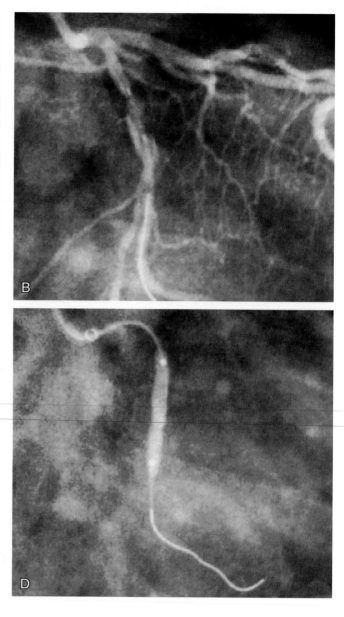

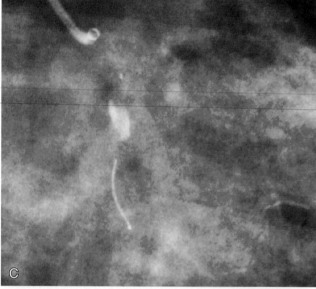

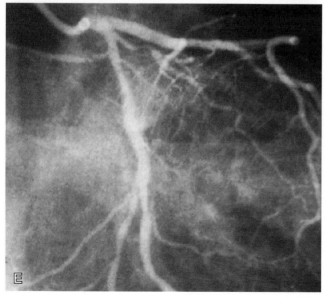

Figure 17–3

An irregular lesion of the midportion of the left circumflex was treated with standard balloon angioplasty *(Panel A)*. Following single-balloon inflation using a 2.5-mm fixed-wire balloon catheter, an extensive spiral dissection developed *(Panel B)*. Contrast medium staining was noted after subsequent balloon inflations failed to resolve the coronary dissection *(Panel C)*. A 0.018-inch wire was advanced across the stenosis, and a 3.0-mm GR stent was advanced across the lesion *(Panel D)*. Following balloon inflation, an excellent anatomic result was obtained with restoration of anterograde flow *(Panel E)*. Stiffer 0.018-inch wires are thought to provide enhanced forward support for deployment of the GR stent and are therefore usually used.

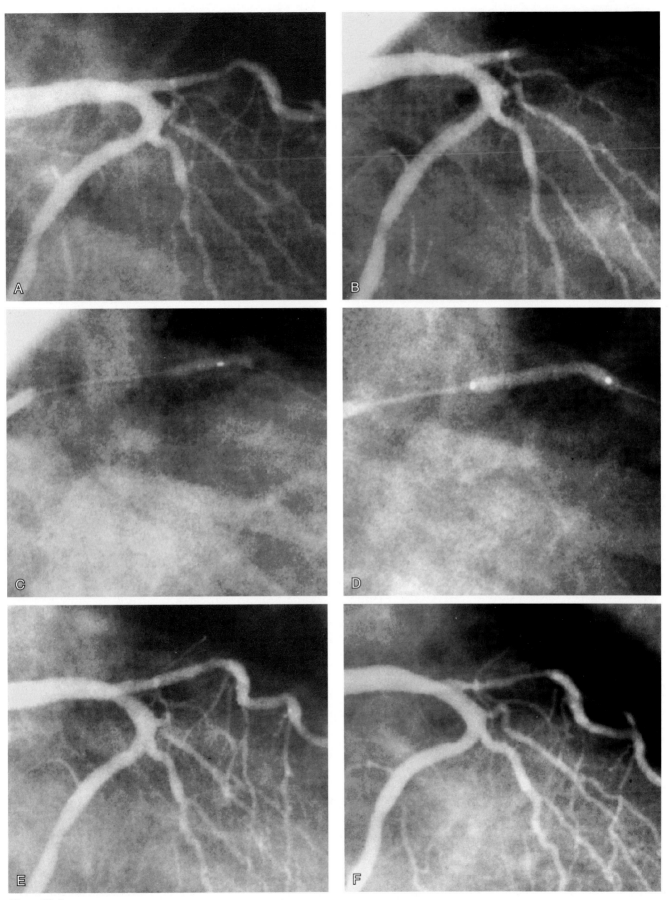

Figure 17–4

A long, concentric stenosis was demonstrated in the proximal portion of the left anterior descending artery *(Panel A)*. Spontaneous abrupt vessel closure developed *(Panel B)*, and emergent balloon angioplasty was performed *(Panel C)*. Owing to marked elastic recoil and a suboptimal initial result, a 2.5-mm GR stent was deployed across the lesion *(Panel D)*. This resulted in marked improvement of the lumen contour and in a 20% residual stenosis *(Panel E)*. Although the patient remained asymptomatic, restenosis within the stent was documented at routine arteriography 6 months later *(Panel F)*.

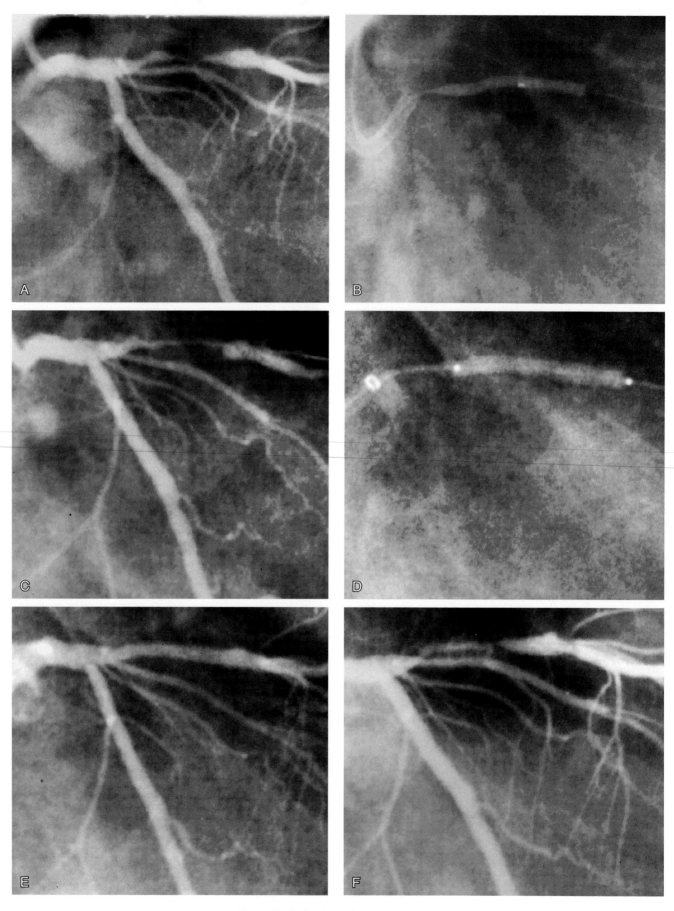

Figure 17–5. *See legend on opposite page*

Figure 17–5

A long (20-mm) stenosis involving the ostium and proximal segment of the left anterior descending artery *(Panel A)* was treated with balloon angioplasty using a 2.5-mm balloon catheter *(Panel B)*. Despite repeated and prolonged balloon inflations, incessant elastic recoil occurred, with eventual reduction in anterograde coronary perfusion *(Panel C)*. A 3.0-mm GR stent was deployed across the long diseased segment and inflated to 4 atm *(Panel D)*, resulting in an excellent initial result *(Panel E)*. Symptom recurrence developed 3 months later, and repeat angiography demonstrated recurrent stenosis along the diffusely diseased segment *(Panel F)*.

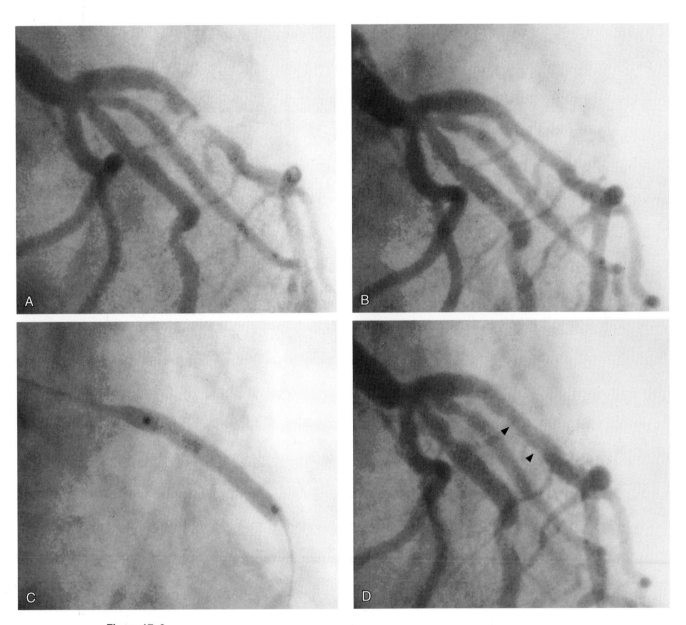

Figure 17–6

The ulcerated lesion of the midportion of the left anterior descending artery *(Panel A)* was treated with standard balloon methods using a 2.5-mm balloon catheter. Following balloon inflation, an irregular 40% residual stenosis persisted *(Panel B)*. A 3.0-mm GR stent was advanced across the stenosis and inflated to 4 atm *(Panel C)*. Following balloon inflation, a 20% residual stenosis as well as a mild degree of coronary scalloping in the region of preprocedural ulceration were observed *(arrowheads, Panel D)*. (Courtesy of C. Pinkerton, MD.)

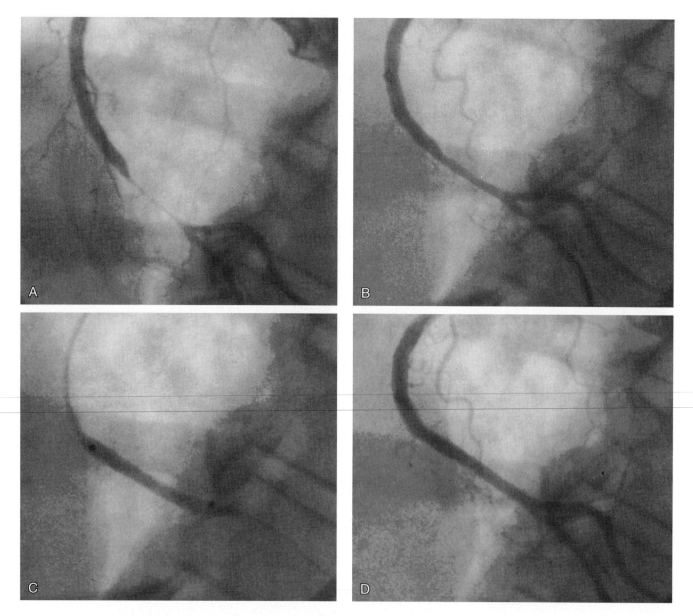

Figure 17–7
A tubular narrowing in the distal portion of the right coronary artery *(Panel A)* was treated with standard balloon angioplasty using a 2.5-mm balloon. Despite multiple inflations, a 40% residual stenosis persisted at the site of dilatation *(Panel B)*. To treat the suboptimal result, a 3.0-mm GR stent was advanced across the stenosis and inflated to 4 atm *(Panel C)*. Following final balloon inflation with a 3.0-mm noncompliant balloon, an excellent anatomic result was obtained without evidence of compromise of the posterior descending or posterolateral branches *(Panel D)*. (Courtesy of C. Pinkerton, MD.)

The GR stent has also been used in selected patients to treat recalcitrant restenosis after standard balloon angioplasty has been performed. However, the value of this stent design in the prevention of restenosis is still under evaluation. Its major value may be in cases in which incomplete dilatation or marked elastic recoil have resulted in suboptimal lumen dimensions after previous conventional balloon angioplasty.

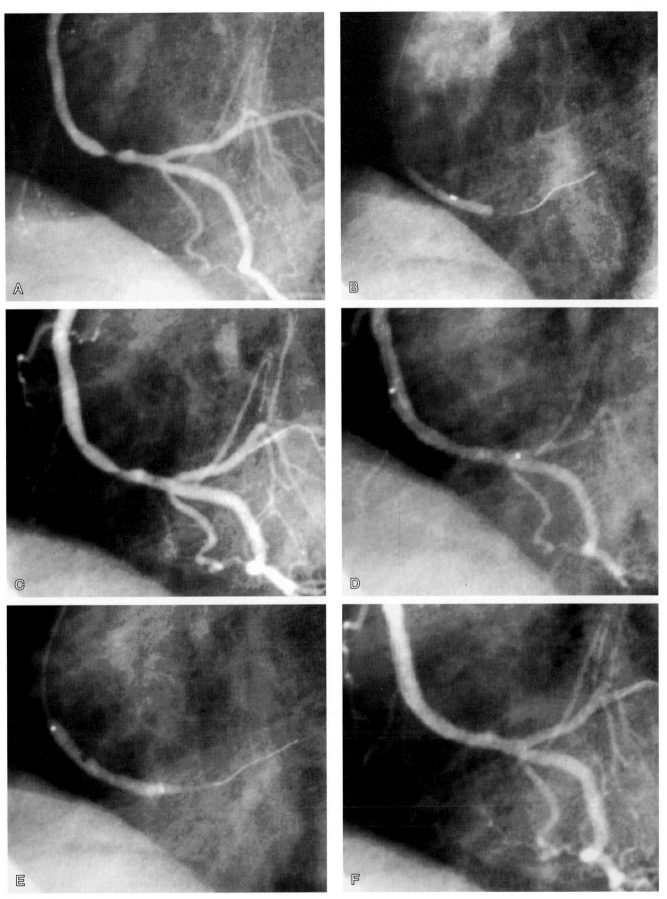

Figure 17–8
The restenotic lesion in the distal portion of the right coronary artery *(Panel A)* was predilated using a 2.5 mm balloon dilatation catheter *(Panel B)*. After initial dilatation, a 30% residual stenosis remained *(Panel C)*. A 3.0 mm GR Stent was positioned using fluoroscopic guidance *(Panel D)* and inflated to 4 atmospheres *(Panel E)*, resulting in an excellent anatomic result *(Panel F)*.

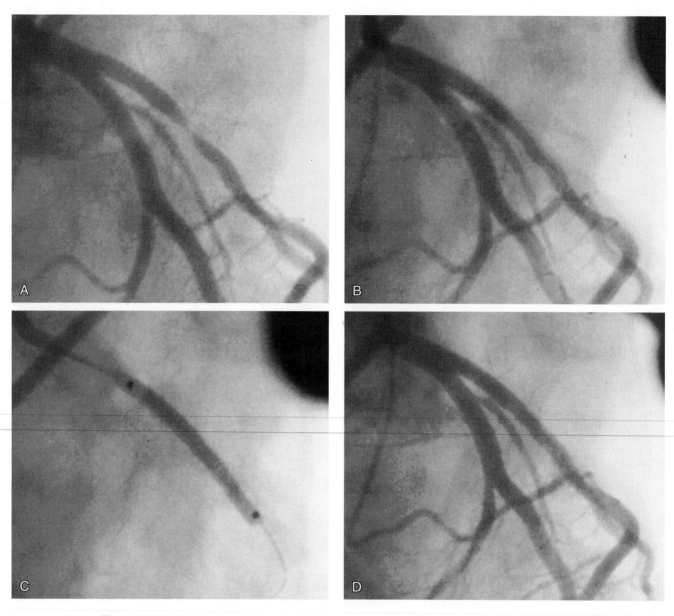

Figure 17–9
A recurrent stenosis in the medial left anterior descending artery *(Panel A)* was predilated with a 2.5-mm balloon catheter, resulting in a 30% residual stenosis *(Panel B)*. A 3.0-mm GR stent was advanced across the residual stenosis and inflated to 4 atm *(Panel C)*. Adjunct balloon inflation was performed with a 3.0-mm noncompliant balloon (not shown), resulting in an excellent angiographic result *(Panel D)*. (Courtesy of C. Pinkerton, MD.)

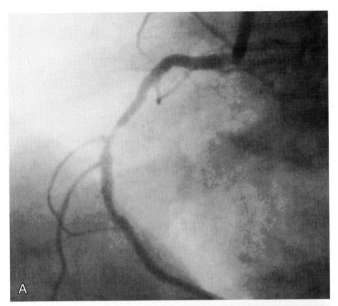

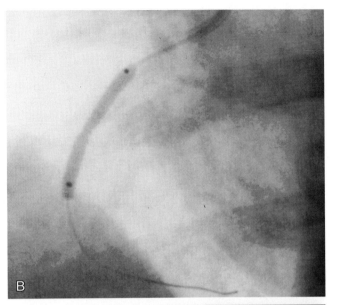

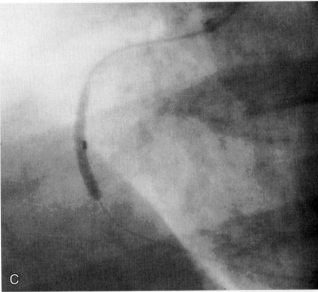

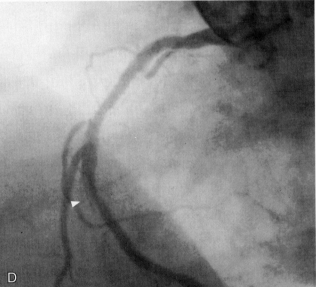

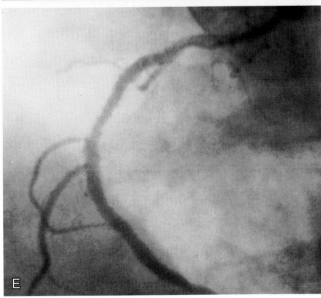

Figure 17–10
A restenotic lesion in the midportion of the right coronary artery *(Panel A)* was predilated with a 2.5-mm balloon catheter (not shown). A 3.0-mm GR stent was deployed across the stenosis and inflated to 4 atm *(Panel B)*. Adjunct angioplasty with a 3.0-mm noncompliant balloon catheter was performed *(Panel C)*. An excellent initial result was obtained; however, a focal dissection developed distal to the site of initial GR stent deployment *(arrow, Panel D)*. A second GR stent was positioned across the distal stenosis (not shown) and resulted in a marked improvement in the distal luminal contour and a "tacking up" of the distal dissection *(Panel E)*. (Courtesy of C. Pinkerton, MD.)

Lesions involving side branches may also be treated with intracoronary stenting using the GR stent. When side branch compromise occurs after primary stent deployment, balloon dilatation across the stent is possible. However, it is preferable to defer side branch angioplasty until the parent vessel has had sufficient time to endothelialize.

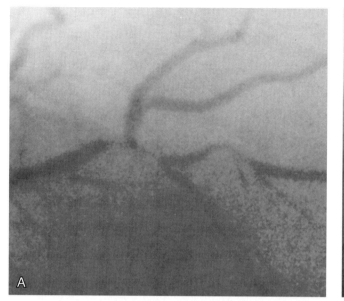

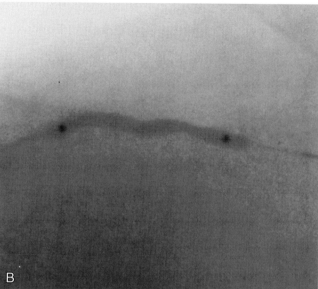

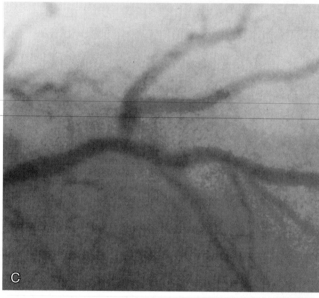

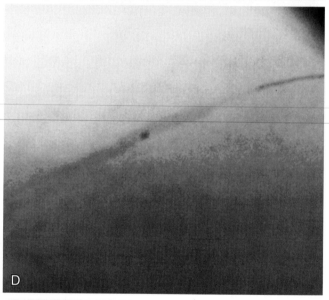

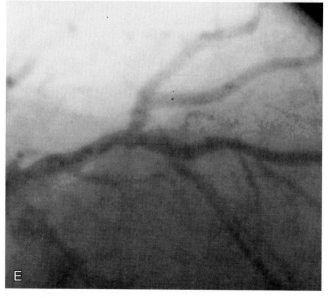

Figure 17–11

A complex bifurcation lesion and distal stenosis involving the midportion of the left anterior descending artery *(Panel A)* was treated with a 2.5-mm GR stent inflated to 4 atm *(Panel B)*. After initial stent deployment, lumen compromise into the diagonal branch was observed *(Panel C)*; a 2.5-mm fixed-wire balloon catheter was used to cross the GR stent and was inflated in the diagonal side branch *(Panel D)*. After parent and side branch dilatation, an excellent angiographic result was obtained *(Panel E)*. (Courtesy of C. Pinkerton, MD.)

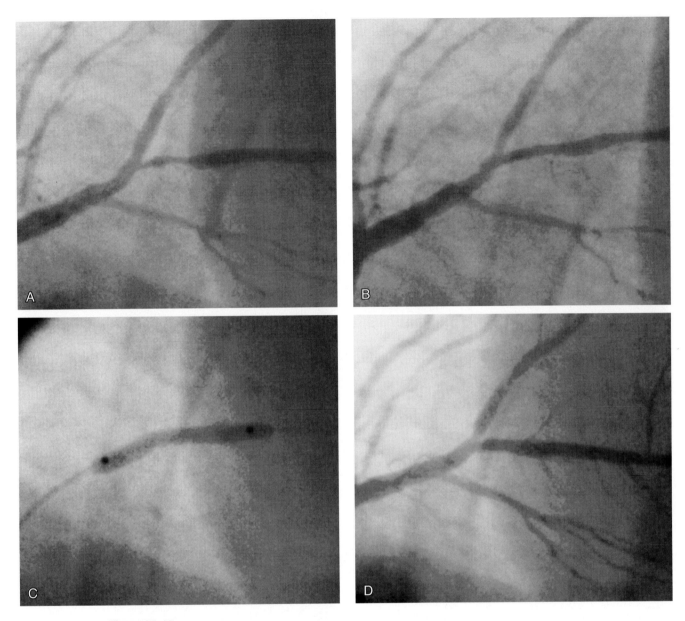

Figure 17–12
A complex restenotic lesion involving the midportion of the left anterior descending artery just distal to the origin of a large diagonal branch *(Panel A)* was predilated with a 2.5-mm balloon catheter. A 30% residual stenosis was obtained *(Panel B)*, and a 3.0-mm GR stent was deployed across the bifurcation *(Panel C)*. A 20% residual stenosis was present after stent deployment, and excellent flow was maintained into the diagonal side branch *(Panel D)*. (Courtesy of C. Pinkerton, MD.)

Limited experience has been gained with the use of the GR stent in SVG lesions.

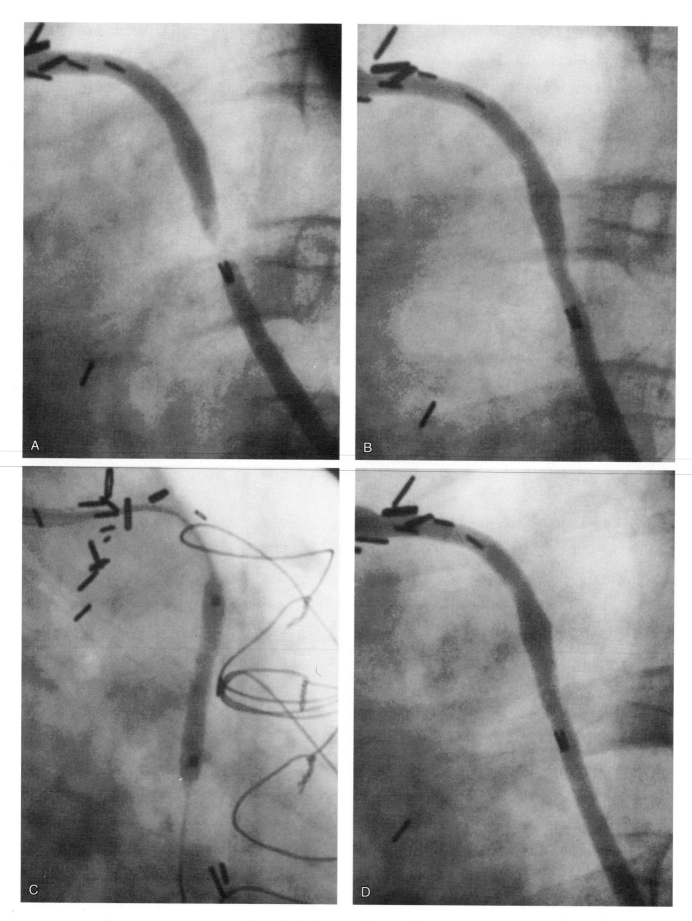

Figure 17–13. *See legend on opposite page*

Figure 17–13
A recalcitrant restenotic lesion in the midbody of the saphenous vein graft to the obtuse marginal branch *(Panel A)* was predilated with a 3.0-mm balloon catheter; this resulted in a 30% residual stenosis *(Panel B)*. A 3.5-mm GR stent was advanced across the lesion and inflated to 4 atm *(Panel C)*. A residual waist was noted within the GR stent balloon, and the stent balloon was exchanged for a 3.5-mm noncompliant balloon; the latter was the inflated to 10 atm *(Panel D)*. Although little change occurred in the angiographic result with adjunct balloon dilatation, the stent struts were presumably more firmly embedded into the SVG wall after dilatation. (Courtesy of C. Pinkerton, MD.)

SELECTED REFERENCES

Anderson P, Bajaj R, Baxley W, Roubin G. Vascular pathology of balloon-expandable flexible coil stents in humans. J Am Coll Cardiol 1992; 19:372–381.

Bilodeau L, Iyer S, Cannon A, et al. Flexible coil stent (Cook, Inc.) in saphenous vein grafts: Clinical and angiographic follow-up (Abstract). J Am Coll Cardiol 1992; 19:264A.

Garratt K, Holmes D, Roubin G. Early outcome after placement of a metallic intracoronary stent: Initial Mayo Clinic experience. Mayo Clin Proc 1991; 66:268–275.

George B, Voorhees W, Roubin G, et al. Multicenter investigation of coronary stenting to treat acute or threatened closure after percutaneous transluminal coronary angioplasty: Clinical and angiographic outcomes. J Am Coll Cardiol 1993; 22:135–143.

Lembo N, Roubin G. Intravascular stents. Cardiol Clin 1989; 7:877–894.

Rab S, King S III, Roubin G, et al. Coronary aneurysms after stent placement: A suggestion of altered vessel wall healing in the presence of anti-inflammatory agents. J Am Coll Cardiol 1991; 18:1524–1528.

Rodgers G, Minor S, Robinson K, et al. The coronary artery response to implantation of a balloon-expandable flexible stent in the aspirin- and non-aspirin–treated swine model. Am Heart J 1991; 122:640–647.

Roubin G, Cannon A, Agrawal S, et al. Intracoronary stenting for acute and threatened closure complicating percutaneous transluminal coronary angioplasty. Circulation 1992; 85:916–927.

Roubin G, King S III, Douglas J, et al. Intracoronary stenting during percutaneous transluminal coronary angioplasty. Circulation 1990; 81(4 Suppl):IV92–100.

Roubin G, Robinson K, King S III, et al. Early and late results of intracoronary arterial stenting after coronary angioplasty in dogs. Circulation 1987; 76:891–897.

Wiktor Stents

Similarly to stents of other designs, the Wiktor stent has been clinically used to treat acute and threatened abrupt closure after coronary angioplasty. The 17-mm long Wiktor stent is composed of 0.125-mm tantalum filaments coiled in a serpentine design and crimped onto a polyethylene angioplasty balloon catheter (Figure 18–1, *Panels A–C*). The potential advantage of this stent is its extreme flexibil-ity, which enables it to reach lesions with marked tortuos-ity. The tantalum filaments render the Wiktor stent radi-opaque, allowing easy visualization of the stent filaments on angiography. Anticoagulation regimens in patients who are to receive Wiktor stents are similar to those for other balloon-expandable stent designs.

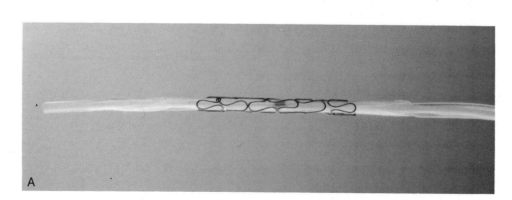

A

Figure 18–1. *See legend on opposite page*

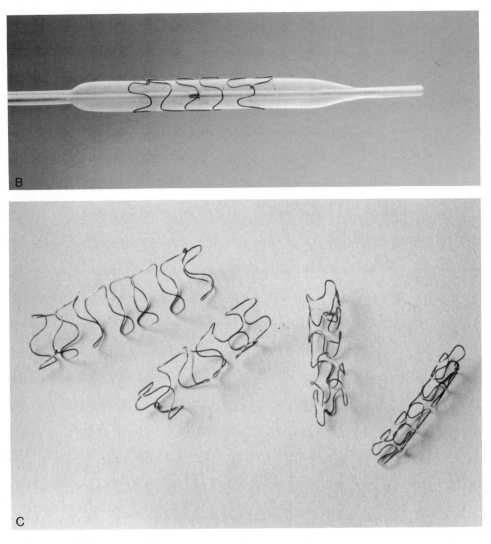

Figure 18–1
The Wiktor stent crimped onto a balloon catheter *(Panel A)*; the same Wiktor stent after inflation of the balloon catheter *(Panel B)*; Wiktor stents expanded to different luminal diameters *(Panel C)*.

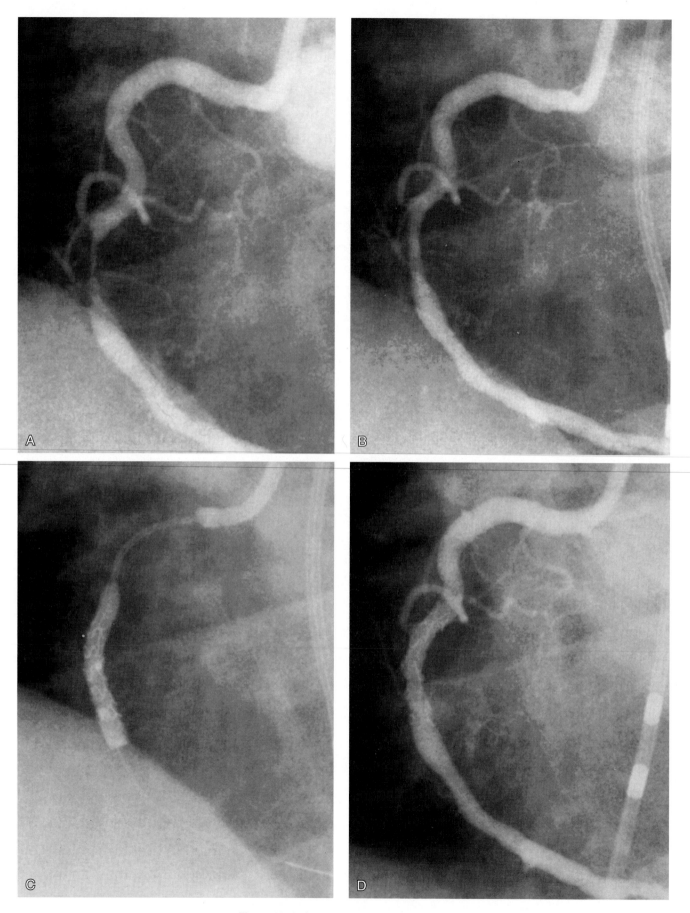

Figure 18–2. *See legend on opposite page*

Figure 18–2
A tubular stenosis of the midportion of the right coronary artery was distal to severe proximal vessel tortuosity *(Panel A)*. Following predilatation with a 2.5-mm balloon catheter, a 40% residual stenosis remained *(Panel B)*. A 3.5-mm Wiktor stent was positioned across the stenosis and inflated to 6 atm *(Panel C)*. Following deployment of the stent, a 20% residual stenosis persisted despite adjunct balloon dilatation *(Panel D)*.

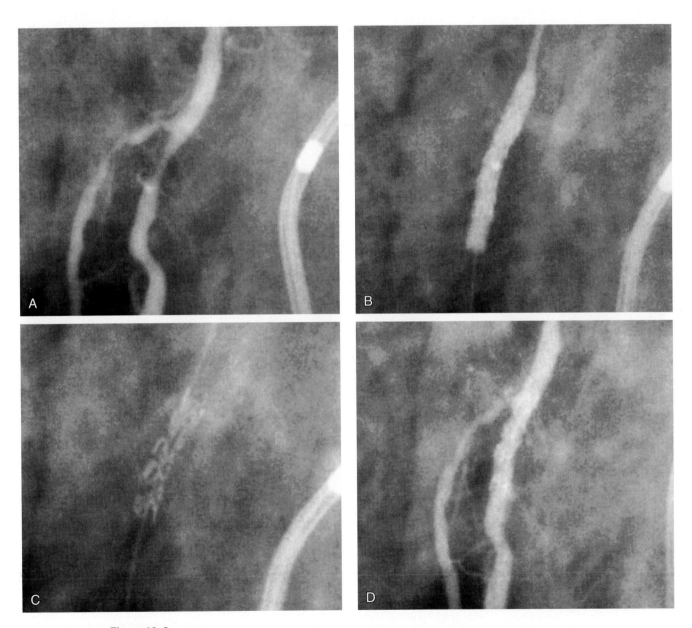

Figure 18–3
A restenotic, tubular stenosis was noted in the midportion of the right coronary artery *(Panel A)*. After predilatation with a 2.5-mm balloon catheter, a 3.0-mm Wiktor stent was deployed across the stenosis *(Panel B)*. The tantalum filaments were visualized fluoroscopically *(Panel C)*, and a 20% residual stenosis was obtained *(Panel D)*. Mild luminal irregularity was noted. The side branch was not approached.

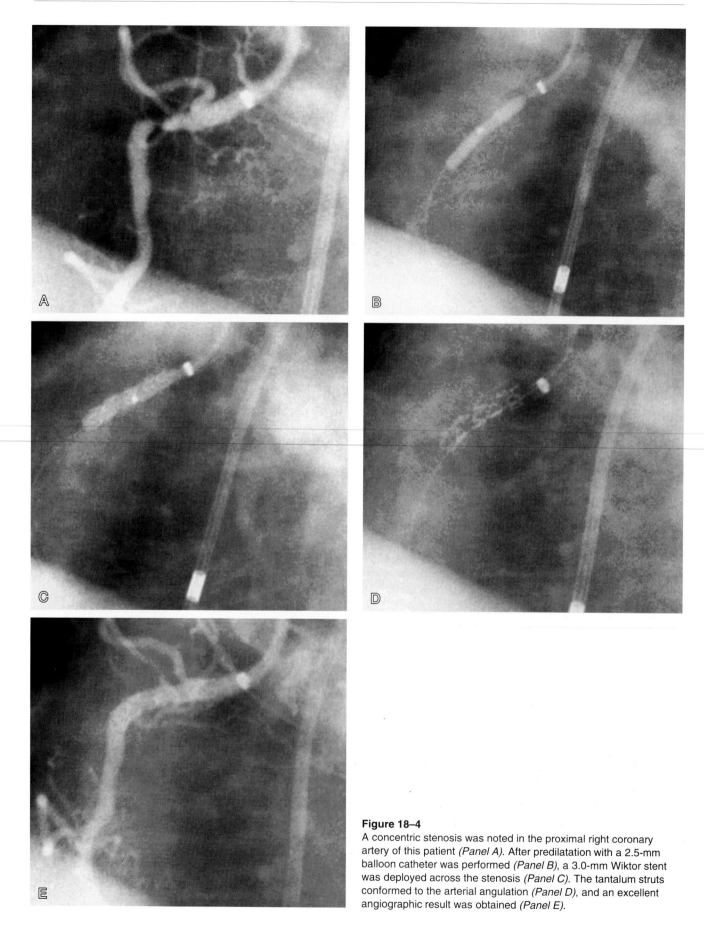

Figure 18–4

A concentric stenosis was noted in the proximal right coronary artery of this patient *(Panel A)*. After predilatation with a 2.5-mm balloon catheter was performed *(Panel B)*, a 3.0-mm Wiktor stent was deployed across the stenosis *(Panel C)*. The tantalum struts conformed to the arterial angulation *(Panel D)*, and an excellent angiographic result was obtained *(Panel E)*.

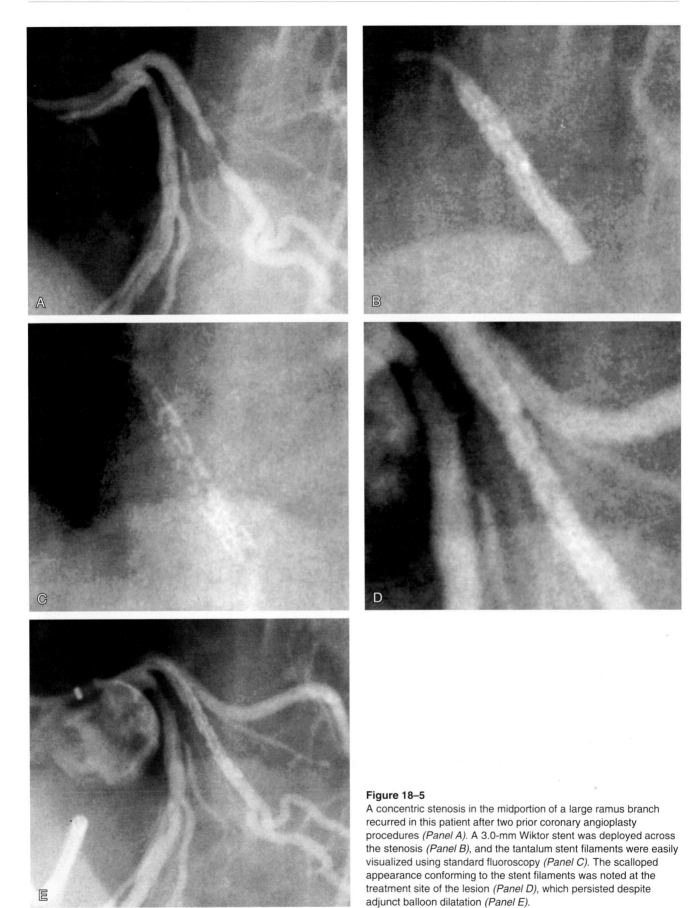

Figure 18–5

A concentric stenosis in the midportion of a large ramus branch recurred in this patient after two prior coronary angioplasty procedures *(Panel A)*. A 3.0-mm Wiktor stent was deployed across the stenosis *(Panel B)*, and the tantalum stent filaments were easily visualized using standard fluoroscopy *(Panel C)*. The scalloped appearance conforming to the stent filaments was noted at the treatment site of the lesion *(Panel D)*, which persisted despite adjunct balloon dilatation *(Panel E)*.

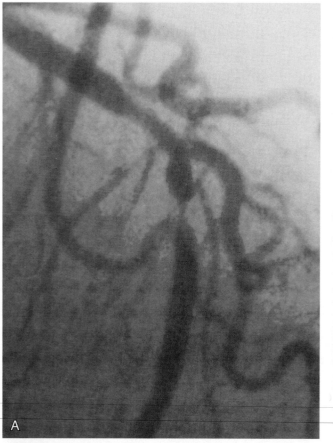

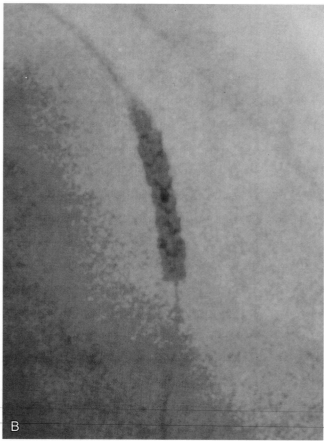

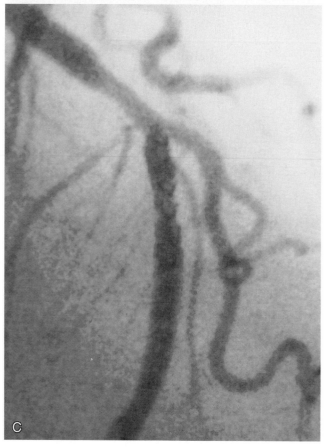

Figure 18–6
A concentric narrowing of the midportion of the left anterior descending artery was noted approximately 5 mm distal to the origin of a large diagonal branch *(Panel A)*. A 3.5-mm Wiktor stent was placed across the lesion with care to avoid crossing the diagonal side branch *(Panel B)*. Following stent deployment, an excellent anatomic result was obtained with mild luminal irregularity within the stent *(Panel C)*.

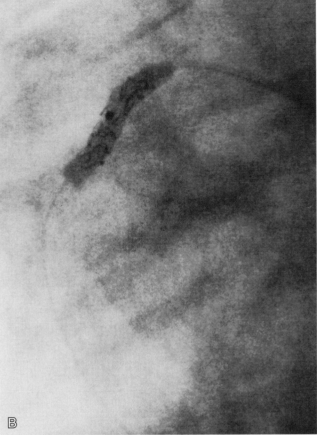

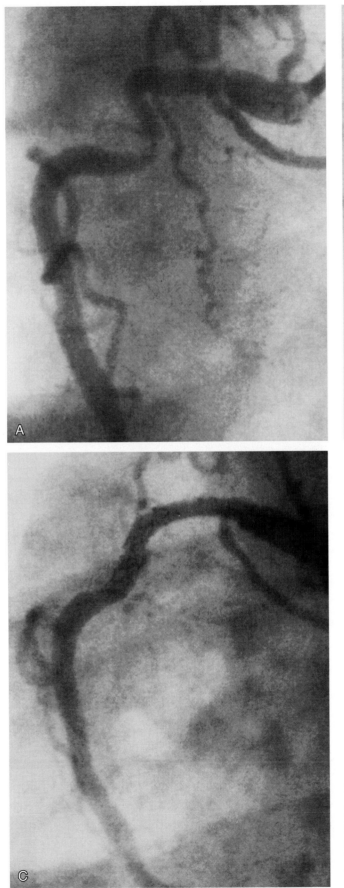

Figure 18–7

A severely angulated, restenotic lesion in the proximal segment of the right coronary artery *(Panel A)* was predilated with a 2.5 mm balloon catheter (not shown). A 3.5 mm Wiktor stent was deployed across the severely angulated lesion *(Panel B)*, resulting in marked improvement in the stenosis severity *(Panel C)*. The proximal right coronary artery was straightened after deployment of the Wiktor stent.

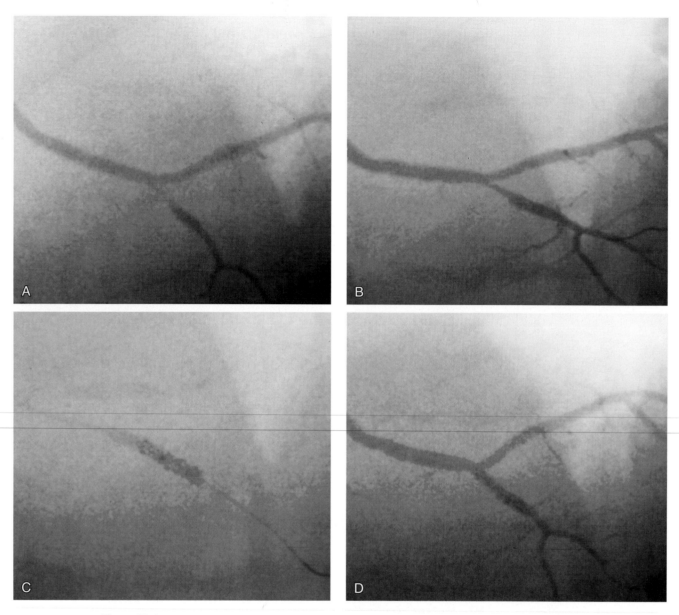

Figure 18–8

A restenotic, ostial lesion of the posterior descending artery *(Panel A)* was predilated with a 2.5-mm balloon catheter (not shown). A 50% residual stenosis was treated with a 3.0-mm Wiktor stent inflated to 6 atm across a side branch *(Panel C)*. An excellent angiographic result *(Panel D)* without side branch compromise resulted. (Courtesy of C. White, MD.)

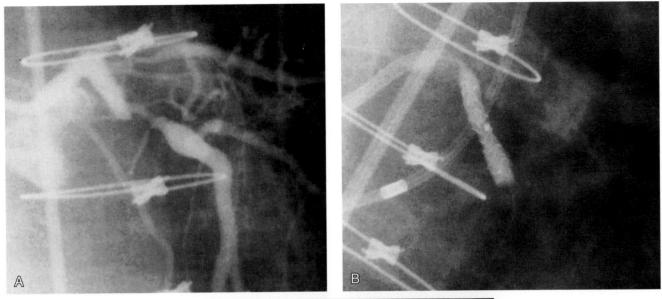

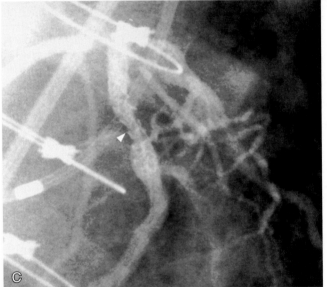

Figure 18–9

A complex recurrent restenosis of the proximal portion of the left circumflex artery *(Panel A)* was predilated with a 2.5-mm balloon catheter. A 3.5-mm Wiktor stent was deployed across the lesion *(Panel B)*, but despite prolonged adjunct balloon inflations with a noncompliant balloon catheter, elastic recoil developed at the treatment site, resulting in a 40% residual stenosis *(Panel C)*.

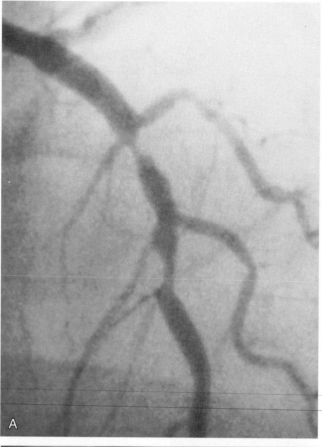

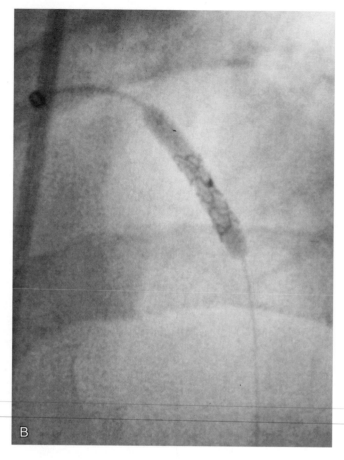

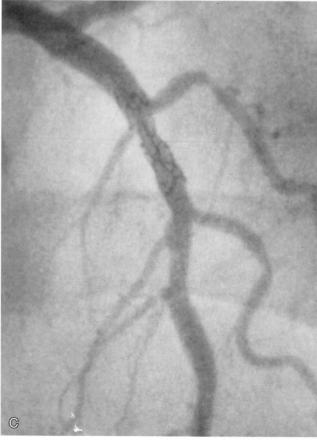

Figure 18–10

A complex, eccentric stenosis just distal to the origin of a diagonal branch was noted in the left anterior descending artery *(Panel A)*. A 3.5-mm Wiktor stent was positioned across the stenosis *(Panel B)* and inflated to 6 atm. Following balloon inflation, a 30% residual stenosis was noted *(Panel C)*. A moderate degree of elastic recoil was observed at the treatment site *(Panel C)*.

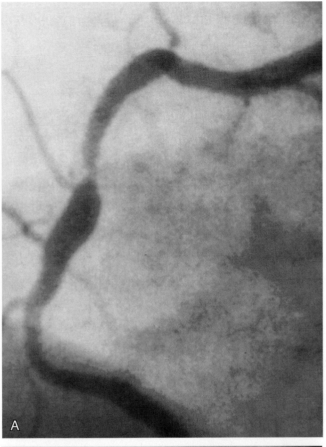

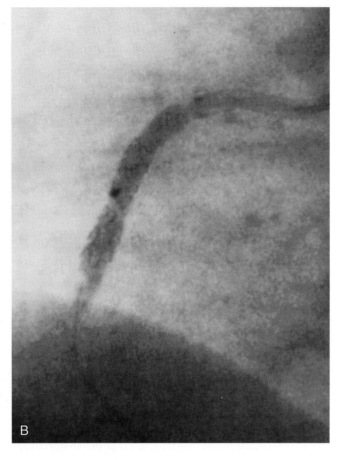

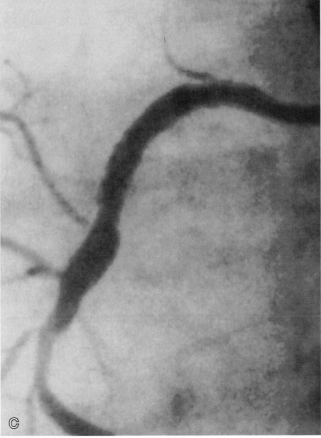

Figure 18–11

The concentric stenosis in the midportion of the right coronary artery *(Panel A)* was treated with a 3.5-mm Wiktor stent *(Panel B)*. Following balloon inflation, a mild degree of vascular recoil was observed, and a 20% residual stenosis persisted after balloon dilatation *(Panel C)*.

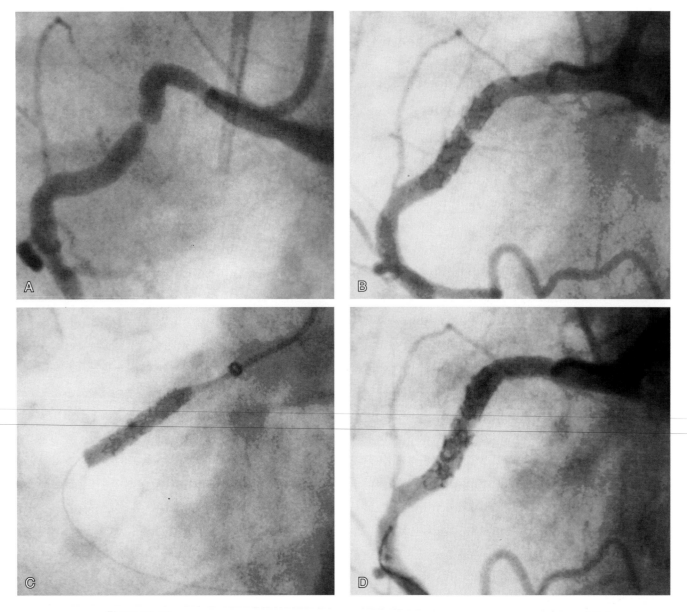

Figure 18–12
A concentric stenosis of the midsegment of the right coronary artery *(Panel A)* was treated with a 3.5-mm stent (not shown). After stent deployment, a focal region of atherosclerotic plaque appeared to extrude into the lumen through the stent struts *(Panel B)*. Adjunct balloon dilatation was performed using a noncompliant balloon *(Panel C)*. This resulted in overall improvement of the lumen contour, but a 20% stenosis persisted at the treatment site *(Panel D)*.

Wiktor stents have also been used to treat patients with coronary artery dissection and to improve suboptimal results after balloon angioplasty.

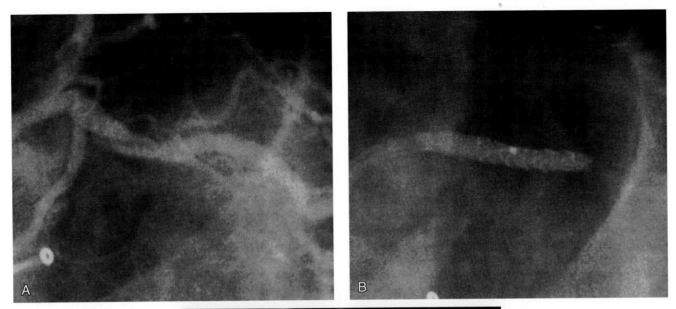

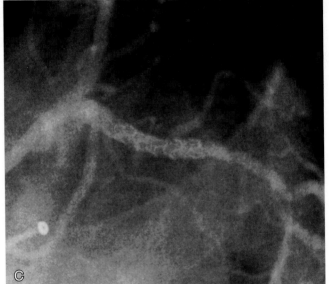

Figure 18–13
Coronary angioplasty of the midportion of the left circumflex resulted in an intimal flap that was refractory to prolonged balloon inflation *(Panel A)*. A 3.5-mm Wiktor stent was positioned across the intimal flap and inflated to 6 atm *(Panel B)*. Following stent deployment, the intimal flap was successfully "tacked up," and a minimal residual stenosis was noted at the lesion treatment site *(Panel C)*.

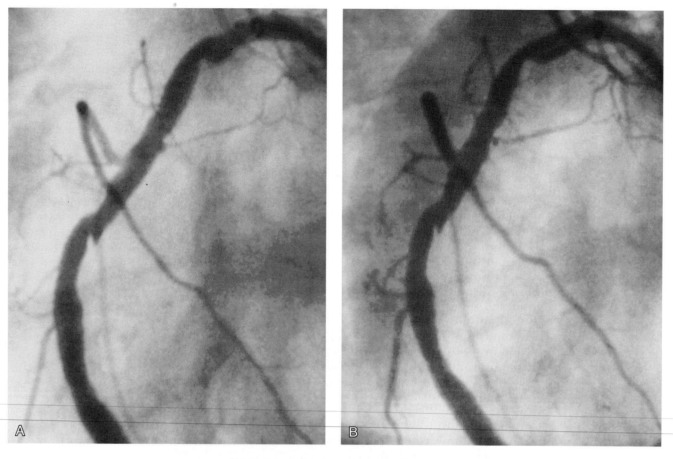

Figure 18–14. *See legend on opposite page*

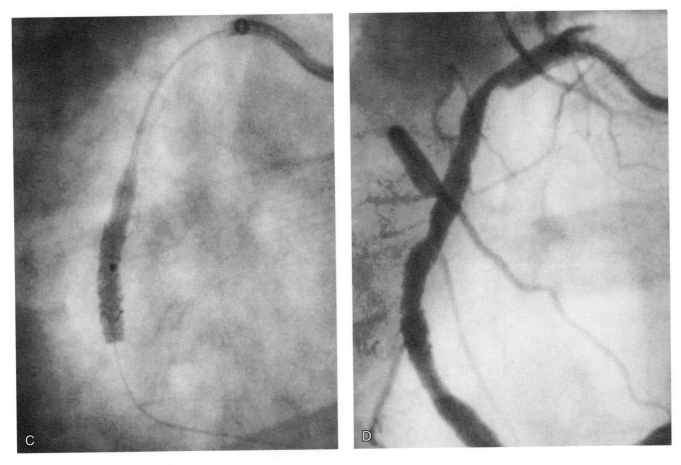

Figure 18–14
Following standard balloon angioplasty, a residual intimal flap was noted in the midportion of the right coronary artery *(Panel A)*. After dilatation with a 3.0-mm balloon catheter, the intimal flap persisted *(Panel B)*. Deployment of a 3.5-mm Wiktor stent *(Panel C)* resulted in obliteration of the intimal flap and smoothing of the lumen contour *(Panel D)*.

As with the use of other stent designs, subacute thrombosis may occur after Wiktor stent placement; thus, meticulous attention to anticoagulation therapy is mandatory.

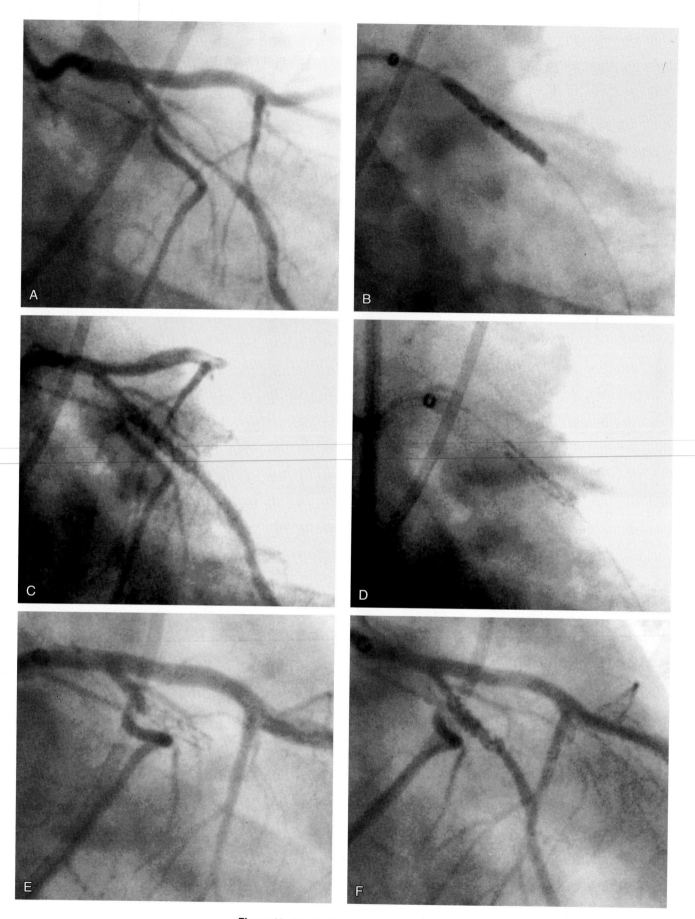

Figure 18–15. *See legend on opposite page*

Figure 18–15

A tubular, restenotic lesion was noted in a large obtuse marginal branch *(Panel A)*. A 3.0-mm Wiktor stent was positioned across the lesion *(Panel B)* and inflated to 6 atm. After stent deployment, an excellent anatomic result was obtained, and a mild degree of lesion ectasia was observed *(Panel C)*. The stent was easily visualized with the use of standard fluoroscopy *(Panel D)*. Forty-eight hours following stent deployment, the patient developed chest pain and posterolateral ST segment elevation despite the administration of adequate anticoagulation therapy. Emergent coronary arteriography demonstrated stent thrombosis *(Panel E)*. Balloon angioplasty was performed emergently, resulting in restoration of the anterograde flow *(Panel F)*.

SELECTED REFERENCES

de Jaegere P, Serruys P, Bertrand M, et al. Wiktor stent implantation in patients with restenosis following balloon angioplasty of a native coronary artery. Am J Cardiol 1992; 69:598–602.

Popma J, Ellis S. Intracoronary stents: Clinical and angiographic results. Herz 1990; 15:307–318.

Scott N, King S III. Coronary stents. Coron Artery Dis 1992; 3:901–907.

Serruys P, de Jaegere P, Bertrand M, et al. Morphologic change in coronary artery stenosis with the Medtronic-Wiktor stent: Initial results from the Core Laboratory for quantitative angiography. Cathet Cardiovasc Diagn 1991; 24:237–245.

van der Giessen W, Serruys P, van Beusekom H, et al. Coronary stenting with a new, radiopaque, balloon-expandable endoprosthesis in pigs. Circulation 1991; 83:1788–1798.

White C, Ramee S, Banks A, et al. A new balloon-expandable tantalum coil stent: Angiographic patency and histologic findings in an atherogenic swine model. J Am Coll Cardiol 1992; 19:870–876.

CHAPTER 19

The Wallstent

The Wallstent was developed jointly in the mid-1980s by Medinvent SA, a Swiss manufacturer, and the University Hospital at Lausanne, Switzerland. The woven, wire mesh tube design was selected chiefly because of its availability, flexibility, elasticity, and radial expansivity. Indicated for the treatment of patients with abrupt closure or recurrent restenosis or for the primary therapy of patients with lesions involving saphenous vein grafts, the Wallstent intracoronary stent underwent clinical evaluation in Europe in March 1986. A multicenter series by Serruys and coworkers summarizing initial procedural results reported high rates of subacute closure with the use of the device (24%); however, the anticoagulation regimens and criteria for patient selection were variable, and selected single-center series reported lower complication rates. Notably, in those patients who did not develop acute complications, the restenosis rate (defined as a follow-up diameter stenosis of >50%) was 14%. Potentially, with alterations in the Wallstent design (including heparin coating), the application of a more aggressive, early anticoagulation regimen, and further modifications in patient selection criteria, better initial results would be anticipated.

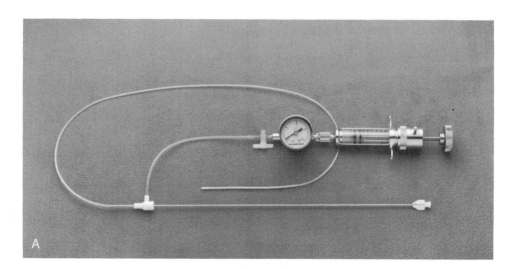

Figure 19–1. *See legend on opposite page*

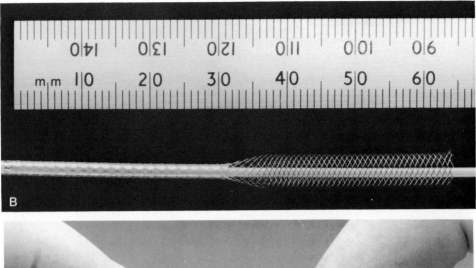

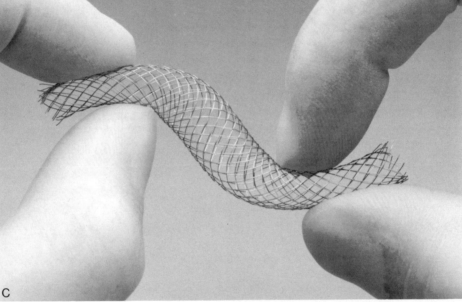

Figure 19–1

As currently designed, the Wallstent comprises a 5-French coaxial delivery catheter onto which a compressed stainless stent composed of 16 0.07- to 0.09-mm filaments is mounted *(Panel A)*. The outer diameter of the loaded catheter system is 1.57 mm, and most 8- to 9-French guiding catheters (≥0.072-inch internal diameter) may be used for stent deployment. The self-expanding stent is held in place within the delivery sheath by a tight doubled-over wrapping membrane *(Panel B)*. Two radiopaque metal markers are attached to the delivery catheter to aid in precise positioning of the stent. These proximal and distal markers indicate the proximal and distal ends of the compressed stent, and a third middle marker is used to estimate the degree of shortening of the stent during implantation. The fully expanded Wallstent may vary in length from 15 to 29 mm *(Panel C)* and constitute approximately 20% of the lumen surface area. In general, the Wallstent that should be selected to be 15% to 20% larger in its unconstrained diameter than the reference arterial diameter. Currently available Wallstents range from 3.0 to 6.0 mm in diameter in their fully expanded state.

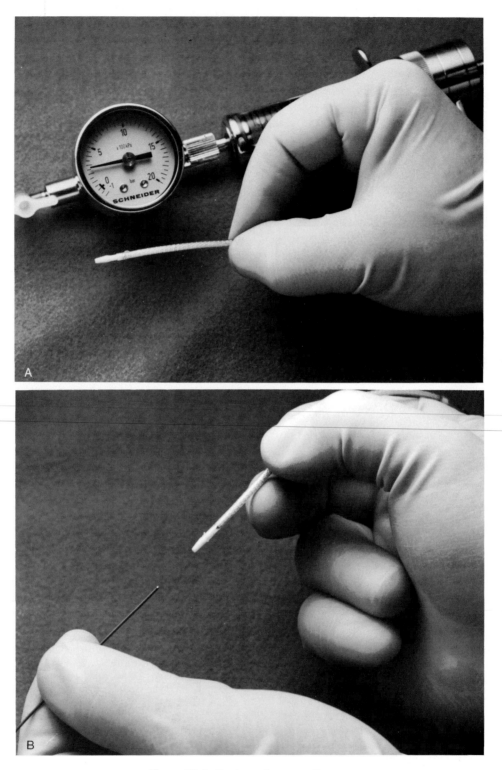

Figure 19–2. *See legend on opposite page*

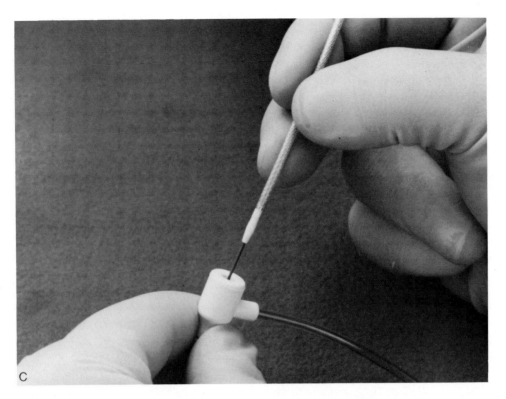

Figure 19–2
The central lumen of the delivery catheter is flushed with heparinized saline in a manner similar to that for over-the-wire balloon expandable systems *(Panel A)*. To minimize friction between the outer and inner retaining membranes, the space between them is filled with fluid (e.g., contrast medium) at 3 to 4 atm; the use of contrast medium aids in the fluoroscopic visualization of the delivery sheath. To avoid the trapping of bubbles, a microscopic perforation is created at the end of the membrane, allowing air to vent while the delivery catheter is filled with contrast medium. The wire is backloaded onto the stent *(Panel B)* and advanced through the hemostatic valve for positioning across the coronary artery or graft lesion *(Panel C)*.

Following coronary intubation with an adequately sized, supportive guiding catheter, a 0.014- or 0.018-inch coronary guide wire is used to cross the lesion. In most circumstances, predilatation with standard balloon angioplasty is performed to provide a sufficient lumen for passage of the delivery catheter. If a balloon dilatation is performed, the wire may be extended or exchanged for a 300-cm coronary guide wire. The over-the-wire delivery catheter is then positioned at the level of the stenosis, and the wrapping membrane is pulled proximally. While the wrapping membrane is fully retracted proximally, the self-expanding stent is gradually displaced. This exerts radial force against the inner surface of the arterial lumen that has the potential to scaffold dissection flaps and compress ulcerated atheromas.

In most circumstances, some degree of residual stenosis persists following initial stent deployment. Residual stenoses may be treated with additional balloon inflations using a slightly oversized compliant balloon. This technique, the so-called "Swiss kiss," results in an additional 10% to 15% improvement in quantitative coronary dimensions. The additional gains in luminal diameter may result in a reduction of the rate of early thrombotic complications and restenosis. As with the use of other stents, adherence to a strict anticoagulation protocol is mandatory.

Current studies suggest that the Wallstent may be useful in three clinical situations: (1) abrupt closure after coronary angioplasty; (2) suboptimal angiographic results after coronary angioplasty; and (3) primary treatment of saphenous vein graft lesions.

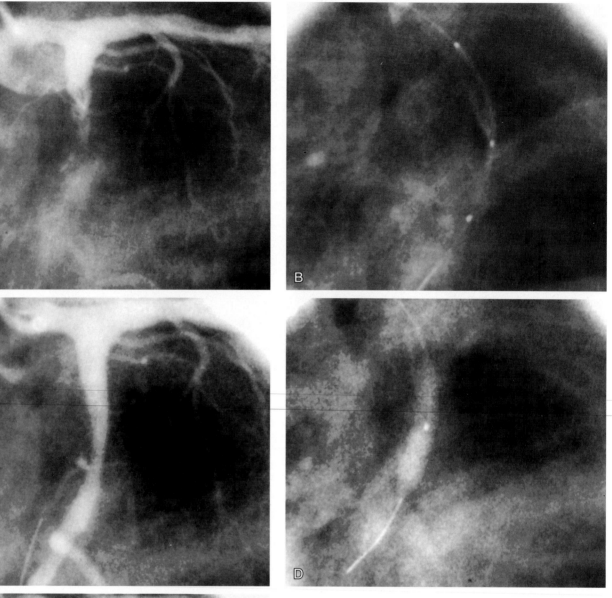

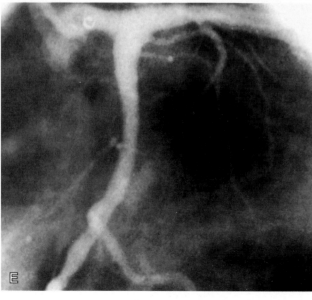

Figure 19–3

Following standard balloon angioplasty, a total occlusion developed in the proximal portion of the left circumflex artery of this patient *(Panel A)*. A 0.014-inch guide wire was positioned across the coronary obstruction and was advanced into the distal vessel. A 3.5-mm Wallstent was positioned across the occluded segment *(Panel B)*, and the retaining membrane of the stent was withdrawn. Stent deployment resulted in restoration of anterograde coronary perfusion. A 40% residual stenosis was effectively treated with repeat balloon dilatation *(Panel C)* using a 3.5-mm balloon catheter (the Swiss kiss technique) *(Panel D)*. After the final balloon inflation, an excellent anatomic result was obtained *(Panel E)*. (Courtesy of U. Sigwart, MD.)

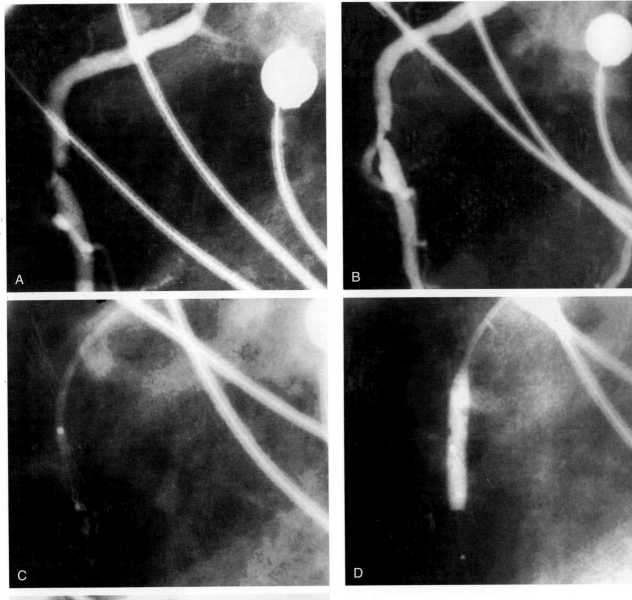

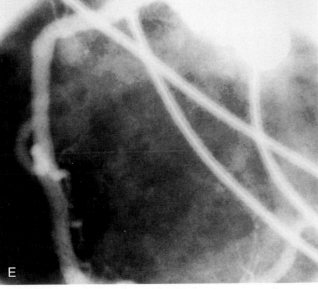

Figure 19–4

A severe (90%) obstruction of the midsegment of the right coronary artery *(Panel A)* was treated with a 2.5-mm balloon catheter (not shown). This approach resulted in a 50% residual stenosis despite additional balloon dilatations *(Panel B)*. A 3.0-mm Wallstent was positioned across the residual coronary stenosis *(Panel C)*; this stent deployment resulted in an improved angiographic result (not shown). An additional balloon inflation using a 3.5-mm balloon catheter *(Panel D)* resulted in an excellent angiographic result *(Panel E)*. The additional linear opacities represent electrocardiographic leads overlying the chest wall. (Courtesy of U. Sigwart, MD.)

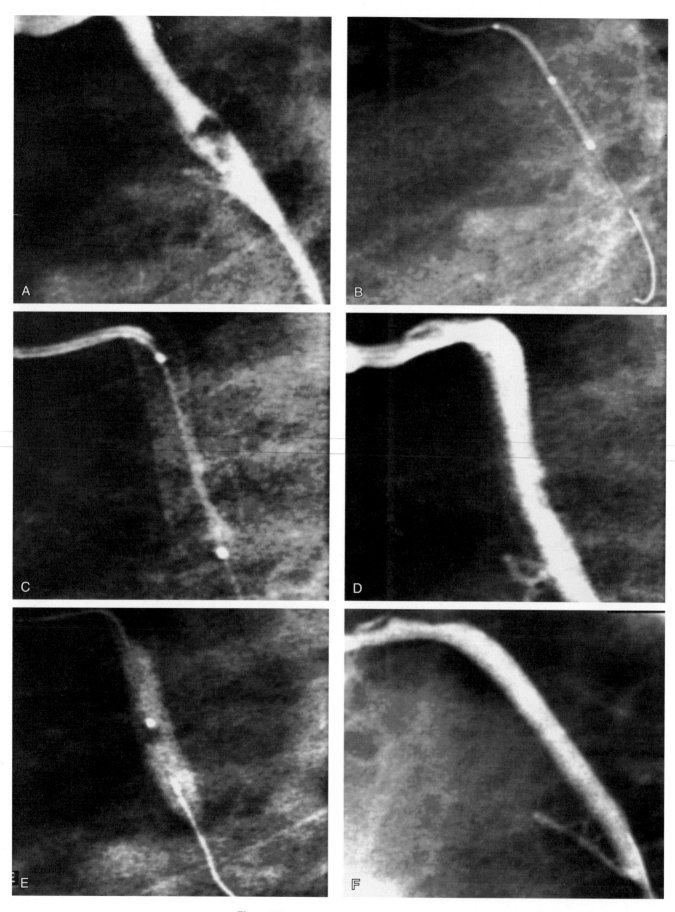

Figure 19–5. *See legend on opposite page*

Figure 19–5
A severely ulcerated lesion in the midportion of the saphenous vein graft to the circumflex coronary artery *(Panel A)* was crossed with a 0.014-inch high-torque floppy wire. A 3.5-mm Wallstent was then positioned across the ulcerated stenosis *(Panel B)*, and the stent was expanded within the vein graft segment *(Panel C)*. A 40% residual stenosis was demonstrated *(Panel D)*; subsequently, a 4.0-mm balloon *(Panel E)* was inflated, resulting in an excellent angiographic result *(Panel F)*. (Courtesy of U. Sigwart, MD.)

SELECTED REFERENCES

de Feyter PJ, DeScheerder I, van den Brand M, et al. Emergency stenting for refractory acute coronary artery occlusion during coronary angioplasty. Am J Cardiol 1990; 66:1147–1150.

Kaufmann U, Sigwart U. Resolution of residual pressure gradients after angioplasty by stenting. J Interven Cardiol 1989; 2:5–8.

Puel J, Juilliere Y, Bertrand M, et al. Early and late assessment of stenosis geometry after coronary arterial stenting. Am J Cardiol 1988; 61:546–553.

Serruys P, Beatt K, Strauss B, et al. Quantitative angiographic follow-up of coronary stents: Report on the initial 105 patients from March 1986 to January 1988. N Engl J Med 1991; 324:13–17.

Sigwart U, Puel J, Mirkovitch V, et al. Intravascular stents to prevent occlusion and restenosis after transluminal angioplasty. N Engl J Med 1987; 316:701–706.

Sigwart U, Urban P, Golf S, et al. Emergency stenting for acute occlusion after coronary balloon angioplasty. Circulation 1988; 78:1121–1127.

Sigwart U, Urban P. Use of coronary stents following balloon angioplasty. Heart Dis 1989; 111–120.

Sigwart U. The self-expanding mesh stent. *In* Textbook of Interventional Cardiology. Topol EJ (ed). Philadelphia, WB Saunders, 1990, pp 605–622.

Strauss B, Leborgne O, DeScheerder I, Serruys P. Implantation of an endoluminal prosthesis at the distal anastomosis of a bypass graft for abrupt closure following balloon angioplasty. Cath Cardiovasc Diagn 1990; 21:271–274.

Urban P, Sigwart U, Golf S, et al. Intravascular stenting for stenosis of aortocoronary venous bypass grafts. J Am Coll Cardiol 1989; 13:1085–1091.

Excimer Laser Angioplasty

Pulsed 308-nm xenon chloride excimer laser systems with optimal characteristics for laser coronary angioplasty have been approved by the Food and Drug Administration Advisory Panel for clinical use. The pulsed laser energy ablates tissue through a combination of photochemical and controlled photothermal effects. In addition, high-pressure acoustic photoacoustic transients resulting from laser ablation generate vapor bubbles that may play a role in plaque fragmentation.

Currently available concentric excimer laser catheters are highly efficient, have a minimum "dead space," and range in diameter from 1.3 to 2.2 mm. Lesions deemed amenable to excimer laser angioplasty include those ≥20 mm in length, total occlusions, aorto-ostial lesions, diffuse saphenous vein graft lesions, moderately calcified lesions, and lesions that are undilatable with the use of conventional methods. Because of an infrequently reported risk of coronary perforation (1–2%), the use of concentric laser catheters should be avoided in patients with bifurcation lesions, highly eccentric lesions, angulated lesions, and lesions with prior coronary dissection.

Stand-alone excimer laser angioplasty was often performed early in the clinical evaluation period. Although a channel equivalent to the size of the laser fiber was created, the excimer laser fibers were generally undersized (1.6 mm) relative to the underlying vessel, and a significant residual stenosis typically persisted. Given the initial procedural results, restenosis rates for stand-alone excimer laser angioplasty were generally high (>50%), and this technique was subsequently supplemented with the use of adjunct balloon dilatation in the event of the occurrence of residual stenosis >40%.

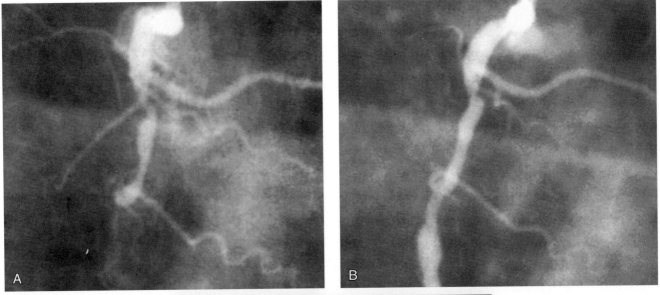

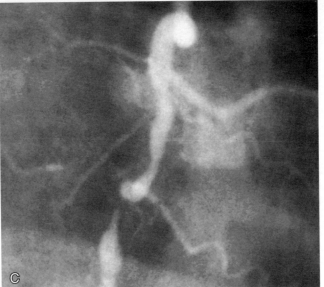

Figure 20–1
A total occlusion of the distal portion of the right coronary artery *(Panel A)* was crossed with a 0.014-inch wire and treated with a 1.6-mm excimer laser catheter (not shown). Several passes were performed, and a 40% stand-alone result was obtained *(Panel B)*. The patient's symptoms recurred 2 months later, and repeat angiography demonstrated a subtotal occlusion at the site of laser angioplasty *(Panel C)*.

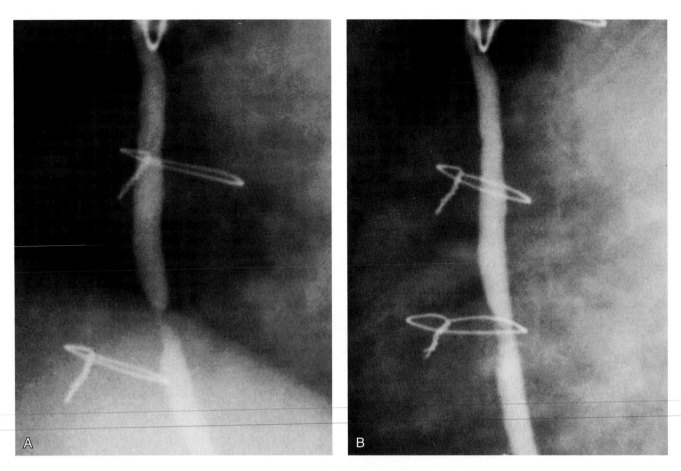

Figure 20–2

A concentric stenosis in the midportion of the saphenous vein graft to the right coronary artery *(Panel A)* was treated with a 2.2-mm stand-alone excimer laser catheter. After four passes were performed, a 40% residual stenosis was obtained *(Panel B)* without evidence of distal embolization or dissection.

The excimer laser catheter may have particular benefit in the ''debulking'' of total occlusions, thereby rendering them more amenable to adjunct balloon dilatation using long and overlapping balloon inflations. As with standard balloon techniques, a guide wire must first be passed across the total occlusion; however, once it is positioned in the distal vessel, the laser catheter crosses the segment of occlusion in most instances. The combination of plaque ''fracturing'' and ''debulking'' and adjunct balloon dilatation is a commonly employed strategy for excimer laser angioplasty in the management of patients with total occlusions.

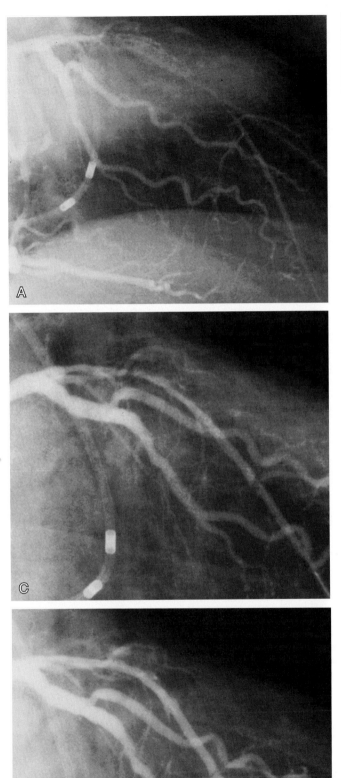

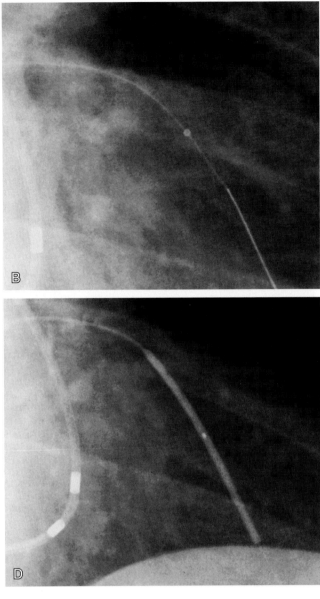

Figure 20–3

A total occlusion of the proximal segment of the left anterior descending artery *(Panel A)* was crossed with a 0.014-inch intermediate wire. A 1.3-mm excimer laser catheter was advanced across the total occlusion at 3 mm/s using 60 mJ/mm^2 of energy *(Panel B)*. After a single pass, the left anterior descending artery was recanalized *(Panel C)*, and adjunct balloon angiography was performed with a 2.5-mm long (40-mm) balloon catheter. After final balloon deflation, an excellent anatomic result was obtained, and normal flow was re-established into the left anterior descending artery *(Panel E)*.

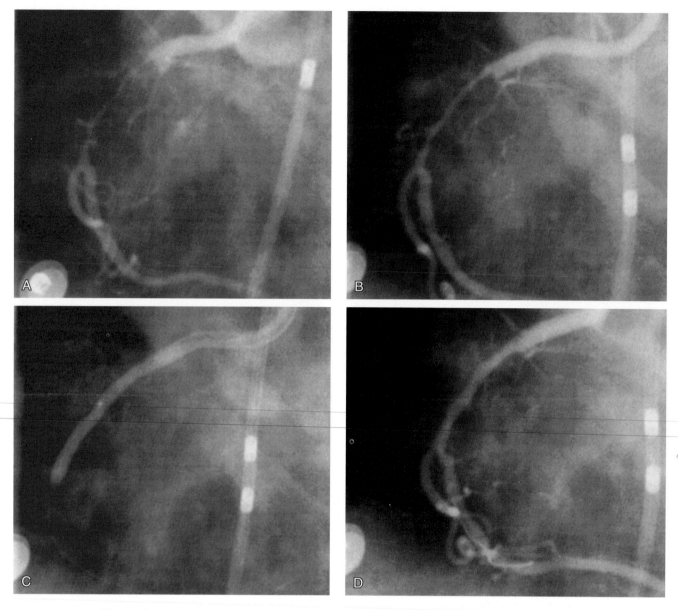

Figure 20–4
A long (30-mm) segment of total occlusion in the midsegment of the right coronary artery *(Panel A)* was crossed with a 0.014-inch intermediate wire. After a single pass with a 1.3-mm high-density laser catheter operating at 60 mJ/mm², a channel was created and the vessel was recanalized *(Panel B)*. A 3.0-mm long (40-mm) balloon was inflated across the residual stenosis *(Panel C)*, and a 20% residual stenosis was obtained *(Panel D)*.

Excimer laser angioplasty may also be used in diffusely (>20 mm) diseased segments. Pulsed laser plaque ablation partially debulks or disrupts the atherosclerotic plaque, allowing more controlled adjunct balloon dilatation to maximize the residual lumen dimensions.

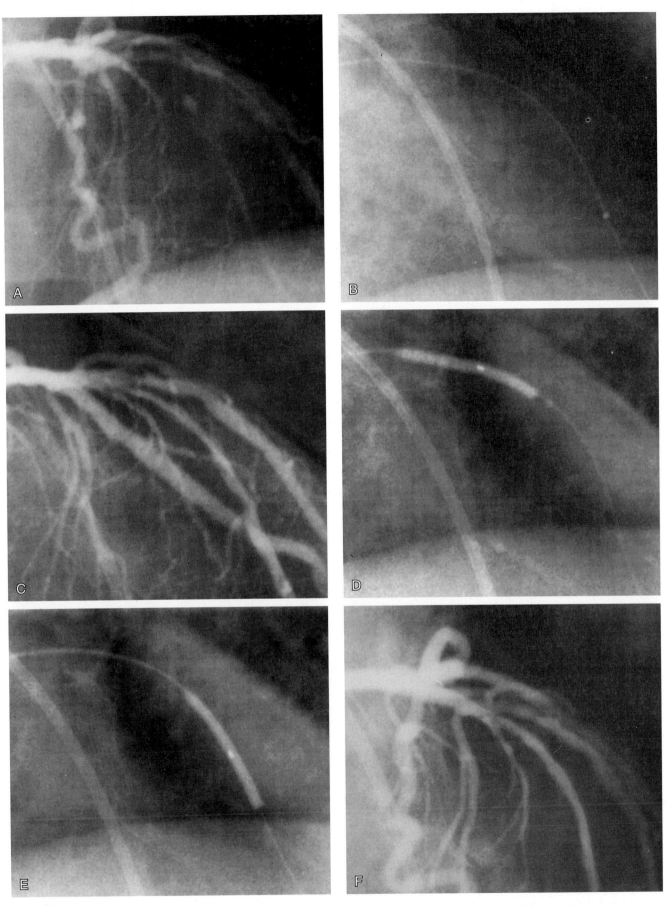

Figure 20–5
A total occlusion of the midsegment of the left anterior descending artery *(Panel A)* was crossed with a 0.014-inch intermediate guide wire. A single pass of the 1.3-mm excimer laser catheter was performed at 60 mJ/mm² *(Panel B)* and resulted in recanalization of the left anterior descending artery *(Panel C)*. Sequential inflations in the proximal *(Panel D)* and midsegments *(Panel E)* of the left anterior descending artery resulted in an excellent anatomic result *(Panel F)*.

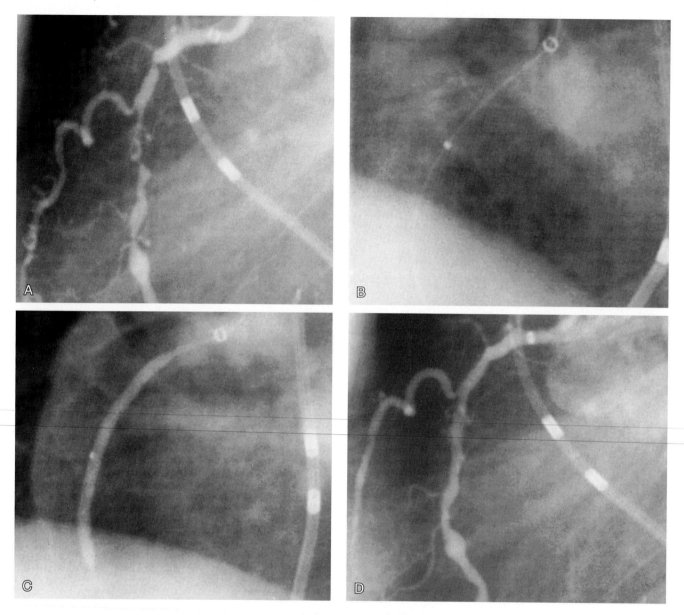

Figure 20–6
A diffusely diseased midsegment of the right coronary artery *(Panel A)* was treated with a 1.3-mm excimer laser catheter *(Panel B)*. A 1.0-mm channel was created using the excimer laser catheter, and adjunct balloon dilatation with a 2.5-mm long (40-mm) balloon was performed to treat the residual stenosis *(Panel C)*. After adjunct balloon dilatation, a marked improvement in the lumen contour was obtained; however, the segment remained diffusely diseased *(Panel D)*.

Several angiographic complications have been noted in patients who have undergone excimer laser angioplasty. Coronary vasospasm may occur distal to the treatment site and is generally reversed with intracoronary administration of nitroglycerin or with adjunct balloon dilatation. In a multicenter Registry report by Litvack and colleagues (1993), minor coronary dissections occurred in 16% of patients, and occlusions occurred in 7%, one-half of which were corrected with balloon angioplasty. Coronary perforation has been reported in 1.2% of cases and is principally related to lesion angulation, bifurcation lesion location, multiple laser passes, use of oversized laser catheters, and lasing at a site of dissection. It has been suggested that saline infusion may reduce the degree of photoacoustic effects; a "fast-pass" technique that diminishes energy exposure may also be of value.

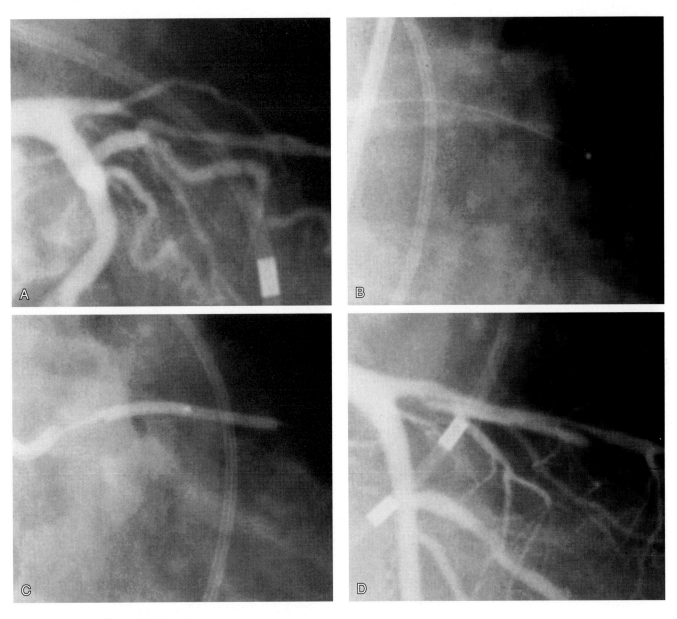

Figure 20–7
A diffuse lesion involving the proximal segment of the left anterior descending artery *(Panel A)* was treated with a 1.3-mm excimer laser catheter *(Panel B)*. After a single pass, reduced flow into the distal left anterior descending artery was demonstrated, and adjunct balloon dilatation with a 2.5-mm long (30-mm) balloon was performed *(Panel C)*. After balloon deflation, a long (30-mm) dissection was demonstrated *(Panel D)*.

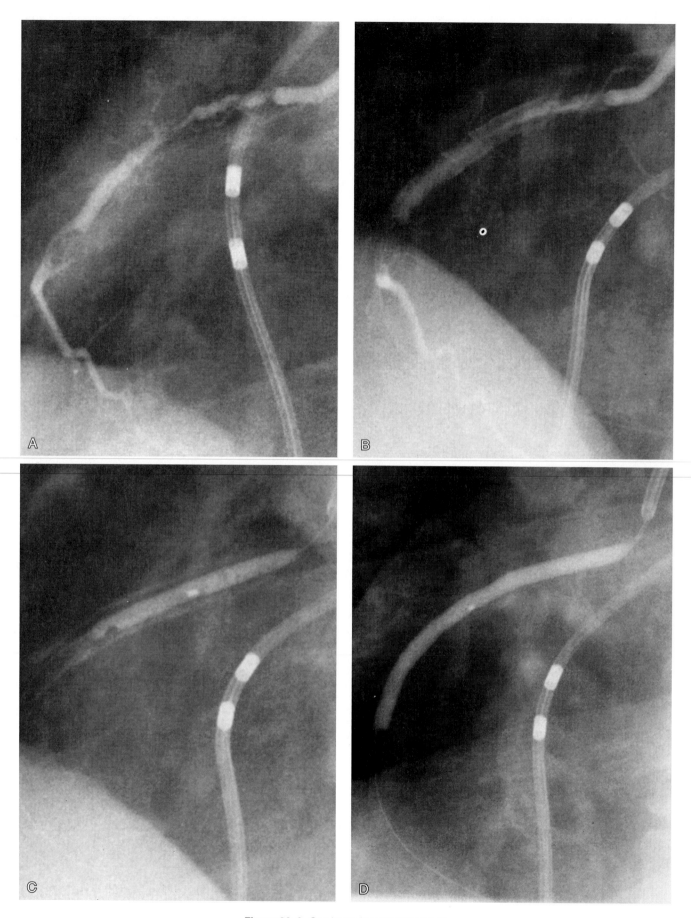

Figure 20–8. *See legend on opposite page*

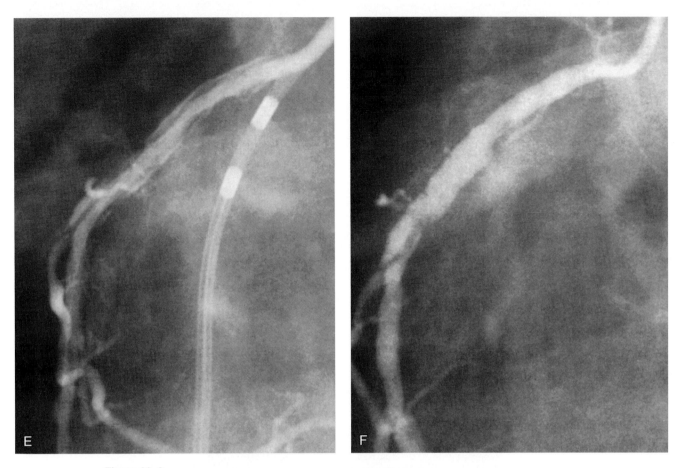

Figure 20–8
A diffusely diseased segment of the right coronary artery *(Panel A)* was treated with a single pass of a 1.3-mm excimer laser catheter *(Panel B)*. After passage of the laser catheter, a deep dissection in the right coronary artery was noted, and adjunct balloon dilatation with a 2.5-mm long (30-mm) balloon catheter was performed *(Panel C)*; this was followed by inflation of a 40-mm balloon *(Panel D)*. After final balloon deflation, normal flow into the distal myocardial bed was observed; however, a significant residual dissection remained *(Panel E)*. The patient received oral warfarin (Coumadin) therapy, and 3 months later, repeat angiography demonstrated persistent coronary patency and remodeling of the arterial dissection *(Panel F)*.

To overcome the limitations of concentric laser ablation, a 1.8-mm directional excimer laser catheter with a 1-cm extension tip has been developed. This apparatus ablates plaque eccentrically owing to the unilateral positioning of the laser fibers. The directional laser catheter is useful in the treatment of patients with bifurcation lesions, eccentric lesions, and lesions on a bend point.

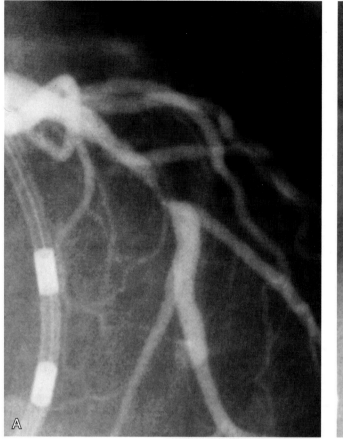

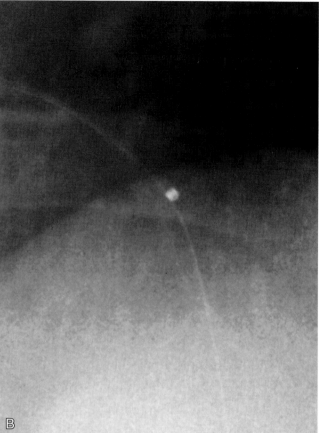

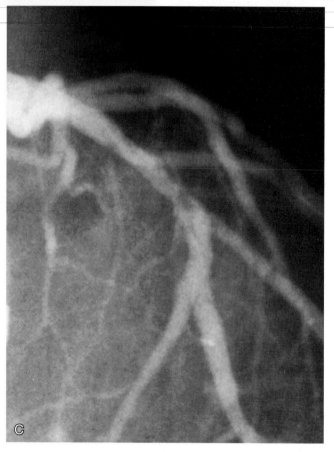

Figure 20–9. *See legend on opposite page*

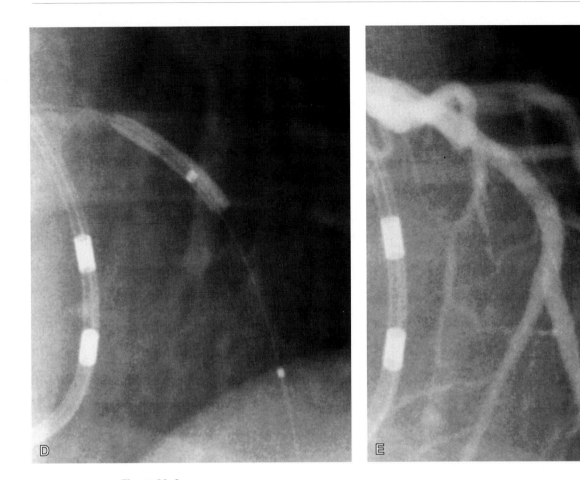

Figure 20–9

An eccentric lesion was noted in the midportion of the left anterior descending artery just proximal to the origin of a medium-sized diagonal branch *(Panel A)*. A 1.8-mm directional laser catheter was aligned to directionally ablate the plaque *(Panel B)*. Note the location of the guide wire within the arterial lumen. After three directed passes, a 20% residual stenosis was obtained; however, a mild degree of intraluminal haziness and possible dissection were observed *(Panel C)*. Adjunct dilatation was performed with a 3.0-mm balloon catheter *(Panel D)*, and a <10% residual stenosis was obtained *(Panel E)*.

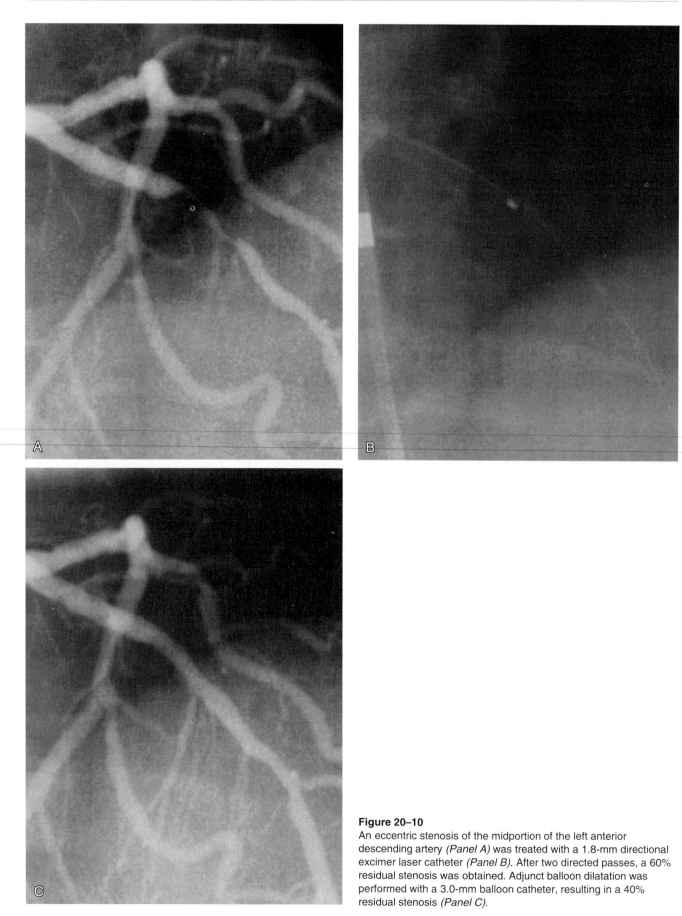

Figure 20–10
An eccentric stenosis of the midportion of the left anterior descending artery *(Panel A)* was treated with a 1.8-mm directional excimer laser catheter *(Panel B)*. After two directed passes, a 60% residual stenosis was obtained. Adjunct balloon dilatation was performed with a 3.0-mm balloon catheter, resulting in a 40% residual stenosis *(Panel C)*.

SELECTED REFERENCES

Bittl J, Sanborn T. Excimer laser-facilitated coronary angioplasty: Relative risk analysis of acute and follow-up results in 200 patients. Circulation 1992; 86:71–80.

Cook S, Eigler N, Shefer A, et al. Percutaneous excimer laser coronary angioplasty of lesions not ideal for balloon angioplasty. Circulation 1991; 84:632–643.

Ghazzal Z, Hearn J, Litvack F, et al. Morphologic predictors of acute complications after percutaneous excimer laser coronary angioplasty. Results of a comprehensive angiographic analysis: Importance of the eccentricity index. Circulation 1992; 86:820–827.

Israel D, Marmur J, Sanborn T. Excimer laser-facilitated balloon angioplasty of a nondilatable lesion. J Am Coll Cardiol 1991; 18:1118–1119.

Karsch K, Haase K, Mauser M, Voelker W. Initial angiographic results in ablation of atherosclerotic plaque by percutaneous coronary excimer laser angioplasty without subsequent balloon dilatation. Am J Cardiol 1989; 64:1253–1257.

Karsch K, Haase K, Voelker W, et al. Percutaneous coronary excimer laser angioplasty in patients with stable and unstable angina pectoris: Acute results and incidence of restenosis during 6-month follow-up. Circulation 1990; 81:1849–1859.

Litvack F, Eigler N, Margolis J, et al. Percutaneous excimer laser coronary angioplasty. Am J Cardiol 1990; 66:1027–1032.

Litvack F, Eigler NL, Forrester JS. In search of the optimized excimer laser angioplasty system. Circulation 1993; 87:1421–1422.

Litvack F, Grundfest W, Goldenberg T, et al. Percutaneous excimer laser angioplasty of aortocoronary saphenous vein grafts. J Am Coll Cardiol 1989; 14:803–808.

Margolis J, Mehta S. Excimer laser coronary angioplasty. Am J Cardiol 1992; 69:3F–11F.

Reeder G, Bresnahan J, Holmes DR, Litvack F. Investigators ELCA. Excimer laser coronary angioplasty: Results in restenosis versus de novo coronary lesions. Cathet Cardiovasc Diagn 1992; 25:195–199.

Sanborn T, Alexopoulos D, Marmur J, et al. Coronary excimer laser angioplasty: Reduced complications and indium-111 platelet accumulation compared with thermal laser angioplasty. J Am Coll Cardiol 1990; 16:502–506.

Sanborn T, Bittl J, Hershman R, Siegel R. Percutaneous coronary excimer laser-assisted angioplasty: Initial multicenter experience in 141 patients. J Am Coll Cardiol 1991; 17:169B–173B.

Watson L, Gantt S. Excimer laser coronary angioplasty for failed PTCA. Cathet Cardiovasc Diagn 1992; 26:285–290.

CHAPTER 21

Thermal Angioplasty

Laser balloon angioplasty and other heat-assisted angioplasty techniques may be useful as alternative methods of coronary revascularization owing to their ability to thermally alter plaque compliance, thereby reducing vascular elastic recoil. These effects may permit a more favorable initial angiographic result, which has been shown to correlate with late clinical and angiographic outcome in patients who have undergone angioplasty with the use of other new devices. Moreover, thermal fusion of dissection flaps may permit treatment of acute and threatened abrupt closure after standard balloon angioplasty, restoring anterograde perfusion in those patients who may otherwise require emergency coronary bypass surgery.

As a representative prototype of thermal balloon angioplasty, the Spears laser balloon underwent clinical evaluation in the late 1980s. Continuous-wave neodymium-yttrium-aluminum-garnet laser irradiation (1064-nm) was delivered within the central shaft of the balloon, heating the surrounding tissues to approximately 100° C. With the balloon materials transparent to the laser energy, the arterial surface was heated directly by the radiation energy, and the inflated balloon scaffolded the artery during laser thermal injury. Clinical and experimental models have demonstrated that better lumen dimensions were achieved with laser balloon angioplasty than those that were obtained after conventional balloon angioplasty due to the reduction of passive vascular recoil.

Laser balloon angioplasty was initially tested to treat restenosis and to manage abrupt closure after balloon angioplasty. Although the initial results with prototype devices were encouraging, the clinical protocol was terminated in 1991 because of the occurrence of delayed subacute thrombosis in some patients and to a high rate of restenosis. However, other thermal balloon devices that utilize radiofrequency current to heat balloon and angioplasty treatment sites are undergoing evaluation in clinical trials.

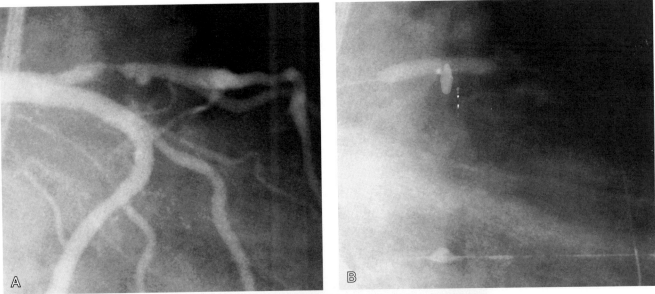

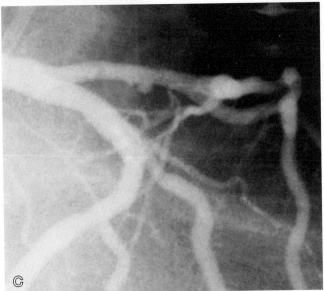

Figure 21–1

Primary laser balloon angioplasty was used for the treatment of an eccentric, ulcerated stenosis in the proximal segment of the left anterior descending artery *(Panel A)*. A 3.0-mm laser balloon was inflated for 60 seconds *(Panel B)*. After balloon deflation, an excellent anatomic result was obtained with a smooth lumen contour *(Panel C)*. Notably, a minimal degree of elastic recoil occurred after balloon deflation.

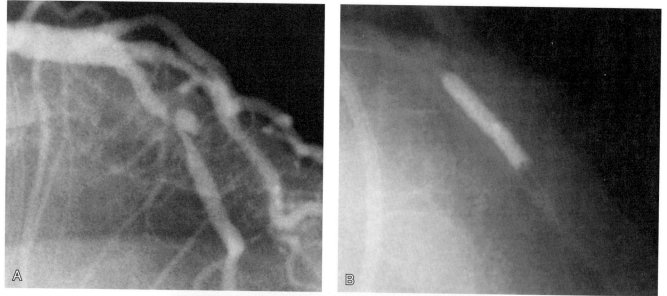

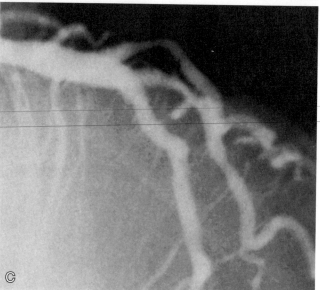

Figure 21–2
A complex, ulcerated stenosis of the midportion of the left anterior descending artery was treated with primary laser balloon angioplasty *(Panel A)*. A 3.0-mm laser balloon was inflated for 60 seconds across the lesion *(Panel B)*, resulting in a <10% residual stenosis *(Panel C)*. Again, the degree of elastic recoil was minimal after balloon deflation. The diagonal lesion was not addressed during this intervention.

Laser balloon angioplasty may also be useful in treating patients with complications after standard balloon angioplasty. Heat and pressure applied to an internal dissection flap may ''tack up'' the flap and smooth the lumen contour.

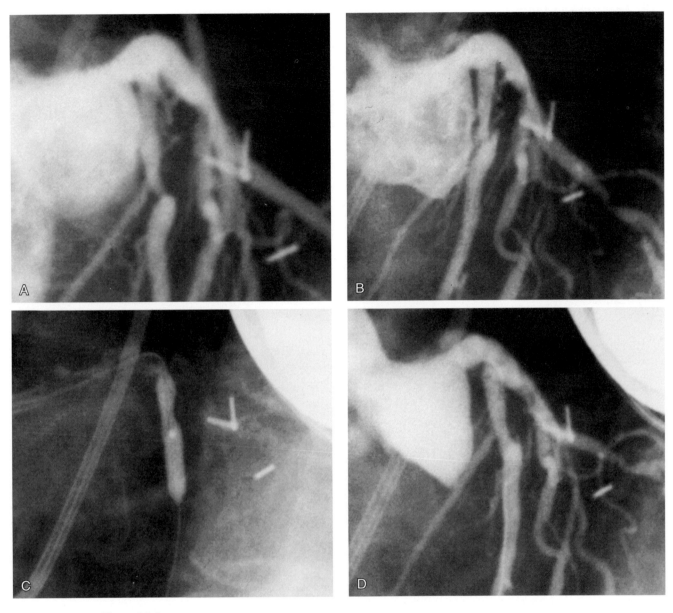

Figure 21–3
An eccentric stenosis of the midportion of the left anterior descending artery *(Panel A)* was treated with a 3.0-mm balloon. After a single balloon inflation, a linear dissection occurred at the site of dilatation *(Panel B)*. After compromise of anterograde coronary perfusion occurred, a 3.0-mm laser balloon catheter was inflated across the lesion for 60 seconds *(Panel C)*. After balloon deflation, a 20% residual stenosis was demonstrated; however, the linear dissection was repaired and anterograde coronary perfusion was re-established, although a moderate residual stenosis remained *(Panel D)*.

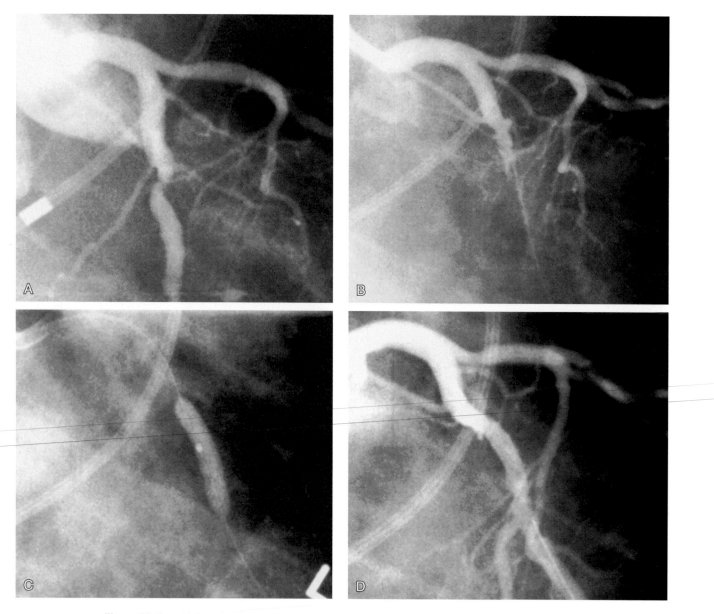

Figure 21–4
A complex lesion of the proximal left circumflex *(Panel A)* was treated with standard balloon angioplasty, which resulted in abrupt closure of the vessel *(Panel B)*. A 3.5-mm laser balloon catheter was advanced across the lesion, and heat was applied repetitively for a total of 20 seconds *(Panel C)*. After laser balloon angioplasty, anterograde flow was re-established, and a minimal residual stenosis was obtained *(Panel D)*.

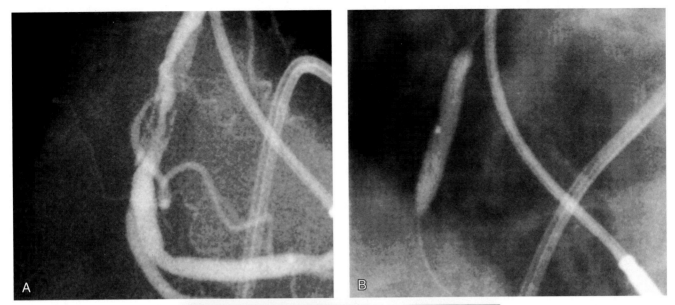

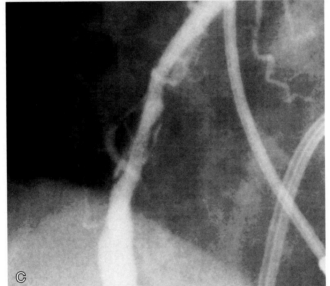

Figure 21–5
Coronary angioplasty performed for treatment of a complex stenosis involving the midportion of a
diffusely diseased right coronary artery was complicated by a spiral dissection *(Panel A)*. A 3.5-mm
laser balloon catheter was advanced across the dissection and inflated for 60 seconds *(Panel B)*.
After balloon deflation, an improvement in the lumen contour was obtained; however, a 40% residual
stenosis persisted *(Panel C)*.

SELECTED REFERENCES

Jenkins R, Spears J. Laser balloon angioplasty: A review of the technique
and clinical applications. J Invasive Cardiol 1990; 2:246–254.

Spears J, Kundu S, McMath L. Laser balloon angioplasty: Potential for
reduction of the thrombogenicity of the injured arterial wall and for
local application of bioprotective materials. J Am Coll Cardiol 1991;
17:179B–188B.

Spears J, Reyes V, Wynne J, et al. Percutaneous coronary laser balloon
angioplasty: Initial results of a multicenter experience. J Am Coll Cardiol 1990; 16:293–303.

Appendix

Throughout the text of *Atlas of Interventional Cardiology,* the identification of specific angioplasty balloon manufacturers and their product brand names has been minimized in an effort to simplify the case presentations and to avoid conflicts of interest for specific product endorsement. Manufacturers of new angioplasty devices and the abbreviations used to reference specific new devices within the text are listed:

Atherectomy Devices

Directional Coronary Atherectomy

- Devices for Vascular Intervention, Inc. (DVI),
   Redwood City, CA

   DVI EX Atherectomy Device (Polyethylene
      terephthalate balloon)
   DVI SCA Atherectomy Device (Surlyn balloon)

Rotational Coronary Atherectomy

- Heart Technologies (HT), Bellevue, WA

Transluminal Extraction Atherectomy

- InterVentional Technologies (IVT), San Diego, CA

Intracoronary Stents

Tubular Slotted Stent (Palmaz-Schatz [PS] stent)

- Johnson & Johnson Interventional Systems, Warren, NJ

Gianturco-Roubin Stent (FlexStent)

- Cook Cardiology, Bloomington, IN

Wiktor Stent

- Medtronic Interventional Systems, San Diego, CA

Wallstent (Medinvent Stent)

- Schneider Corporation, Minneapolis, MN

Excimer Laser Angioplasty

- Advanced Interventional Systems [AIS], Irvine, CA
- Spectranetics, Inc., Colorado Springs, CO

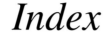

Index

Note: Numbers followed by an i indicate illustrations; those followed by a t indicate tables.

"Accordion" effect, 195
Algorithm, for balloon angioplasty, 184i
  for coronary occlusion, 42i
  for dissection, 184i
  for ostial lesions, 20i
  for saphenous vein graft lesions, 94i
Amplatz catheter, 48i, 192i
  for eccentric lesion, 21i, 164i
Anastomotic lesion(s), 133i, 136i, 137i
  angioplasty for, 102
  concentric, 135i
  eccentric, 134i
  saphenous vein graft with, 103i–108i
Aneurysm, 3t, 14, 214i. *See also* Dissection *and* Pseudoaneurysm.
Aneurysmal dilatation, 14, 214i
Angioplasty, atherectomy with, 248
  balloon. *See* Balloon angioplasty.
  benefits from, 175
  complications of, 175–196, 176i–198i, 226
  direct, 49, 183i
  for left mainstem lesions, 165–166
  for mammary artery, 132–138, 133i–139i
  for "protected" artery, 169
  for saphenous vein graft, 94
  for thrombus-containing lesion, 140, 142, 144
  for tortuous vessels, 161i–164i, 161–163
  laser. *See* Excimer laser angioplasty.
  registry for, 175, 229
  risk of, 167i, 169, 176i, 177i, 185
  thermal. *See* Thermal angioplasty.
Angulated lesion(s), 65–72, 66i–76i, 163i, 230t
  calcified, 66i, 73i, 74i, 76i
  concentric, 75i
  eccentric, 68i, 72i
  restenotic, 313i
  saphenous vein graft with, 98i
  treatment of, 69
  tubular, 189i
Anterior descending artery lesion(s), angulated, 66i, 73i, 189i
  atherectomy for, 207i, 213i, 225i
  bifurcation, complex, 224i, 246i–247i, 302i
    eccentric, 88i
    type D, 80i, 83i, 84i
    type F, 90i
  calcified, 236i
  complex, 191i
  concentric, 198i, 312i
    calcified, 14i
    long, 295i
  diffuse, 339i
  discrete, 205i

Anterior descending artery lesion(s) *(Continued)*
  eccentric, 6i, 15i, 276i, 342i–344i
    angulated, 233i
    calcified, 8i, 16i, 89i, 232i
    complex, 316i
    tubular, 109i, 158i
  long, 296i
  ostial, 29i, 33, 40i–41i
    calcified, 239i
    eccentric, 34i
    long, 35i
    noncalcified, 33i, 275i
  restenotic, 300i, 303i
  sequential, 72i, 244i
  thrombus-containing, 51i
  tubular, 10i
  ulcerated, 10i, 11i, 13i, 297i
    complex, 347i
    eccentric, 347i
    tubular, 215i
Anterior descending artery occlusion, chronic, 47i
  subtotal, 223i
  total, 43i, 53i, 335i, 337i
Aorto-ostial lesion, 20i, 20–21, 98, 332. *See also* Ostial lesion(s).
Arteries. *See named arteries, e.g.,* Left main coronary artery.
Arteriography, 167i, 212i
Atherectomy, directional. *See* Directional coronary atherectomy.
  extraction. *See* Transluminal extraction atherectomy.
  for branch vessel lesions, 37
  for intimal flap, 17i
  for long lesion, 35i
  for ostial lesion, 36i, 124i–125i
  rotational. *See* Rotational coronary atherectomy.
Atherectomy devices, 353
Atherosclerosis, accelerated, 266i

Balloon angioplasty, 3–4, 33. *See also* Angioplasty.
  algorithm for, 184i
  atherectomy with, 158, 159i
  bypass surgery and, 95, 107
  complications of, 15, 45, 47, 221
  for anastomotic lesion, 102, 103i–108i, 133i–137i
  for angulated lesion, 5i, 65–72, 66i–76i, 98i, 187i, 189i
  for aorto-ostial lesion, 20i, 20–21, 98
  for bifurcation lesion, 78i, 80i–84i, 92i
  for calcified lesion, 22i, 59i, 60i, 66i
  for complex lesion, 191i
  for concentric lesion, 100i, 122i, 135i 198i
  for coronary occlusion, 43i–58i, 177i, 196i